Personalizing Breast Cancer Care

Editor

MELISSA PILEWSKIE

SURGICAL ONCOLOGY CLINICS OF NORTH AMERICA

www.surgonc.theclinics.com

Consulting Editor
TIMOTHY M. PAWLIK

October 2023 • Volume 32 • Number 4

ELSEVIER

1600 John F. Kennedy Boulevard • Suite 1800 • Philadelphia, Pennsylvania, 19103-2899

http://www.theclinics.com

SURGICAL ONCOLOGY CLINICS OF NORTH AMERICA Volume 32, Number 4
October 2023 ISSN 1055-3207, ISBN-13: 978-0-443-18175-7

Editor: John Vassallo (j.vassallo@elsevier.com)
Developmental Editor: Malvika Shah

Surgical Oncology Clinics of North America (ISSN 1055-3207) is published quarterly by Elsevier Inc., 360 Park Avenue South, New York, NY 10010-1710. Months of publication are January, April, July, and October. Business and Editorial Offices: 1600 John F. Kennedy Blvd., Ste. 1800, Philadelphia, PA 19103-2899. Customer Service Office: 3251 Riverport Lane, Maryland Heights, MO 63043. Periodicals postage paid at New York, NY and additional mailing offices. Subscription prices are $335.00 per year (US individuals), $651.00 (US institutions) $100.00 (US student/resident), $374.00 (Canadian individuals), $823.00 (Canadian institutions), $100.00 (Canadian student/resident), $484.00 (foreign individuals), $823.00 (foreign institutions), and $205.00 (foreign student/resident). Foreign air speed delivery is included in all *Clinics* subscription prices. All prices are subject to change without notice. **POSTMASTER**: Send address changes to *Surgical Oncology Clinics of North America*, Elsevier Health Science Division, Subscription Customer Service, 3251 Riverport Lane, Maryland Heights, MO 63043. **Customer Service: 1-800-654-2452 (US and Canada). 314-447-8871 (outside US and Canada). Fax: 314-447-8029. E-mail: journalscustomerservice-usa@elsevier.com (for print support); journalsonline support-usa@elsevier.com (for online support).**

Reprints. For copies of 100 or more, of articles in this publication, please contact the Commercial Reprints Department, Elsevier Inc., 360 Park Avenue South, New York, New York 10010-1710. Tel. 212-633-3874; Fax: 212-633-3820; E-mail: reprints@elsevier.com.

Surgical Oncology Clinics of North America is covered in *MEDLINE/PubMed (Index Medicus)* and *EMBASE/ Excerpta Medica, Current Contents/Clinical Medicine, and ISI/BIOMED.*

Contributors

CONSULTING EDITOR

TIMOTHY M. PAWLIK, MD, PhD, MPH, MTS, MBA, FACS, FRACS (Hon)
Professor and Chair, Department of Surgery, The Urban Meyer III and Shelley Meyer Chair for Cancer Research, Professor of Surgery, Oncology, Health Services Management and Policy, The Ohio State University, Wexner Medical Center, Columbus, Ohio

EDITOR

MELISSA PILEWSKIE, MD, FACS
Associate Professor, Department of Surgery, Director of Breast Care Center, University of Michigan, Ann Arbor, Michigan

AUTHORS

ROBERT J. ALLEN JR, MD
Associate Attending, Plastic and Reconstructive Surgery Service, Department of Surgery, Memorial Sloan Kettering Cancer Center, New York, New York

ANDREA V. BARRIO, MD
Breast Service, Department of Surgery, Memorial Sloan Kettering Cancer Center, New York, New York

JUDY C. BOUGHEY, MD
W.H. Odell Professor of Individualized Medicine, Professor of Surgery, Chair, Division of Breast and Melanoma Surgical Oncology, Rochester, Minnesota

LIOR Z. BRAUNSTEIN, MD
Program Director, Department of Radiation Oncology, Memorial Sloan Kettering Cancer Center, New York, New York

ABIGAIL S. CAUDLE, MD
Professor, Breast Surgical Oncology, MD Anderson Cancer Center, Office of Chief Operating Officer, Houston, Texas

AKIKO CHIBA, MD
Assistant Professor, Department of Surgery, Duke University Medical Center, Duke Cancer Institute, Department of Surgery, Durham VA Medical Center, Durham, North Carolina

AMY E. CYR, MD
Assistant Professor, Department of Medicine, Washington University, St Louis, Missouri

LESLY A. DOSSETT, MD, MPH
Associate Professor, Department of Surgery, Institute for Healthcare Policy and Innovation, University of Michigan, Ann Arbor, Michigan

STEPHANIE DOWNS-CANNER, MD, FACS
Breast Service, Department of Surgery, Memorial Sloan Kettering Cancer Center, New York, New York

LEISHA C. ELMORE, MD, MPHS
Assistant Professor, Department of Surgery, University of Pennsylvania, Perelman School of Medicine, Philadelphia, Pennsylvania

OLUWADAMILOLA M. FAYANJU, MD, MA, MPHS, FACS
Helen O. Dickens Presidential Associate Professor, Chief, Division of Breast Surgery, University of Pennsylvania, Perelman School of Medicine, Philadelphia, Pennsylvania

EUN-SIL SHELLEY HWANG, MD, MPH
Mary and Deryl Hart Distinguished Professor, Department of Surgery, Duke University Medical Center, Duke Cancer Institute, Durham, North Carolina

KAITLYN KENNARD, MD
Breast Surgical Oncology Fellow, Department of Surgery, Washington University, St Louis, Missouri

SEEMA AHSAN KHAN, MD
Professor, Department of Surgery, Northwestern University Feinberg School of Medicine, Chicago, Illinois

MINJI KIM, BS
Research Fellow, Plastic and Reconstructive Surgery Service, Department of Surgery, Memorial Sloan Kettering Cancer Center, New York, New York

MARLA LIPSYC-SHARF, MD
Fellow, Department of Medical Oncology, Dana-Farber Cancer Institute, Boston, Massachusetts

ELIZABETH A. MITTENDORF, MD, PhD, FACS
Professor, Division of Breast Surgery, Department of Surgery, Brigham and Women's Hospital, Breast Oncology Program, Dana-Farber Brigham Cancer Center, Harvard Medical School, Boston, Massachusetts

GIACOMO MONTAGNA, MD, MPH
Breast Service, Department of Surgery, Memorial Sloan Kettering Cancer Center, New York, New York

MONICA MORROW, MD
Breast Service, Department of Surgery, Anne Burnett Windfohr Chair of Clinical Oncology, Memorial Sloan Kettering Cancer Center, Professor of Surgery, Weill Medical College of Cornell University, New York, New York

JONAS A. NELSON, MD, MPH
Assistant Attending, Plastic and Reconstructive Surgery Service, Department of Surgery, Memorial Sloan Kettering Cancer Center, New York, New York

ANN H. PARTRIDGE, MD, MPH
Vice Chair, Department of Medical Oncology, Founder and Director of the Program for Young Adults with Breast Cancer, Director of the Adult Survivorship Program, Eric P. Winer Chair in Breast Cancer Research, Dana-Farber Cancer Institute, Professor of Medicine, Harvard Medical School, Boston, Massachusetts

SYDNEY M. RECORD, BA
Department of Surgery, Duke University Medical Center, Durham, North Carolina

DANIELLE ROCHLIN, MD
Clinical Fellow, Plastic and Reconstructive Surgery Service, Department of Surgery, Memorial Sloan Kettering Cancer Center, New York, New York

JENNA L. STURZ, DO
Department of Surgery, Mayo Clinic, Rochester, Minnesota

PERRI S. VINGAN, BS
Research Fellow, Plastic and Reconstructive Surgery Service, Department of Surgery, Memorial Sloan Kettering Cancer Center, New York, New York

TON WANG, MD, MS
Department of Surgery, Cedars-Sinai Medical Center, Los Angeles, California

ASHLEY A. WOODFIN, MD
MD Anderson Cancer Center, Breast Surgical Oncology, Houston, Texas

Contents

The primary prevention of breast cancer is a worthwhile goal for which the efficacy of antiestrogens is well established. However, implementation has been problematic related to low prioritization by providers and the reluctance of high-risk women to experience medication side effects. Emerging solutions include improved risk estimation through the use of polygenic risk scores and the application of radiomics to screening mammograms; and optimization of medication dose to limit toxicity. The identification of agents to prevent estrogen receptor negative or HER2-positive tumors is being pursued, but personalization of medical risk reduction requires the prediction of tumor subtypes.

Multiple tools exist to assess a patient's breast cancer risk. The choice of risk model depends on the patient's risk factors and how the calculation will impact care. High-risk patients–those with a lifetime breast cancer risk of $\geq 20\%$–are, for instance, eligible for supplemental screening with breast magnetic resonance imaging. Those with an elevated short-term breast cancer risk (frequently defined as a 5-year risk $\geq 1.66\%$) should be offered endocrine prophylaxis. High-risk patients should also receive guidance on modification of lifestyle factors that affect breast cancer risk.

DCIS detection has increased dramatically since the introduction of screening mammography. Current guidance concordant care recommends surgical intervention for all patients with DCIS, followed by radiation and/or endocrine therapy for some. Adjuvant therapies after surgical excision have reduced recurrence rates but not breast cancer mortality. Given the lack of evidence of current treatment regimens and the morbidity associated with these treatments, there is concern that DCIS is over-treated. Active surveillance may be a favorable alternative for selected patients and is currently being investigated through four international clinical trials.

This article reviews the incidence of nodal metastases in early-stage breast cancer and the need for axillary staging to maintain local control in the axilla or to determine the need for adjuvant systemic therapy across the spectrum of patients with breast cancer, and reviews clinical trials addressing this question. At present, sentinel lymph node biopsy should be omitted in women age ≥70 years with cT1–2 N0, HR+/HER2− cancers. The importance of nodal status in selecting patients for radiotherapy remains the main reason for axillary staging in younger postmenopausal women with cT1–2N0, HR+/HER2− cancers.

De-escalation of axillary management after neoadjuvant chemotherapy in clinically node-positive patients is feasible. The current literature shows this may be accomplished by sentinel lymph node biopsy (SLNB) with the use of dual tracer and removal of at least 2 sentinel lymph nodes, or by targeted axillary dissection (TAD). The accuracy of TAD has been consistently shown as better than that of SLNB. However, these techniques should only be offered to select patients without extensive axillary disease, understanding that long-term outcomes of minimal axillary surgery in this population are limited at this time.

In the setting where breast cancer-related lymphedema (BCRL) remains a feared and common complication of breast cancer, here we review important factors for the development, diagnosis, prevention, and treatment of BCRL. We find that race/ethnicity affect BCRL development risk, that future studies should focus on understanding the biological reasons behind the increased susceptibility of certain racial minorities to BCRL, that surveillance, early detection, exercise programs, and arm compression can reduce the risk of BCRL, and that surgical techniques to preserve and restore lymphatic drainage being evaluated in randomized trials may become transformative in reducing BCRL risk for high-risk patients.

Although adjuvant breast radiotherapy has long been a universal component of breast conservation therapy (BCT), it is now clear that "breast cancer" is a broad class of many disparate diseases with varying natural histories and risk profiles. In turn, some breast conservation patients enjoy exceedingly favorable outcomes following surgery alone. Ongoing trials seek to identify such low-risk patient populations, hypothesizing that some may safely forego radiotherapy. Whereas prior-generation trials focused on clinicopathologic features for risk stratification, contemporary studies are employing molecular biomarkers to identify those patients who are unlikely to benefit significantly from radiotherapy.

Breast cancer treatment, timeliness of care, and clinical outcomes are inferior for patients of Black race and Hispanic ethnicity, and the origin of these inequities is multifactorial. Owing to aggregate reporting of data in the United States for patients of Asian, Native Hawaiian, and Pacific Islander ancestry, disparities within and across these groups are difficult to appreciate. In large part due to low prevalence, male breast cancer remains understudied, and treatment algorithms are primarily extrapolated from research conducted in female patients.

The COVID-19 pandemic was an unprecedented time that placed unique challenges on the screening and treatment of breast cancer in the United States. Collaboration among medical disciplines and societies provided guidelines and strategies to mitigate the exposure of patients and medical providers to the virus and provide optimal care. We discuss the changes that the pandemic had on the multidisciplinary management of breast cancer.

SURGICAL ONCOLOGY CLINICS OF NORTH AMERICA

SERIES OF RELATED INTEREST

Advances in Surgery
https://www.advancessurgery.com
Surgical Clinics of North America
https://www.surgical.theclinics.com
Thoracic Surgery Clinics
https://www.thoracic.theclinics.com

THE CLINICS ARE AVAILABLE ONLINE!
Access your subscription at:
www.theclinics.com

Foreword

Personalizing Breast Cancer Care

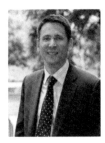

Timothy M. Pawlik, MD, MPH, PhD, FACS, FRACS (Hon.)
Consulting Editor

This issue of the *Surgical Oncology Clinics of North America* focuses on Personalizing Breast Cancer Care. Breast cancer is among the most common cancers diagnosed among women in the world and is the second leading cause of death among women.[1] In fact, the incidence of breast cancer between 2015 and 2019 was 128.1 per 100,000, age adjusted to the 2000 US standard population, with an estimated 43,700 deaths in 2023.[1] Breast cancer is a cancer in which there is effective screening, and there have been significant technological advances in imaging over the last decade improving screening and early detection. William S. Halsted[2] initially proposed that breast cancer was a local disease that spread locally and regionally and could be treated largely with "radical" surgery alone. More than 50 years later, Fisher and others[3] challenged that paradigm and suggested that breast cancer was often a systemic disease that required systemic therapy—in addition to resection—to achieve optimal results. Today, we know that a true multidisciplinary approach to patients with breast cancer is needed to define personalized treatment strategies and achieve better outcomes. In particular, care of breast cancer patients should include broad multidisciplinary input, as treatment often involves surgery, chemotherapy, radiation, hormone therapy, and targeted therapy. In turn, it is important that providers who care for patients with breast cancer are familiar with the most recent treatment approaches to breast cancer in order to personalize and tailor care. To that end, this current issue of *Surgical Oncology Clinics of North America* is an important practical resource that offers a timely update on the topic. We are fortunate to have Melissa Pilewskie, MD as our Guest Editor. Dr Pilewskie is Associate Professor and Director of the Breast Care Center at the University of Michigan. She received her BS in biology from the University of Michigan, a medical degree from The Ohio State University, completed her general surgical residency training at Northwestern Memorial Hospital in Chicago, and received additional fellowship training in surgical breast oncology at Memorial Sloan Kettering Cancer Center. During her training, Dr Pilewskie was the recipient of the

https://doi.org/10.1016/j.soc.2023.06.002
1055-3207/23/© 2023 Published by Elsevier Inc.

Breast Cancer Achievement Award from the Lynn Sage Breast Cancer Symposium and was a two-time recipient of the Conquer Cancer Foundation of the American Society of Clinical Oncology Merit Award. Dr Pilewskie's clinical practice is devoted to the management of breast cancer and surgical breast diseases. She performs all aspects of surgery for breast cancer and high-risk breast lesions. Dr Pilewskie has an active role in clinical research, which has focused broadly on breast cancer risk and safely minimizing surgery for breast cancer patients. Her work has included accurate risk assessment for high-risk populations, optimal imaging strategies for high-risk women, studying novel risk-reduction therapies, and investigating the safety of minimizing axillary lymph node surgery.

The issue covers multiple important topics, including breast cancer risk reduction, individualizing breast cancer risk assessment, as well as how to navigate the treatment spectrum of multimodality therapy versus observation of DCIS. Other important topics, such as evidenced-based strategies to minimize likelihood of axillary lymph node dissection, as well as managing the morbidity of lymphedema, are covered. Furthermore, key subjects, including the role of radiation therapy, immunotherapy, and how to address fertility and sexual health concerns, are discussed. Also, health care delivery issues, such as addressing inequalities, value-based care, and the impact of COVID-19, are also examined.

I want to thank Dr Pilewskie for putting together a great group of coauthors to contribute to this issue of *Surgical Oncology Clinics of North America*. The authors did a wonderful job highlighting the important clinical topics related to breast cancer care. This issue of *Surgical Oncology Clinics of North America* will provide surgeons and all health care providers with important information to advance the treatment of patients with breast cancer. Again, thank you to Dr Pilewskie and all the contributing authors.

Timothy M. Pawlik, MD, MPH, PhD, FACS, FRACS (Hon.)
Professor and Chair
Department of Surgery
The Urban Meyer III and Shelley Meyer Chair for Cancer Research
The Ohio State University
Wexner Medical Center
395 West 12th Avenue, Suite 670
Columbus, OH 43210, USA

E-mail address:
tim.pawlik@osumc.edu

REFERENCES

1. Available at: https://www.cancer.org/research/cancer-facts-statistics/breast-cancer-facts-figures.html. Accessed June 14, 2023.
2. Halsted WSI. The results of radical operations for the cure of carcinoma of the breast. Ann Surg 1907;46:1–19.
3. Fisher ER. The interrelationship of hematogenous and lymphatic tumor cell dissemination. Surg Gynecol Obstet 1966;122:791–8.

Preface

Personalizing Breast Cancer Care

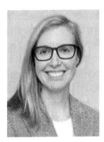

Melissa Pilewskie, MD, FACS
Editor

There are currently over 290,000 cases of invasive and over 50,000 cases of noninvasive breast cancer diagnosed annually in the United States. While cases of breast cancer continue to increase with the growing population, the mortality from the disease continues to decline, resulting in a growing number of breast cancer survivors, highlighting the importance of not only optimizing cancer care but also focusing on long-term treatment morbidity and survivorship issues. The current series reviews approaches to individualize breast cancer care through the spectrum of risk assessment through cancer care and symptom management. As breast cancer is the most prevalent cancer among American women, there is growing interest in expanding both patient and provider knowledge on risk assessment and options for risk reduction, as these interventions have the potential to impact cancer risk for millions of unaffected individuals and are currently underutilized.

An underlying theme remains the need to use evidence-based medicine to counsel patients on best practices while minimizing potential side effects. This desire is driving the work to develop novel options for risk reduction and is a cornerstone in assessing the safety of treatment de-escalation. Incorporation of tumor biology and genomic profiling is a crucial aspect of multidisciplinary breast cancer care and drives decision making for care escalation and de-escalation, as discussed in articles focusing on DCIS treatment options, axillary management, considerations for radiation omission, and advances in systemic therapy for triple-negative disease. Counseling individuals on appropriate de-escalation techniques remains a pillar of value-based care, vital at the patient and population level.

Unfortunately, breast cancer treatments may be associated with significant morbidity, including lymphedema, upper-extremity dysmotility, cosmetic alterations, and a decrease in quality of life. With the growing population of breast cancer survivors, attention to strategies to improve outcomes and quality of life is imperative. In addition to the above-mentioned strategies to personalize treatment recommendations, additional

Surg Oncol Clin N Am 32 (2023) xv–xvi
https://doi.org/10.1016/j.soc.2023.06.001
1055-3207/23/© 2023 Published by Elsevier Inc.

efforts, such as optimizing breast reconstruction and addressing sexuality and fertility-preservation concerns, are essential for patient well-being.

Emerging data identify both treatment modalities and patient-related factors as important risks for long-term side effects. Racial and ethnic disparities exist in both breast cancer survival outcomes and long-term morbidity development. As providers, we must work to minimize gaps in access and outcomes across the cancer care delivery spectrum. The COVID-19 pandemic brought new challenges and disparities in breast cancer care, and we are now identifying the long-term repercussions of care modifications during this time as well as opportunities for streamlining care with growth in outpatient surgery and telemedicine. The accompanying articles take an in-depth look at these important concepts in personalizing breast cancer care in 2023 and touch on outstanding questions and emerging techniques to further refine care for our patients in the years to come.

Melissa Pilewskie, MD, FACS
Department of Surgery
University of Michigan
1500 East Medical Center Drive
3306 Rogel Cancer Center
Ann Arbor, MI 48109, USA

E-mail address:
mpilewsk@umich.edu

Breast Cancer Risk Reduction

Current Status and Emerging Trends to Increase Efficacy and Reduce Toxicity of Preventive Medication

Seema Ahsan Khan, MD

KEYWORDS

- Breast cancer • Primary prevention • Antiestrogens • Risk estimation

KEY POINTS

- The primary prevention of breast cancer with antiestrogen agents is effective but has performed poorly at the level of implementation.
- Recent approaches have focused on dose reduction to achieve improved acceptance and adherence by high-risk women.
- Improved precision in risk estimation through the use of polygenic risk scores and radiomics to better identify high-risk women can increase the impact of primary prevention strategies.
- Novel approaches are under investigation, including drugs targeting the progesterone receptor pathway, vaccines, and others.

Although "chemoprevention" is a revered term … it is time for the word to be retired from the clinic for it conveys the wrong message, that of toxic chemotherapy. The terminology needs to be updated and to enter the mainstream of medicine as risk reduction" Frank Meyskens editorial JNCI 2012.

INTRODUCTION

Cancer prevention has long been recognized as an endeavor that will yield significant dividends in the improvement of health in society and a reduction in treatment-related morbidity. Debates around the notion of cancer prevention that were based on the lack of observed survival benefit in participants receiving preventive medication in clinical trials have largely been quenched, and research on preventive interventions has risen in the national research agenda. Recent stimuli for the prioritization of cancer prevention include the explosion in genetic susceptibility research over the past 2

Department of Surgery, Feinberg School of Medicine of Northwestern University, 303 East Superior Street, Chicago, IL 60614, USA
E-mail address: s-khan2@northwestern.edu

Surg Oncol Clin N Am 32 (2023) 631–646
https://doi.org/10.1016/j.soc.2023.05.001
1055-3207/23/© 2023 Elsevier Inc. All rights reserved.
surgonc.theclinics.com

decades and the validation and wide availability of statistical models for risk estimation that allow identification of women at increased risk who do not have an identifiable monogenic susceptibility. These developments have pushed breast cancer risk estimation into the mainstream workflow of breast clinics and breast imaging centers, leading to the identification of increasing numbers of women who can be included in the "high risk" group.

A widely accepted principle in implementation strategies is that interventions must be tailored to risk. Surgery only for the highest risk, medication for those at intermediate risk, and lifestyle modifications for those at modestly increased or standard risk (**Fig. 1**). This review will focus on the moderate risk group, which will benefit from medical prevention. Because these women are identified largely through a process of risk estimation, a discussion of methods of estimating risk is also necessary. However, the implementation of breast cancer prevention with medications has been a challenge, related partly to the variability in the output of currently available risk estimation tools and to the reluctance of at-risk women to use medications with adverse impacts on quality of life (QOL) and quality of health.

THE PRESENT
Landmark Prevention Trials

In the early 1990s, a growing body of evidence documented the reduced frequency of contralateral breast cancer (CBC) in women treated with adjuvant tamoxifen. These data, from several trials, led to the suggestion that primary breast cancer prevention in women at increased risk for breast cancer would be served by the use of "prophylactic" tamoxifen therapy.[1] Several landmark trials followed, showing relative risk reduction of 30% to 50% with the use of a series of antiestrogen medications[2–5] (tamoxifen, raloxifene, aromatase inhibitors summarized in **Table 1**), leading to a consensus that women at increased risk for breast cancer should be offered an antiestrogen agent, with the specific agent selected based on menopausal status and comorbidities.[6,7]

Other benefits of medical risk reduction that are well documented for tamoxifen include a reduction in breast density, which was first demonstrated in a nested

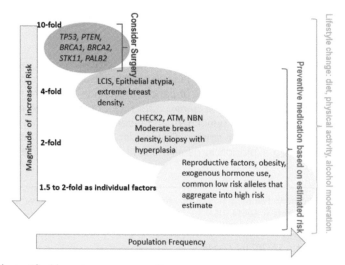

Fig. 1. Risk-stratified breast cancer prevention.

Table 1
Major randomized clinical trials of antiestrogens for breast cancer risk reduction

Trial	Agent	Risk Level of Population	N	Hazard Ratio (95% CI)
NSABP P-1	Tamoxifen vs placebo	5 y Gail risk ≥1.7	13,388	0.57 (0.46–0.70)
IBIS-1	Tamoxifen vs placebo	Increased 2-fold for age 45–70, 4-fold for 40–44, 10-fold for 35–39.	7154	0.71 (0.60–0.83)
Italian RCT	Tamoxifen vs placebo	Healthy hysterectomized women	5408	0.24 (0.10–0.59)[a]
Royal Marsden	Tamoxifen vs placebo	Family history of breast cancer	2471	0.24 (0.10–0.59)[b]
MORE	Raloxifene 120 mg vs 60 mg vs placebo	Postmenopausal with osteoporosis	7705	0.24 (0.13–0.44)
RUTH	Raloxifene vs placebo	Postmenopausal with cardiac risk		0.56 (0.38 = 0.83)
STAR	Tamoxifen vs. raloxifene	Postmenopausal, Gail risk ≥1.7	19,747	1.24 (1.05–1.47)[c]
MAP-3	Exemestane vs placebo	Postmenopausal, Gail risk ≥1.7[d]	4560	0.35 (0.18–0.70)
IBIS-II	Anastrozole vs placebo	Increased 4-fold for age 40–45, 2-fold for 45–60, 1.5-fold for 60–70	3864	0.51 (0.39–0.66)
PEARL	Lasofoxifene 0.5 mg vs. 0.25 mg vs placebo	Postmenopausal with osteoporosis	2740	0.21 (0.08–0.55)

[a] Risk reduction in high-risk women only.
[b] Risk reduction for ER+ cancer only.
[c] Long-term results favor tamoxifene.
[d] Several other inclusion criteria (age > 60, history of epithelial atypia or DCIS).

case-control analysis of the IBIS-I trial and was associated with a larger risk reduction than in the overall trial population (odds ratio [OR] 0.32, 95% confidence interval [CI] 0.14–0.72) compared with tamoxifen-treated women showing no change in density.[8] An additional benefit of breast density reduction is anticipated to be increased sensitivity of mammograms because of the decrease in the masking effect of breast density.[9] Women in the tamoxifen arm of the National Surgical Adjuvant Breast and Bowel Project (NSABP) P1 trial also experienced significantly fewer benign biopsies[10], and favorable effects on bone health are reported for essentially all selective estrogen receptor modulators (SERMs).[11] Improvements in lipid profiles are also a regular feature of most SERMs,[12,13] and have been observed in the breast cancer prevention trials.

Importantly, the duration of the protective benefit of antiestrogens is long-lived, continuing after cessation of therapy for at least 15 years for tamoxifen[14] and at least 10 years for anastrozole.[15] This longevity of benefit is a particular advantage to younger women; a woman initiating tamoxifen in her early to mid-forties can expect to experience protection against breast cancer until about age 60. Longer follow-up data are not available, but it is possible that the benefit extends even longer.

Uptake of preventive medication

The Achilles heel of this wealth of evidence supporting the risk-reducing value of an-tiestrogens has been the low levels of uptake of these agents by women at increased risk. A meta-analysis of the published experience in this regard, involving over 23,000 women who were included in 26 randomized and non-randomized studies.[16] Esti-mated overall uptake was 16%, and factors associated with increased likelihood of uptake included an abnormal biopsy, a physician recommendation, higher objective risk, fewer side-effect or trial concerns, and older age. Factors associated with lower adherence included allocation to tamoxifen (vs placebo or raloxifene), depression, smoking, and older age. Although individual institutions have reported better-than-average uptake, the proportion of risk-eligible women who are persuaded to initiate therapy remains below 20%. Multiple solutions have been suggested for this, with the greatest weight being placed on education (of physician providers and of the at risk population), alleviation of toxicity through new paradigms for dosing and delivery, and the introduction of new, better tolerated agents.[17]

Attempts to alleviate the QOL effects of antiestrogens have included a range of stra-tegies, control of vasomotor symptoms with a variety of medical interventions (SSRIs,[18] gabapentin,[19] oxybutynin[20]) or alternative therapies (acupuncture[21]). The impact of these on improving acceptance or maintaining adherence to medical pre-vention agents has not been well studied, but they are useful for women who are committed to the idea of risk reduction through medication. A second strategy (dis-cussed in greater depth in the "Future" section below) is that of using the minimal effective dose for cancer prevention, in contrast to the strategy of the "maximal toler-ated dose" that is commonly followed in the therapeutic setting. For women who are willing to "take a pill" to avoid future problems, dose reduction is likely to be a persua-sive addition to the preventive armamentarium.

Risk Estimation

Because quantitative risk estimates should guide most recommendations for preven-tive medication, a discussion of the methods available and their application is appropriate.

Strengths and limitations of calculated risk estimates

Widely used and easily available risk models include the National Cancer Institute (NCI) Breast Cancer Risk Assessment Tool, initially developed by Gail and col-leagues,[22] the Tyrer-Cuzick model developed from the IBIS-I trial population[23]; and the Breast Cancer Surveillance Consortium (BCSC) model, based on US nation-wide screening mammography data.[24] All are well-validated with good calibration (how many women in a given population will develop breast cancer) but only fair discrimination (can the model distinguish those who develop breast cancer from those who do not).

A cautionary note is required in terms of the certainty that is attributed to specific risk estimates using these models; a recent review of model performance demon-strates that the degree of calibration is variable and the risk of bias is high.[25] Neverthe-less, the highest risk groups are generally identified with most tools. Some tools generate extremely high numerical estimates (over 50% lifetime risk in the absence of heritable cancer susceptibility); this may prompt questions regarding the need for surgical risk reduction. However, CIs around risk estimates widen progressively as the time interval over which they are applied lengthens, since data become sparse af-ter intervals of more than 10 years. As a result, evidence enabling the evaluation of a long risk-prediction intervals on observed cancer incidence is extremely limited.[25]

Therefore, use of 5 to 10 year risk estimates provides the best evidence basis for recommendations, and lifetime estimates are of questionable value. This uncertainty in long-term estimates is important to convey to patients, with the explanation that an extremely high lifetime risk estimate derived from a statistical model may simply mean that the individual is at substantially higher risk than an average risk peer and should give serious consideration to medical risk reduction.

Major contributors to breast cancer risk
The main target group for medical prevention is those at moderately increased risk, identified largely through the use of statistical risk estimation models, or carriers of moderate penetrance susceptibility genes. Women with a suggestive family history but without an explanatory germline finding on testing of the appropriately selected family members form the bulk of this group. The other major contributor to this group is women who have had diagnostic biopsies revealing epithelial atypia. Although extreme breast density carries a risk on par with epithelial atypia, and breast density (either extreme or heterogeneous) has been incorporated into several risk estimation tools, including Tyrer-Cuzick and BCSC, the incremental improvement in accuracy of risk estimation with this addition is marginal.[26,27] Women at high risk (carriers of highly penetrant variants in cancer susceptibility genes) may also consider risk reducing medication, but for them, efficacy data are limited and surgical risk reduction is also a consideration.

Risk thresholds for recommending preventive medication
The magnitude of increased risk required for inclusion in the randomized trials varied somewhat, but a commonly used threshold was a 5 year risk estimate of 1.67% using the model developed by Gail and colleagues[28] This threshold was equivalent to the 5 year probability that an average 60 year old US woman would develop breast cancer. Subsequent analysis that included considerations of the risk of adverse effects of antiestrogens and risk–benefit ratios based on comorbidities resulted in an upward revision of the risk threshold that justifies the use of antiestrogens, to a 5 year risk of 3% or greater.[6] However, the application of this threshold may only be reasonable for women of European descent, whose background risks are derived from robust population-based data. Similarly robust data are not available for women of non-European descent. This limitation is recognized in the recent guidelines from the American Society of Clinical Oncology,[29] where consideration of risk-reducing medication is encouraged based on a fold-increase in estimated risk compared with average-risk peers (2-fold increase for women over 45 and 4-fold increase for women 45 and under).[30]

Predictors of protective benefit
A breast biopsy demonstrating epithelial atypia or lobular carcinoma in situ is associated with a larger risk reduction in women at risk for other reasons.[2] Another promising predictor is that of a reduction in mammographic density, as demonstrated in tamoxifen-treated women in the IBIS-I trial.[8] Although subsequent studies have documented breast density reduction related to tamoxifen use,[29] none have reported on quantitative density reduction and its relation to the subsequent occurrence of breast cancer in a population. In breast cancer survivors, a marginal relationship was observed in the reduction of CBCs and breast density reduction (OR 0.63, 95% CI 0.40, 1.01).[31] A recent Cochrane review concludes that there is low confidence in the evidence supporting breast density reduction as an indicator of tamoxifen benefit.[32] Some have suggested that the occurrence of tamoxifen-related QOL side

effects is related to prevention efficacy, but a recent analysis of data from the IBIS-1 trial testing tamoxifen 20 mg daily against, suggests otherwise.[33]

THE FUTURE

New directions in the implementation of medical risk reduction are summarized in **Table 2**.

Preventive Medication

Optimizing dose

The large-scale prevention trials initiated in the 1990s were not preceded by any attempts to define the minimal effective dose required for successful cancer prevention. The experience of the following 2 decades has made it clear that the QOL and health side effects of full dose antiestrogens are not acceptable to the majority of women who would benefit from them. The notion of dose reduction for preventive therapy was pioneered by Decensi and co-workers through a long series of investigations showing that low-dose tamoxifen led to similar biomarker modulation as standard dose therapy.[34–36] These studies culminated in a randomized trial of tamoxifen 5 mg daily versus placebo (the TAM-01 study) that enrolled women with duct carcinoma in situ (DCIS) or epithelial atypia and treated them for 3 years.[37] Thus, dose and duration of tamoxifen treatment were de-escalated, but the resultant hazard ratio for all breast events (ipsilateral, contralateral, invasive, and DCIS) was 0.48 (95% CI, 0.26–0.92), similar to that seen in the NSABP P1 trial. QOL side effects were minimal, consisting mainly of a marginal increase in hot flashes, but the population of 500 women randomized was not sufficient to assess health effects such as uterine neoplasia or thromboembolic disease in a meaningful way. The study population included just under 200 premenopausal women, and in this group, the risk reduction was not significant (HR = 0.73; 95% CI, 0.30–1.76).[38] Because tamoxifen is the only preventive agent available to premenopausal women, this area needs more work, but the paradigm-shifting value of this seminal work is clear.

Decensi and colleagues have gone further in a subsequent trial of intermittent dosing of exemestane, tested in a cancer population randomized to daily versus 3 doses/wk versus one dose/wk, with a primary endpoint of non-inferiority in reduction of serum estradiol.[39] They enrolled postmenopausal women with ER-positive breast cancer; 173 were evaluated for response. The median percent change of estradiol was −98%, −98%, and −70% for daily, thrice-weekly, and weekly groups ($P = .9$ comparing daily to thrice-weekly dosing). Among the secondary endpoints, Ki-67

Table 2
Factors driving the selection of individuals who would benefit from breast cancer prevention strategies

Current	Opportunities for Personalization	Timeframe to the Clinic
Inherited susceptibility to breast cancer	Inherited susceptibility informed by polygenic risk	Next few years
Epithelial atypia	Informed by the molecular profile of atypical lesions	Next decade or more
Risk estimate more than 2-fold peer group	Informed by the risk of non-indonent cancer	Next decade
Method of risk estimation based on classical risk factors	Risk estimated based on radiomics and genomics	Next decade

and PgR were reduced in all arms. Adverse events and menopausal symptoms were similar in all arms over the short treatment time in this trial. Additional studies are planned in the prevention and adjuvant settings. This important work shows that dose optimization should be an integral step in the introduction of any new agents for the purposes of preventing cancer in healthy populations.

New selective estrogen receptor modulators with no agonist activity in the uterus
Later generation SERMS have been tested to varying degrees in postmenopausal women, with larger trials having endpoints of bone mass, menopausal symptoms, or breast cancer therapy. Of these, lasofoxifene has a bone protective effect and a breast cancer prevention effect. It is now approved for use in the United States for advanced breast cancer because of its demonstrated activity in tumors that have acquired *ESR1* gene mutations.[40] It is not approved for breast cancer prevention, and the cost of treatment is high; therefore, it is not currently used for this purpose. Bazedoxifene, a drug with SERM and SERD (selective estrogen receptor degrader) activity, in combination with Premarin, is marketed as Duavee and is approved for relief of menopausal symptoms in women with an intact uterus. The inclusion of Premarin alleviates the QOL effects of bazedoxifene and may also contribute to breast cancer protective effects, as seen in the Women's Health Initiative trial among women who had undergone hysterectomy and were randomized to Premarin versus placebo.[41] Another promising SERM with no uterotrophic activity is acolbifene[42]; it also has favorable effects on the lipid profile and serum cholesterol.[43] In a single arm trial that enrolled 25 premenopausal women at increased risk for breast cancer, Fabian and colleagues showed that this is a well-tolerated agent with a significant antiproliferative effect on breast cells.[44] A new, randomized, and placebo-controlled phase 2 trial will be launched soon to confirm these findings and potentially lead the way to larger trials of this potent SERM, which has significant potential for breast cancer risk reduction and will likely extend to premenopausal and postmenopausal women.

Alternative delivery methods
A potential solution to the problem of systemic toxicity of oral agents is the use of alternative drug delivery methods that allow targeted local delivery to the breast if they preserve efficacy but minimize toxicity because of low systemic exposure. Transdermal drug delivery through the breast skin has been tested since 1986,[45] using 4-hydroxytamoxifen (4-OHT), one of the major active metabolites of tamoxifen,[46–48] with efficacy similar to that of the other major tamoxifen metabolite, endoxifen.[49] A gel formulation of 4-OHT when applied to the breast skin showed good retention of 4-OHT in breast tissue with low systemic exposure,[50] leading to studies of this agent for women with mastalgia.[51] Subsequently, 2 presurgical window studies in women with ER-positive invasive cancer and ER-positive DCIS provided encouraging data that suggested transdermal 4-OHT can suppress tumor cell proliferation to a similar degree as that achieved with oral tamoxifen,[52,53] with far lower plasma levels of 4-OHT than seen with 20 mg oral tamoxifen. Changes in circulating markers of estrogenic effect and activation of the coagulation cascade were not observed with transdermal delivery.[53] A confirmatory phase II randomized presurgical window trial has compared oral-TAM to 4OHT-gel applied to breasts of women undergoing surgery for ER positive DCIS (NCT02993159). This was designed to demonstrate the non-inferiority of the 4-OHT gel to oral tamoxifen in terms of the decrease in proliferative index of the DCIS lesion, but failed to do so. A parallel trial of 4-OHT gel versus placebo gel with the primary endpoint of breast density reduction has completed accrual (NCT03063619), and results are expected in late 2023. Newer formulations potentially containing the other

important tamoxifen metabolite (endoxifen) should therefore be tested because trans-dermally delivered agents penetrate deep into the breast,[54] and show biological effect even at low concentrations.

Progesterone receptor as a breast cancer prevention target

Progesterone exposure through repetitive luteal phase cycles during reproductive life and as uterus-protective additions to postmenopausal estrogen therapy has long been recognized as a risk factor for breast cancer development. However, the proges-terone receptor (PR) has never been targeted for cancer prevention. Recent preclinical data document the important role of progesterone in creating a pro-tumorigenic envi-ronment in the breast,[55,56] as well as the possibility of breast cancer prevention through the use of PR modulators.[57,58] Intriguingly, there is a possibility that PR antag-onists will also be protective against ER negative breast cancers.[57] However, the clas-sical PR antagonist, mifepristone has off-target effects on the glucocorticoid receptor and a toxicity profile that is not compatible with long-term use in a healthy population, and the more selective PR modulators such as ulipristal, although promising, have had their development interrupted because of rare but serious idiosyncratic liver injury.[59] Therefore, until alternative delivery methods or novel drug modifications that avoid liver injury are developed, anti-PR agents are not an option for further clinical develop-ment. Alternative dosing regimens may also alleviate some toxicity concerns, such as cyclical use for 2 to 3 months every few years.

Targeting the receptor activator of nuclear factor kappa beta ligand for breast cancer prevention

The RANK (receptor activator of nuclear factor kappa beta) and RANK ligand path-ways were first reported to be important in the development of BRCA1-associated breast cancer by Lindemann and colleagues,[60] leading quickly to the realization that the antibody to RANKL (denosumab), already approved for therapy for osteoporosis, was a potential preventive strategy for carriers of pathogenic variants of the BRCA1 gene. An international placebo-controlled trial is now ongoing to test this hypothesis (NCT04711109). It enrolls women without breast cancer history, not planning risk reducing surgery or pregnancy in the next 5 years, and has a primary endpoint of breast cancer occurrence. The incidence of ovarian and other cancers will also be tracked, and it will measure patient reported QOL outcomes as well as adverse events. In addition to its role in BRCA1-associated breast cancer, data from noncarrier populations implicate the RANK/RANKL pathway in breast cancer occurrence, showing that levels are increased prior to cancer diagnosis.[61] Postmenopausal women undergoing screening mammography showed a linear relationship between volumetric breast density and gene expression for estrogen receptor alpha, RANK, and TNFRSF18 (a member of the same receptor family as RANKL).[62] These data have led to a clinical trial of denosumab versus placebo to test the hypothesis that RANKL inhibition with denosumab will decrease mammographic density in high-risk premenopausal women with dense breasts. Additional breast tissue biomarkers of RANKL inhibition and effects on breast tissue, including RANKL pathway genes, pro-gesterone pathway genes, and cell proliferation, will also be evaluated. Studies like this will build a case for the testing of RANKL inhibitors for the prevention of sporadic breast cancer.

Vaccines for cancer prevention or interception

Vaccines are an attractive option for cancer prevention, even though the therapeutic performance of some vaccines has been disappointing when tested in patients with advanced disease, where patients are often immunosuppressed. On the other hand, target populations for cancer prevention are generally healthy and can mount a robust immune response, presenting an excellent opportunity for prevention or interception of evolving malignancies in the cancer-initiation phase of healthy individuals. Because the driver oncogenes of a tumor yet to come are not known, the diagnosis of preinvasive disease allows an opportunity to intercept future invasive disease through the antigen profile of the preinvasive lesion. This concept has been applied to HER2 over-expressing DCIS, where anti-HER2 vaccines have been tested. One such vaccine is the HER2 peptide pulsed dendritic cell vaccine, which produces a strong anti-HER2 immune response and sensitizes CD4+ and CD8+ T cells.[63] HER2 positive DCIS patients received intralesional and intranodal injections; 80% of patients had an increased immune response postinjection regardless of the delivery route; and 28% of patients had no residual DCIS in the surgical specimen, compared with approximately 15% in clinical practice when no HER2 therapy is used. Although promising, this approach has not advanced further in the prevention arena.

Another HER2 vaccine (NeuVax) is a combination of E75 (Nelipepimut-S), an immunogenic peptide that is derived from the HER2 protein, and GM-CSF (sargramostim).[64] This vaccine has been compared with GM-CSF alone in DCIS patients who are HLA-A2 positive in a single-blind multicenter study (NCT02636582, paper in press). The trial analyzed the CD8+ response, cell proliferation, apoptosis, and infiltration of the DCIS lesion with immune cells, as well as vaccine safety and toxicity. In 13 participants randomized to NeuVax (n = 9) or GM-CSF alone (n = 4), vaccination was well tolerated. Cytotoxic T lymphocytes specific to Nelipepimut-S increased in arms between baseline (pre-vaccination) and 1 month post-op. The increase was non-significantly greater in the vaccine arm, suggesting that 2 inoculations with NeuVax + GM-CSF can induce in vivo immunity and a continued antigen-specific T-cell response 1 month post-surgery.

Recognition that partial elimination of cells expressing a single antigen may result in alternative clones emerging has led to the idea that multiple-antigen vaccines may be more effective. Preclinical testing of a multiple antigen vaccine to intercept high-risk lesions in the breast has been performed by Disis and colleagues.[65] This targets HER2, insulin-like growth factor receptor-1, and insulin-like growth factor binding protein-2, proteins that are upregulated in high-risk and preinvasive breast lesions and overexpressed in multiple types of poor-prognosis breast cancer. A multi-epitope vaccine derived from these 3 antigens was tested in transgenic mice and was shown to be highly effective, preventing mammary tumors in 65% of mice. A recently completed phase I clinical trial (NCT02780401) in breast patients with cancer shows favorable toxicity and immunogenicity,[65] and additional studies are likely to follow.

Additional antigens that are highly expressed in early lesions and are potential targets for breast cancer prevention vaccines include MUC1, lactalbumin, and mammaglobin, but these are still in early therapeutic trials. The utility of these for cancer prevention and interception could be the next step, once safety and immunogenicity are well established.

Recent Innovations in Risk Estimation Tools

Polygenic risk scores

Apart from the monogenic cancer susceptibility syndromes, it has been recognized since the early days of genome-wide association studies that there are a large number of common single nucleotide polymorphisms (SNPs) that may carry minimal increased risks for cancer as single events but, when inherited together, might lead to meaningful risk increases.[66] Significant advances have occurred in this area, as exemplified by a recent validation study applying the BOADICEA (Breast and Ovarian Analysis of Disease Incidence and Carrier Estimation Algorithm) model and a validated panel of 303 SNPs to an independent mammography cohort in Sweden.[67] They were able to assess the improvement in predictive accuracy of a model when the 303 gene polygenic risk scores (PRS) were added to models including family history, questionnaire-based risk factors, breast density, and pathogenic variant status in 8 breast cancer susceptibility genes (*BRCA1*, *BRCA2*, *PALB2*, *CHEK2*, *ATM*, *RAD51C*, *RAD51D*, and *BARD1*). The joint model yielded an AUC = 0.70 (95% CI: 0.66–0.73), E/O ratio = 0.88 (95% CI: 0.75–1.04), and calibration slope = 0.97 (95% CI: 0.95–0.99). The full multifactorial model classified 3.6% women as high risk (5 year risk ≥3%) and 11.1% as very low risk (5 year risk <0.33%). The improvement was observed mainly at the high end of the risk spectrum, where the addition of PRS enabled the identification of women with a 3% 5 year risk, whereas without the PRS, the highest predicted 5 year risk ranged up to 2% (**Fig. 2**). Importantly, PRS addition to other parameters allows women at the lowest risk to be better identified, opening up the possibility of scaling back on screening recommendations for these women.

Radiomics techniques applied to digital mammography

Breast density as measured on mammography is a well-established breast cancer risk factor. About one-half of US women have heterogeneously or extremely dense breasts on mammogram, and their risk for future breast cancer is increased by 2-fold and 4-

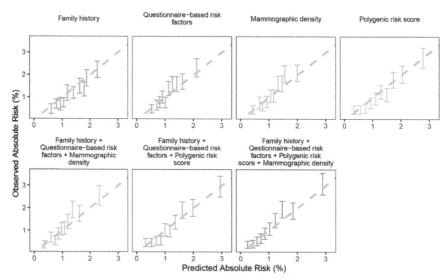

Fig. 2. Observed and predicted 5 year breast cancer risks using the subcohort of participants with polygenic risk score information (n = 15,502) under different risk factor combinations. Women were grouped into grouped into deciles of predicted risks. Each dot represents the mean observed and predicted risk in the decile and the vertical segments represent 95% CIs. The dashed line is the diagonal line with slope equal to 1 (corresponding to expected to observed number of cases ratio of 1 for each decile). When the CI crosses the diagonal, the decile-predicted risk is not significantly different from the observed risk. When a dot and the associated CI fall above the diagonal, there is a suggestion for underprediction of risk; when a dot and associated CI fall below the diagonal, there is a suggestion for overprediction of risk. (Yang X, et al. *J Med Genet* 2022;59:1196-1205. https://doi.org/10.1136/jmg-2022-108806.)

fold, respectively.[68] More recently, with the widespread use of digital mammography, radiomic features of mammograms have been examined using artificial intelligence (AI) approaches to personalize supplemental screening decisions based on estimates of short-term risk.[69,70] These have led to the observation that it is possible to derive risk-related information from screening mammograms; once validated in multiple data sets and operationalized, they will push breast cancer risk estimation into the mainstream workflow of breast imaging centers. Several versions of this approach have been reproduced in cohorts beyond the populations used for model development, with promising results.

A particularly promising approach is a deep-learning model derived only from mammographic features, potentially obviate the patient history or risk factor data.[70] It was trained and validated in all patients undergoing screening, including breast cancer survivors and mutation carriers. Four standard view mammographic images are processed through an image encoder, generating a deep-learning score using architectural details (the code is open-source and available online). When compared with the Tyrer-Cuzick and NCI BCRAT models, it demonstrated superior performance in identifying a group with higher cancer detection rates on screening mammogram than either of the questionnaire-based models. Although not directly relevant to the selection of women for preventive medication as yet, longitudinal data on populations whose mammograms have been assessed in this way may provide an objective and simpler approach to the identification of women who are at increased risk in the future.

Also of great interest is the use of mammographic image data to identify women at risk for aggressive cancers over the next few years, as demonstrated in a multiethnic US cohort.[71] The main utility of this in the near future will be to stratify women with normal screening mammograms into those who either need supplemental imaging or do not; but with longitudinal follow-up, it may also be more informative regarding indications for preventive therapy.

SUMMARY

Several promising avenues under development will provide inexpensive and accessible methods of risk estimation and cancer prevention, the most notable being the application of AI to mammograms without the need for extensive risk factor history, de-escalating dosing of established agents, and the development of new agents. These developments are critical since a recent analysis of breast cancer incidence trends shows increases in 5 of 7 global regions, particularly in women under 50 and over 70.[72] Breast cancer prevention therefore remains an important priority, achievable with affordable interventions that avoid the labor and expense of being sick.

CLINICS CARE POINTS

- Women who are eligible for medication to reduce breast cancer risk should be encouraged to consider it, with detailed counselling regarding proven benefits and risks.
- Eligible women include those with a calculated absolute 5-year risk estimate $\geq 3\%$.
- Also eligible are those aged under 45 with estimated risk ≥ 4-fold that of an average risk peer, and those 45 years or older with estimated risk ≥ 2-fold that of an average risk peer.
- The use of polygenic risk scores and the application of radiomics techniques to mammographic images will improve the selection of candidates for medical risk reduction, but has not entered the clinical care environment as yet.

- Anti-estrogen medications reduce risk for such women by one-half overall, and by two-thirds for those with atypical lesions of the breast.
- For premenopausal women tamoxifen 20 mg daily is the only approved risk-reducing drug, but use at lower doses can be considered for women who are unwilling to take the full dose or cannot tolerate it.
- For postmenopausal women, the choice between aromatase inhibitors and tamoxifen or raloxifene will depend on risk of comorbidity (i.e. bone health versus uterine health versus risk of thromboembolism).

DISCLOSURE

The author has no conflicts of interest to disclose.

REFERENCES

1. Fisher B, Redmond C. New perspective on cancer of the contralateral breast: a marker for assessing tamoxifen as a preventive agent. J Natl Cancer Inst 1991; 83(18):1278–80.
2. Fisher B, Costantino JP, Wickerham DL, et al. Tamoxifen for prevention of breast cancer: report of the National Surgical Adjuvant Breast and Bowel Project P-1 Study. JNatlCancer Inst 1998;90(18):1371–88.
3. Cuzick J, Forbes J, Edwards R, et al. First results from the International Breast Cancer Intervention Study (IBIS-I): a randomised prevention trial. Lancet 2002; 360(9336):817–24.
4. Vogel VG, Costantino JP, Wickerham DL, et al. Update of the National Surgical Adjuvant Breast and Bowel Project Study of Tamoxifen and Raloxifene (STAR) P-2 Trial: Preventing breast cancer. Cancer Prev Res 2010;3(6):696–706.
5. Cuzick J, Sestak I, Forbes JF, et al. Anastrozole for prevention of breast cancer in high-risk postmenopausal women (IBIS-II): an international, double-blind, randomised placebo-controlled trial. Lancet 2014;383(9922):1041–8.
6. Force USPST, Owens DK, Davidson KW, et al. Medication Use to Reduce Risk of Breast Cancer: US Preventive Services Task Force Recommendation Statement. JAMA 2019;322(9):857–67.
7. Freedman AN, Yu B, Gail MH, et al. Benefit/risk assessment for breast cancer chemoprevention with raloxifene or tamoxifen for women age 50 years or older. J Clin Oncol 2011;29(17):2327–33.
8. Cuzick J, Warwick J, Pinney E, et al. Tamoxifen-induced reduction in mammographic density and breast cancer risk reduction: a nested case-control study. JNatlCancer Inst 2011;103(9):744–52.
9. Eriksson M, Czene K, Conant EF, et al. Use of Low-Dose Tamoxifen to Increase Mammographic Screening Sensitivity in Premenopausal Women. Cancers 2021;13(2):302.
10. Tan-Chiu E, Wang J, Costantino JP, et al. Effects of tamoxifen on benign breast disease in women at high risk for breast cancer. JNatlCancer Inst 2003;95(4): 302–7.
11. Goldstein SR. Selective estrogen receptor modulators and bone health. Climacteric 2022;25(1):56–9.
12. Yang F, Li N, Gaman MA, et al. Raloxifene has favorable effects on the lipid profile in women explaining its beneficial effect on cardiovascular risk: A meta-analysis of randomized controlled trials. Pharmacol Res 2021;166:105512.

13. Alomar SA, Gaman MA, Prabahar K, et al. The effect of tamoxifen on the lipid profile in women: A systematic review and meta-analysis of randomized controlled trials. Exp Gerontol 2022;159:111680.
14. Cuzick J, Sestak I, Cawthorn S, et al. Tamoxifen for prevention of breast cancer: extended long-term follow-up of the IBIS-I breast cancer prevention trial. Lancet Oncol 2015;16(1):67–75.
15. Cuzick J, Sestak I, Forbes JF, et al. Use of anastrozole for breast cancer prevention (IBIS-II): long-term results of a randomised controlled trial. Lancet 2020; 395(10218):117–22.
16. Smith SG, Sestak I, Forster A, et al. Factors affecting uptake and adherence to breast cancer chemoprevention: a systematic review and meta-analysis. Ann Oncol 2016;27(4):575–90.
17. Crew KD, Albain KS, Hershman DL, et al. How do we increase uptake of tamoxifen and other anti-estrogens for breast cancer prevention? NPJ Breast Cancer 2017;3:20.
18. Loprinzi CL, Barton D, Rummans T. Newer antidepressants inhibit hot flashes. Menopause 2006;13(4):546–8.
19. Loprinzi CL, Kugler JW, Barton DL, et al. Phase III trial of gabapentin alone or in conjunction with an antidepressant in the management of hot flashes in women who have inadequate control with an antidepressant alone: NCCTG N03C5. J Clin Oncol 2007;25(3):308–12.
20. Leon-Ferre RA, Novotny PJ, Wolfe EG, et al. Oxybutynin vs Placebo for Hot Flashes in Women With or Without Breast Cancer: A Randomized, Double-Blind Clinical Trial (ACCRU SC-1603). JNCI Cancer Spectr 2020;4(1):pkz088.
21. D'Alessandro EG, da Silva AV, Cecatto RB, et al. Acupuncture for Climacteric-Like Symptoms in Breast Cancer Improves Sleep, Mental and Emotional Health: A Randomized Trial. Med Acupunct 2022;34(1):58–65.
22. Rockhill B, Spiegelman D, Byrne C, et al. Validation of the Gail et al. model of breast cancer risk prediction and implications for chemoprevention. JNatlCancer Inst 2001;93(5):358–66.
23. Tyrer J, Duffy SW, Cuzick J. A breast cancer prediction model incorporating familial and personal risk factors. Stat Med 2004;23(7):1111–30.
24. Tice JA, Bissell MCS, Miglioretti DL, et al. Validation of the breast cancer surveillance consortium model of breast cancer risk. Breast Cancer Res Treat 2019; 175(2):519–23.
25. Velentzis LS, Freeman V, Campbell D, et al. Breast Cancer Risk Assessment Tools for Stratifying Women into Risk Groups: A Systematic Review. Cancers 2023; 15(4):1124.
26. Brentnall AR, Cuzick J, Buist DSM, et al. Long-term Accuracy of Breast Cancer Risk Assessment Combining Classic Risk Factors and Breast Density. JAMA Oncol 2018;4(9):e180174.
27. Tice JA, Cummings SR, Ziv E, et al. Mammographic breast density and the Gail model for breast cancer risk prediction in a screening population. Breast Cancer Res Treat 2005;94(2):115–22.
28. Spiegelman D, Colditz GA, Hunter D, et al. Validation of the Gail et al. model for predicting individual breast cancer risk [see comments]. J NatlCancer Inst 1994; 86(8):600–7.
29. Eriksson M, Eklund M, Borgquist S, et al. Low-Dose Tamoxifen for Mammographic Density Reduction: A Randomized Controlled Trial. J Clin Oncol 2021; 39(17):1899–908.

30. Visvanathan K, Fabian CJ, Bantug E, et al. Use of Endocrine Therapy for Breast Cancer Risk Reduction: ASCO Clinical Practice Guideline Update. J Clin Oncol 2019;37(33):3152–65.

31. Knight JA, Blackmore KM, Fan J, et al. The association of mammographic density with risk of contralateral breast cancer and change in density with treatment in the WECARE study. Breast Cancer Res 2018;20(1):23.

32. Atakpa EC, Thorat MA, Cuzick J, et al. Mammographic density, endocrine therapy and breast cancer risk: a prognostic and predictive biomarker review. Cochrane Database Syst Rev 2021;10(10):CD013091.

33. Hale MJ, Howell A, Dowsett M, et al. Tamoxifen related side effects and their impact on breast cancer incidence: A retrospective analysis of the randomised IBIS-I trial. Breast 2020;54:216–21.

34. Decensi A, Robertson C, Guerrieri-Gonzaga A, et al. Randomized double-blind 2 x 2 trial of low-dose tamoxifen and fenretinide for breast cancer prevention in high-risk premenopausal women. J Clin Oncol 2009;27(23):3749–56.

35. Bonanni B, Serrano D, Gandini S, et al. Randomized biomarker trial of anastrozole or low-dose tamoxifen or their combination in subjects with breast intraepithelial neoplasia. Clin Cancer Res 2009;15(22):7053–60.

36. Lazzeroni M, DeCensi A. Alternate dosing schedules for cancer chemopreventive agents. Semin Oncol 2016;43(1):116–22.

37. DeCensi A, Puntoni M, Guerrieri-Gonzaga A, et al. Randomized Placebo Controlled Trial of Low-Dose Tamoxifen to Prevent Local and Contralateral Recurrence in Breast Intraepithelial Neoplasia. J Clin Oncol 2019;37(19):1629–37.

38. DeCensi A, Puntoni M, Johansson H, et al. Effect Modifiers of Low-Dose Tamoxifen in a Randomized Trial in Breast Noninvasive Disease. Clin Cancer Res 2021;27(13):3576–83.

39. Serrano D, Gandini S, Thomas P, et al. Efficacy of Alternative Dose Regimens of Exemestane in Postmenopausal Women With Stage 0 to II Estrogen Receptor-Positive Breast Cancer: A Randomized Clinical Trial. JAMA Oncol 2023;9(5):664–72.

40. Evaluation of Lasofoxifene Versus Fulvestrant in Advanced or Metastatic ER+/HER2- Breast Cancer With an ESR1 Mutation - Full Text View - ClinicalTrials.gov.

41. Chlebowski RT, Anderson GL, Aragaki AK, et al. Association of Menopausal Hormone Therapy With Breast Cancer Incidence and Mortality During Long-term Follow-up of the Women's Health Initiative Randomized Clinical Trials. JAMA 2020;324(4):369–80.

42. Labrie F, Martel C, Gauthier S, et al. Effect of toremifene and ospemifene, compared to acolbifene, on estrogen-sensitive parameters in rat and human uterine tissues. Horm Mol Biol Clin Investig 2010;1(3):139–46.

43. Lemieux C, Phaneuf D, Labrie F, et al. Estrogen receptor alpha-mediated adiposity-lowering and hypocholesterolemic actions of the selective estrogen receptor modulator acolbifene. Int J Obes 2005;29(10):1236–44.

44. Fabian CJ, Kimler BF, Zalles CM, et al. Clinical Trial of Acolbifene in Premenopausal Women at High Risk for Breast Cancer. Cancer Prev Res 2015;8(12):1146–55.

45. Mauvais-Javis P, Baudot N, Castaigne D, et al. trans-4-Hydroxytamoxifen concentration and metabolism after local percutaneous administration to human breast. Cancer Res 1986;46(3):1521–5.

46. Kuiper GG, Carlsson B, Grandien K, et al. Comparison of the ligand binding specificity and transcript tissue distribution of estrogen receptors alpha and beta. Endocrinology 1997;138(3):863–70.

47. Wakeling AE, Slater SR. Estrogen-receptor binding and biologic activity of tamoxifen and its metabolites. Cancer Treat Rep 1980;64(6–7):741–4.
48. Johnson MD, Zuo H, Lee KH, et al. Pharmacological characterization of 4-hydroxy-N-desmethyl tamoxifen, a novel active metabolite of tamoxifen. Breast Cancer Res Treat 2004;85(2):151–9.
49. Lim YC, Desta Z, Flockhart DA, et al. Endoxifen (4-hydroxy-N-desmethyl-tamoxifen) has anti-estrogenic effects in breast cancer cells with potency similar to 4-hydroxy-tamoxifen. Cancer Chemother Pharmacol 2005;55(5):471–8.
50. Pujol H, Girault J, Rouanet P, et al. Phase I study of percutaneous 4-hydroxy-tamoxifen with analyses of 4-hydroxy-tamoxifen concentrations in breast cancer and normal breast tissue. Cancer Chemother Pharmacol 1995;36(6):493–8.
51. Mansel R, Goyal A, Nestour EL, et al. A phase II trial of Afimoxifene (4-hydroxy-tamoxifen gel) for cyclical mastalgia in premenopausal women. Breast Cancer Res Treat 2007;106(3):389–97.
52. Rouanet P, Linares-Cruz G, Dravet F, et al. Neoadjuvant percutaneous 4-hydroxytamoxifen decreases breast tumoral cell proliferation: a prospective controlled randomized study comparing three doses of 4-hydroxytamoxifen gel to oral tamoxifen. J Clin Oncol 2005;23(13):2980–7.
53. Lee O, Page K, Ivancic D, et al. A randomized phase II presurgical trial of transdermal 4-hydroxytamoxifen gel versus oral tamoxifen in women with ductal carcinoma in situ of the breast. Clin Cancer Res 2014;20(14):3672–82.
54. Lee O, Pilewskie M, Karlan S, et al. Local Transdermal Delivery of Telapristone Acetate Through Breast Skin, Compared With Oral Treatment: A Randomized Double-Blind, Placebo-Controlled Phase II Trial. Clin Pharmacol Ther 2021; 109(3):728–38.
55. Tanos T, Sflomos G, Echeverria PC, et al. Progesterone/RANKL is a major regulatory axis in the human breast. Sci Transl Med 2013;5(182):182ra155.
56. Ranjan M, Lee O, Cottone G, et al. Progesterone receptor antagonists reverse stem cell expansion and the paracrine effectors of progesterone action in the mouse mammary gland. Breast Cancer Res 2021;23(1):78.
57. Lee O, Bosland MC, Wang M, et al. Selective progesterone receptor blockade prevents BRCA1-associated mouse mammary tumors through modulation of epithelial and stromal genes. Cancer letters 2021;520:255–66.
58. Bartlett TE, Evans I, Jones A, et al. Antiprogestins reduce epigenetic field cancerization in breast tissue of young healthy women. Genome Med 2022;14(1):64.
59. Donnez J, Arriagada P, Marciniak M, et al. Liver safety parameters of ulipristal acetate for the treatment of uterine fibroids: a comprehensive review of the clinical development program. Expert Opin Drug Saf 2018;17(12):1225–32.
60. Nolan E, Vaillant F, Branstetter D, et al. RANK ligand as a potential target for breast cancer prevention in BRCA1-mutation carriers. Nature medicine 2016; 22(8):933–9.
61. Kiechl S, Schramek D, Widschwendter M, et al. Aberrant regulation of RANKL/OPG in women at high risk of developing breast cancer. Oncotarget 2017;8(3):3811–25.
62. Mintz R, Wang M, Xu S, et al. Hormone and receptor activator of NF-kappaB (RANK) pathway gene expression in plasma and mammographic breast density in postmenopausal women. Breast Cancer Res 2022;24(1):28.
63. Lowenfeld L, Mick R, Datta J, et al. Dendritic Cell Vaccination Enhances Immune Responses and Induces Regression of HER2(pos) DCIS Independent of Route: Results of Randomized Selection Design Trial. Clin Cancer Res 2017;23(12):2961–71.
64. Clifton GT, Peoples GE, Mittendorf EA. The development and use of the E75 (HER2 369-377) peptide vaccine. Future Oncol 2016;12(11):1321–9.

65. Disis ML, Cecil DL. Breast cancer vaccines for treatment and prevention. Breast Cancer Res Treat 2022;191(3):481–9.
66. Ponder BA, Antoniou A, Dunning A, et al. Polygenic inherited predisposition to breast cancer. Cold Spring Harb Symp Quant Biol 2005;70:35–41.
67. Yang X, Eriksson M, Czene K, et al. Prospective validation of the BOADICEA multifactorial breast cancer risk prediction model in a large prospective cohort study. J Med Genet 2022;59(12):1196–205.
68. Boyd NF, Guo H, Martin LJ, et al. Mammographic density and the risk and detection of breast cancer. N Engl J Med 2007;356(3):227–36.
69. McKinney SM, Sieniek M, Godbole V, et al. International evaluation of an AI system for breast cancer screening. Nature 2020;577(7788):89–94.
70. Lehman CD, Mercaldo S, Lamb LR, et al. Deep Learning vs Traditional Breast Cancer Risk Models to Support Risk-Based Mammography Screening. J Natl Cancer Inst 2022;114(10):1355–63.
71. Eriksson M, Destounis S, Czene K, et al. A risk model for digital breast tomosynthesis to predict breast cancer and guide clinical care. Sci Transl Med 2022; 14(644):eabn3971.
72. Lima SM, Kehm RD, Terry MB. Global breast cancer incidence and mortality trends by region, age-groups, and fertility patterns. EClinicalMedicine 2021;38: 100985.

Individualizing Breast Cancer Risk Assessment in Clinical Practice

Amy E. Cyr, MD[a],*, Kaitlyn Kennard, MD[b]

KEYWORDS

- Breast cancer risk • High risk • Risk assessment • Risk models • Risk factors
- Risk reduction • Screening

KEY POINTS

- Multiple tools exist to assess future breast cancer risk for individual patients.
- A risk calculator may depend heavily on family history, the risk of a genetic mutation, prior biopsy results, breast density, lifestyle, and hormonal factors.
- Choice of risk model depends on which risk factors apply to a patient.
- Risk calculations inform both screening and risk-reduction options.
- Although many risk factors are nonmodifiable, patients can reduce their risk to some extent with lifestyle modifications.

INTRODUCTION

Breast cancer (BC) is the most common malignancy in American women.*,[1] Mortality has declined, in part because screening detects cancers at an early stage.[2] For most women, screening means annual mammography, starting at 40 years of age. Mammography improves survival, with the caveat that some women undergo procedures for benign findings or treatment for clinically insignificant cancers.[2,3] For women whose BC risk is above average, the addition of annual breast magnetic resonance imaging (MRI) to mammography is superior to mammography alone.[4] Women identified as high risk (HR) are also eligible for risk-reducing endocrine therapy or surgery.

   This chapter discusses BC risk factors, tools used to identify HR patients, and how to use this information to reduce BC-related morbidity and mortality.

a Department of Medicine, Washington University, Box 8056, 660 South Euclid Avenue, Saint Louis, MO 63110, USA; b Department of Surgery, Washington University, Box 8051, 660 South Euclid Avenue, Saint louis, MO 63110, USA
* Corresponding author.
E-mail address: amycyr@wustl.edu

Surg Oncol Clin N Am 32 (2023) 647–661
https://doi.org/10.1016/j.soc.2023.05.013
surgonc.theclinics.com

DISCUSSION
Nonmodifiable Risk Factors

Age and race
White women have the highest BC rate, followed by Black women, although this gap has narrowed. Hispanic, American Indian, and Pacific Islander women have the lowest incidence. Aging increases risk, but the incidence has increased for women aged 20 to 49 years, while remaining stable or declining for older women.[5]

Although all young women are more likely to have higher stage and more aggressive disease, at all ages, these poor prognostic indicators disproportionately affect Black women. In addition, stage-for-stage, young Black women are twice as likely to die from BC as White women.[6]

Thoracic radiation
For children and young adults treated with thoracic radiation, the incidence of BC by the age of 55 years is as high as 29%.[7] Radiation increases the risk for both estrogen receptor positive (ER+) and negative (ER−) disease. Patient age during therapy, radiation dose, use of alkylating agents, and therapy-related suppression of ovarian function impact the degree of risk attributable to radiation.[7–9] Thoracic radiation is not a variable in any risk model but is a stand-alone indication for HR screening and risk-reducing therapy.[4]

Breast density
Increased breast density is an independent risk factor for BC.[10,11] Women with the highest level of density have a 4-fold increase in risk compared with women with minimal density. Density is, in part, heritable (Asian women, for instance, have the highest breast density), but higher alcohol intake and the use of hormone replacement therapy (HRT) also increase density.[11] Many patients taking endocrine therapy see a decrease in breast density; some studies suggest that this mammographic change is prognostic and predictive.[10]

Pathologies
Benign breast disease comprises nonproliferative lesions, proliferative lesions without atypia, atypical hyperplasia, and lobular carcinoma in situ (LCIS). Nonproliferative pathologies increase risk minimally and only for women with a family history (FHx). Proliferative change without atypia doubles risk, atypical hyperplasia increases risk 4-fold, and LCIS increases risk 8- to 10-fold.[12,13] A younger age at diagnosis of benign disease further increases risk, and for women of any age, the increased risk persists for 2 decades. Although the risk affects both breasts, the ipsilateral breast is twice as likely as the contralateral breast to develop a cancer within the first 5 years after biopsy (within the first 10 years for women with atypia).[12,14]

BC predisposition genes
The widespread use of multigene panel testing identifies cancer-predisposing variants. These pathogenic variants are overall rare, but the incidence of ATM and CHEK2 mutations is 1% to 2% in White Europeans or European descendants, while the incidence of BRCA mutations is about 2.5% in the Ashkenazi Jewish population.[15,16]

High-penetrance genes like *BRCA1*, *BRCA2*, and *TP53* increase lifetime BC risk to at least 50%, while moderate penetrance genes like *ATM, BARD1, CDH1, CHEK2, RAD51 C, RAD51D,* and *STK11* increase lifetime risk to 20% to 50%; the gene, specific variant, and FHx modify the risk. While most pathogenic ATM variants increase lifetime BC risk to under 30%, lifetime risk with the missense variant c.7271 T > G approaches that of *BRCA2*. Lifetime BC risk with PALB2, often classified as moderately penetrant, and with PTEN may exceed 50%.[15–17] Risk with moderately penetrant variants can be further refined with polygenic risk scores (PRSs).[15]

Pathogenic ATM and CHEK2 variants primarily increase the risk of ER+ disease, suggesting a possible role for endocrine prophylaxis. In contrast, *BARD1, RAD51 C,* and *RAD51D* increase ER cancer risk.[15,17]

Risk Models

Risk models incorporate nonmodifiable and modifiable variables to estimate BC risk. Model choice depends on (1) why a patient may be HR and (2) how the information will drive management.

Breast cancer risk assessment tool

Gail and colleagues used data from Caucasian women aged 35 to 74 years to develop a model to calculate invasive and noninvasive BC risk. Their model included age of menarche and first parity, number of biopsies, presence of atypia, and number of affected female first-degree relatives (FDRs).[18]

Other investigators refined the model and limited its prediction to an invasive disease. This modified Gail model, or National Cancer Institute Breast Cancer Risk Assessment Tool (BCRAT), calculates risk over the next 5 years and by the age of 90 years (**Box 1**).[19,20]

The BCRAT performs well at the population level, measured by the expected-to-observed (E/O) event ratio, but this varies by subpopulation: Although modifications to the BCRAT incorporated data from African American, Asian, Pacific Islander, and Hispanic women, BCRAT performance is poorer in non-White populations.[21–23]

The model underestimates risk in general. In one study evaluating model performance in women with atypia, investigators expected 34.9 cancers but observed 58 (E/O 0.6). For individual women, the concordance statistic (or area under the curve [AUC]) was 0.50 (95% confidence interval [CI] 0.44–0.55), no better than the flip of a coin.[24] A meta-analysis showed that the BCRAT performs poorly at the individual level for women without atypia as well.[25] In addition, female FDRs are the only included FHx, so the model underestimates risk for patients with an extended or paternal FHx or affected male relatives.

The BCRAT is more likely to underestimate, rather than overestimate, lifetime risk, so it is best used to determine eligibility for endocrine therapy (as it was used in chemoprevention trials), but not for screening MRI.

Breast Cancer Surveillance Consortium

Tice and colleagues assessed density alone to predict BC risk and calculated an AUC of 0.67 (95% CI 0.66–0.70), equivalent to the AUC calculated using BCRAT variables.

Box 1
BCRAT (Gail model)

- Available online at https://bcrisktool.cancer.gov/
- Calculates risk at 5 years and by the age of 90 years
- Cannot be used for patients younger than 35 years or with a BRCA mutation or LCIS
- Underestimates lifetime risk for patients with atypia and those with extended or paternal family history
- Better used to determine endocrine therapy eligibility rather than to direct screening recommendations

Adding density to BCRAT variables modestly improved the AUC.[26] They further refined and validated their risk model using data from the Breast Cancer Surveillance Consortium (BCSC) registries, limiting FHx of affected FDR to yes/no, and adding categories of benign disease (nonproliferative, proliferative without atypia, proliferative with atypia, and LCIS) (**Box 2**).[27]

The final model underestimates the risk for young women, those with fatty density, Asian and Hispanic women, and Black women, while overpredicting risk overall (E/O 1.04, 95% CI 1.03–1.06); AUC was 0.665. Only 3% of women had a 5-year risk over 3%, and about 7% had a 10-year risk over 5%. For women with proliferative disease, the addition of that pathology to the risk calculation identifies 3 times as many as HR.[28,29]

Because BCSC provides 5- and 10-year risk but not lifetime BC risk, it is best used to determine eligibility for endocrine prophylaxis.[30]

International Breast Cancer Intervention Study model

Developed with the data from the International Breast Cancer Intervention Study (IBIS), the Tyrer-Cuzick, or IBIS model (**Box 3**), calculates the likelihood of having a BRCA-related cancer and refines that calculation with risk attributable to personal factors. The software is downloadable, and there is an online platform. Although not a default setting with the most recent software (version 8), IBIS creators recommend inclusion of competing mortality.[31–33]

Unlike BCRAT, IBIS incorporates diverse risk factors, including hormonal history, BRCA status, and breast density. Body mass index (BMI) refines the risk attributable to density. An elevated BMI independently adds risk for postmenopausal women; the protective effect of increased BMI in premenopausal women is not addressed in the model.[32,33]

FHx includes bilateral breast, ovarian, and male BCs. Unaffected relatives and their current age (or age at death) further refine results.[32,33]

Biopsy history includes benign/nonproliferative disease, hyperplasia, atypia, and LCIS. Pathologies such as adenosis, apocrine change, and mild usual ductal hyperplasia (UDH) are considered nonproliferative. Proliferative disease includes moderate or florid UDH, sclerosing adenosis, and papillomas. Atypia includes atypical ductal and lobular hyperplasia, but not flat epithelial atypia. The calculated relative risk attributed to atypia is 4-fold, while that for LCIS is 8-fold.[31,32]

IBIS overestimates risk for women with LCIS and atypia, however.[34–36] In one study, the AUC for women with LCIS was only 0.493.[29] Another reported an E/O ratio of 1.48 in patients with LCIS and an AUC of 0.54 (95% CI 0.48–0.62).[36]

IBIS performs well across ethnic populations but may overestimate the risk for Hispanic women while underestimating that for African Americans. It also overestimates

---

Box 2
BCSC Risk Model

- Available online at https://tools.bscs-scc.org/BC5yearRisk/calculator.htm
- Calculates invasive breast cancer risk at 5 and 10 years
- Incorporates personal risk factors, including breast density, biopsy history, and limited family history but is not validated in women with implants
- Underestimates risk in younger women, non-Caucasian women, and women with minimal breast density
- Can be used to determine eligibility for endocrine prophylaxis

---

Box 3
IBIS (Tyrer-Cuzick model)

- Available online at https://ibis.ikonopedia.com or at https://www.ems-trials.org/riskevaluator/
- Calculates breast cancer risk at 5 or 10 years and by the age of 85 years and calculates the likelihood of carrying a BRCA mutation
- Incorporates personal risk factors, including breast density, biopsy history, and extensive family history
- Overestimates lifetime risk with extended follow-up and for patients with atypia or LCIS
- Can be used to determine eligibility for high-risk screening or for endocrine prophylaxis

---

the risk for women with the highest risk, for BRCA carriers, and with longer follow-up.[37,38] PRS data can be added and improve model performance.[39]

CanRisk

CanRisk (**Box 4**), previously known as Breast and Ovarian Analysis of Disease Incidence and Carrier Estimation Algorithm, was developed using a cohort of women diagnosed with BC before the age of 55 years.[40]

It incorporates diverse variables, such as hormonal and lifestyle risk factors, breast density, personal cancer history, and risk-reducing surgery, but not biopsy history. Relevant FHx includes breast, ovarian, male breast, and pancreatic cancers, along with BC receptor information.[40–42] Like IBIS, a PRS can be included.[43]

CanRisk is time-consuming but valuable in some situations. *BRCA1, BRCA2, ATM, PALB2, CHEK2, RAD51 C, RAD51D, BARD1*, and *BRIP1* mutations are included, so it is helpful for calculating risk with moderately penetrant genes and for women who do not have a familial moderate penetrance gene. CanRisk provides 5- or 10-year and lifetime BC risk, ovarian cancer risk, and contralateral BC risk for patients with a personal history of cancer.[44]

CanRisk, available online,[44] is frequently updated and performs better than other models at both population and individual levels. In one study, E/O ratios ranged from 0.88 to 1.12, depending on the thoroughness of the variable input, with AUCs ranging from 0.61 to 0.70.[45]

Claus

Claus and colleagues assumed a dominant allele could explain hereditary cancer and proposed a model using data from Caucasian BC patients (age 20–54 years) and

---

Box 4
CanRisk

- Available online at https://canrisk.org
- Calculates breast, ovarian, and contralateral breast cancer risk at 5 or 10 years and by the age of 80 years
- Incorporates personal risk factors, including breast density, extensive family history, and various cancer predisposition genes
- Frequently updated and able to refine risk due to moderately penetrant genes
- Results determine eligibility for high-risk screening

---

matched controls (**Box 5**). Input includes up to 2 relatives (FDR and second-degree relatives with BC and FDRs with ovarian cancer) and age at diagnosis. Risk estimates are available in table form or online.[46]

In one cohort, Claus underpredicted cancers (E/O ratio 1.69, 95% CI 1.48–1.87), and the AUC was lower than that for other models evaluated in the same study (AUC 0.59, 95% CI 0.56–0.62).[47]

BRCAPRO

BRCAPRO (**Box 6**) shares many features with IBIS and CanRisk. It incorporates unaffected FDR and second-degree relatives and those with bilateral breast and ovarian cancer. Cancer receptors, race, ethnicity, and risk-reducing surgery can be included. Like IBIS, it determines cancer risk based on the likelihood of having a BRCA gene. It provides an estimated risk of breast, ovarian, or contralateral BC.[48,49] Unlike IBIS, BRCAPRO does not include competing mortality, and there is no free online tool.

At the population level, BRCAPRO overestimates risk for older women and those without a significant FHx, while underestimating risk overall, especially for younger women and for those with a more extensive FHx. Discrimination at the individual level is similar, but somewhat inferior, to that of IBIS and BCRAT.[37,47]

Ask2Me

Although several of these risk calculators incorporate germline mutations, management guidelines, including those provided by testing companies and the National Comprehensive Cancer Network (NCCN), report broad lifetime cancer risks.[16] The online All Syndromes Known to Man Evaluator (Ask2Me) provides an age-adjusted estimate of cancer risk associated with any of almost 3-dozen genes. It also provides risk in 5-year intervals, which can guide the timing of risk-reducing interventions.[50,51]

The website is updated less frequently than others, including CanRisk and NCCN. For instance, NCCN currently recommends consideration of HR screening for women with BARD1 and reports no increase in ovarian cancer risk, while Ask2Me continues to show an increased ovarian cancer risk. Ask2Me references NCCN and other professional society guidelines, but as of the date of this writing, that information is outdated.[49,50]

Artificial intelligence

Deep learning–based convolutional neural networks improve cancer detection and refine mammographic breast density classification. These and other artificial intelligence tools also use mammographic images to provide risk stratification. The AUCs reported with deep learning are equivalent or superior to those of the tools discussed in this chapter. However, minority women are underrepresented in many data sets used to develop this technology, and tools need to be validated in diverse screening populations.[52]

Box 5
Claus

- Determines breast cancer risk using published risk tables
- Calculates breast cancer risk in 10-year increments, up to the age of 79 years
- Incorporates up to 2 first- or second-degree relatives with breast or ovarian cancer
- Less robustly validated and may underestimate breast cancer risk
- Results determine eligibility for high-risk screening

| Box 6 |
| BRCAPRO |

- Available with a commercial software package
- Calculates breast, ovarian, and contralateral breast cancer risk
- Incorporates a complex family history of breast or ovarian cancer
- May underestimate breast cancer risk, especially for young patients
- Results determine eligibility for high-risk screening

Polygenic risk scores

While some BCs are attributable to highly or moderately penetrant genes, most result from common alleles. Individually these minimally affect risk. For patients with many HR alleles, though, the increase in BC risk may be significant and is reflected in a PRS.

PRS data are applicable to non-White populations, help predict contralateral BC risk, and refine risk with moderately penetrant genes.[53-55] Addition of PRS to standard risk factors improves model performance over that with either PRS or standard risk factors alone. Such refinements to risk calculations may in the future not only identify women as HR but identify those with low risk who may not need yearly mammography. PRS may even determine risk for certain types of BC (for instance ER+ disease), informing management.[54,56] Outside of their inclusion in models like IBIS and CanRisk; however, PRS are not yet routinely used to make clinical decisions.

Choosing a model

Table 1 summarizes the variables included in these frequently used models, which represent only a proportion of available models. As with those discussed here, others were developed and validated using different sets of data and incorporate variable risk factors. Model performance, therefore, varies by patient subpopulation (age, risk factors, ethnicity, etc).[37]

Investigators have compared the population-level calibration and individual-level discrimination of these models. Discrimination is best for CanRisk and IBIS. All models, with the exception of CanRisk, underestimate risk in patients with the lowest risk and overestimate in patients with the highest risk.[57] IBIS identifies the highest proportion of HR women.[58] Most models predict risk better for luminal than for nonluminal cancers.[59]

Based on performance, ease of use, accessibility, and utility for directing management, we recommend BCRAT, BCSC, or IBIS for identifying patients eligible for endocrine prophylaxis and the FHx-based models (especially IBIS and CanRisk) to determine eligibility for HR screening.[60-62]

Modifiable Risk Factors

Modifiable risk factors impact BC risk to a lesser degree than most nonmodifiable factors but remain important. Addressing these empowers patients while lowering their risk for diseases beyond BC.

Physical activity

Increasing physical activity lowers BC risk. Regular exercise may delay the onset of menarche, increase the length of the menstrual cycle, and increase the number of anovulatory cycles, decreasing exposure to sex hormones. Studies, though, show the benefit of exercise in the absence of menstrual cycle changes.[63] Aerobic exercise may also induce changes in insulin sensitivity, antioxidant defense, epigenetic mechanisms, and intracellular signaling pathways.[64]

Table 1
Variables included in selected risk models

Risk Factor	BCRAT	IBIS	CanRisk	BRCAPRO	Claus	BCSC
Age	•	•	•	•	•	•
Race/ethnicity	•			•		•
Ashkenazi Jewish		•	•	•		
Menarche	•	•	•	•		
First parity	•	•	•	•		
Menopause		•	•			
Atypia	•	•				•
LCIS	NA	•				•
Prior biopsy	•	•				•
Breast density		•	•			•
PRS		•	•			
BRCA status	NA	•	•	•		
Other genes			•			
History of breast cancer	NA	NA	•	•		
BMI		•	•			
Family history variables						
Affected FDR	•	•	•	•	•	•
Non–FDR		•	•	•	•	
Male relatives		•	•	•		
Bilateral cancers	NA	•	•	•		
Cancer receptors	NA		•	•		
Ovarian cancer		•	•	•	•	
Other cancers			•			

Abbreviations: BCRAT, Breast Cancer Risk Assessment Tool; BCSC, breast cancer surveillance consortium; BMI, body mass index; FDR, first-degree relative; IBIS, breast cancer intervention study; LCIS, lobular carcinoma in situ; NA, not applicable (the model is not applicable to patients with this factor); PRS, polygenic risk score.

Moderate to vigorous activity reduces risk by an average of 25% in premenopausal and postmenopausal women, both lean and obese. There is a dose-dependent relationship, but the optimal level of physical activity for risk reduction remains unclear.[65]

Hormonal
Women using estrogen plus progestin have a higher risk of both ER+ and ER− disease. Combination HRT also interferes with mammographic sensitivity. The risk is most pronounced with longer HRT use and with current or recent use.[66,67]

Data on estrogen replacement therapy (ERT) are less clear. While some observational studies reported higher BC incidence and mortality, randomized trials showed that ERT lowered incidence and mortality compared with placebo, with the greatest reduction in ER+ cancers. ERT did not appear to interfere with cancer detection by mammography.[66–69] Given these high-level data, ERT appears to be safe, even for HR women.

Diet and alcohol
The Mediterranean diet (excluding alcohol) is protective, especially for postmenopausal women, independent of body weight and BMI.[70] Conversely, a diet high in refined sugar and fat increases BC risk, which may result from inflammatory processes.[71]

Despite the concern about the pro-estrogen effect of soy, studies consistently show its protective effects. Phytoestrogens are structurally similar to estradiol and bind to ER-alpha in the breast and uterus and ER-beta in the cardiovascular system, urogenital tract, and bone. Soy binds to ER more weakly than does estradiol and has a higher affinity for ER-beta. Soy may therefore act as a selective ER modulator, lowering the risk of an ER+ disease and reducing recurrence risk in women with a personal history of cancer.[72,73]

Dairy products may lower BC risk. Breast tissue has receptors for vitamin D, which moderates cell proliferation, malignant cell differentiation, apoptosis, and angiogenesis. The impact of dairy depends, however, on the dairy product, its fat content, and a patient's menopausal status.[74]

Alcohol use contributes to a significant proportion of BCs, especially ER+ tumors. It increases risk in a dose-dependent fashion, likely though ER-dependent pathways. This seems to be independent of alcohol type. The most susceptible period for carcinogenesis is likely the period after menarche and before first pregnancy.[75,76]

Weight

A higher BMI in early adulthood lowers BC risk.[77] However, weight gain and postmenopausal obesity increase BC risk: Each 5-kg/m^2 increase in BMI may increase risk by 12%. The increase in risk is most pronounced for nonusers of HRT. Even a 2-kg weight loss, though, reduces the risk of postmenopausal BC.[77–79] The benefit extends beyond BC risk reduction: Even a modest weight loss reduces the risk of other chronic diseases. Importantly, women who are aware of the link between elevated BMI and BC risk are more likely to participate in weight loss interventions.[80]

The Impact of Risk Assessment on Management Options

Endocrine prophylaxis reduces the risk of ER+ disease by 50% to 86%. It also reduces the risk of benign disease and biopsy frequency. Endocrine therapies, however, have side effects and adverse events. The American Society of Clinical Oncology and the United States Preventive Services Task Force note that the women most likely to benefit are those with a 5-year risk of at least 3%, usually calculated with the BCRAT, or a 10-year risk of at least 5% using IBIS.[62,81] Patient uptake of endocrine prophylaxis is low, but women who are aware of their risk status are more likely to opt in.[82]

These risk calculations also drive screening, which reduces mortality and morbidity. Those with a lifetime risk of 20% or higher, for instance benefit from the addition of breast MRI to annual mammography. The FHx-dependent calculators, especially IBIS, BRCAPRO, and CanRisk, are excellent tools for identifying women eligible for HR screening.[4,83,84]

CHALLENGES AND OPPORTUNITIES

We need to identify HR women before they should start screening, to optimize early detection and utilize the opportunity for risk-reducing therapy. Some women, including Ashkenazi Jews who (have a 1 in 40 chance of carrying a BRCA mutation) and Black women (who are significantly more likely to be diagnosed with BC before the age of 40 years), need risk assessment well before the age of 40 years.[4]

While it is beyond the scope of this chapter to discuss barriers to enhanced screening and risk-reducing therapies, a few points deserve mention. People of color are more likely to present with advanced disease, less likely to participate in screening, less likely to be offered genetic assessment, and more likely to die from cancer. Beyond race, other factors related to disparities include geography, socioeconomic status, insurance status, and gender identity. Unfortunately, HR screening may be out of financial reach for patients with substantial out-of-pocket costs or those limited by barriers like transportation needs. Nonbinary individuals may not be offered assigned sex-appropriate screening or may be unwelcome in those environments.[3,85,86]

SUMMARY

Patients can only benefit from HR screening and management if they are aware of their risk status and their options and can access those options. We have excellent tools for identifying HR patients, but we need to reach traditionally underserved populations and ensure their access to these services.

*We recognize that gender identity may differ from sex assigned at birth. For the purposes of this chapter, "women" refers to individuals assigned female sex at birth.

CLINICS CARE POINTS

- Women with a lifetime breast cancer risk of ≥20% are considered "high risk" and benefit from the addition of screening breast MRI to annual mammography. Family history-based tools like IBIS, BRCAPRO, and CanRisk are the best risk models to assess a patient's eligibility for high-risk screening.

- Women with a 5-year breast cancer risk of ≥1.7% are eligible for endocrine prophylaxis; those with a 5-year risk of ≥3% or a 10-year risk ≥5% are most likely to benefit. Based on professional society guidelines and their use in clinical trials, BCRAT, BCSC, and IBIS are the best risk models to assess a patient's eligibility for endocrine prophylaxis.

- Patient awareness of high-risk status improves their adherence to screening recommendations.

- Women can lower their breast cancer risk by maintaining a healthy BMI, being physically active, eating a healthy diet, and limiting alcohol use.

DISCLOSURE

The authors have nothing to disclose.

REFERENCES

1. NCI. National Cancer Institute: Cancer Statistics. Available at: https://www.cancer.gov/about-cancer/understanding/statistics#:~:text=The%20most%20common%20cancers%20(listed,endometrial%20cancer%2C%20leukemia%2C%20pancreatic%20cancer. Accessed January 29, 2023.
2. Duffy SW, Tabár L, Yen AM, et al. Mammography screening reduces rates of advanced and fatal breast cancers: Results in 549,091 women. Cancer 2020; 126(13):2971–9.
3. Monticciolo DL, Malak SF, Friedewald SM, et al. Breast cancer screening recommendations inclusive of all women at average risk: update from the ACR and Society of Breast Imaging. J Am Coll Radiol 2021;18(9):1280–8.
4. Monticciolo DL, Newell MS, Moy L, et al. Breast cancer screening in women at higher-than-average risk: recommendations from the ACR. J Am Coll Radiol 2018;15(3 Pt A):408–14.
5. Ellington TD, Miller JW, Henley SJ, et al. Trends in breast cancer incidence, by race, ethnicity, and age among women aged ≥20 years - United States, 1999-2018. MMWR Morb Mortal Wkly Rep 2022;71(2):43–7.

6. Baquet CR, Mishra SI, Commiskey P, et al. Breast cancer epidemiology in blacks and whites: disparities in incidence, mortality, survival rates and histology. J Natl Med Assoc 2008;100(5):480–8.

7. Travis LB, Hill D, Dores GM, et al. Cumulative absolute breast cancer risk for young women treated for Hodgkin lymphoma. J Natl Cancer Inst 2005;97(19): 1428–37.

8. Inskip PD, Sigurdson AJ, Veiga L, et al. Radiation-related new primary solid cancers in the childhood cancer survivor study: comparative radiation dose response and modification of treatment effects. Int J Radiat Oncol Biol Phys 2016;94(4):800–7.

9. Veiga LH, Curtis RE, Morton LM, et al. Association of breast cancer risk after childhood cancer with radiation dose to the breast and anthracycline use: a report from the Childhood Cancer Survivor Study. JAMA Pediatr 2019;173(12): 1171–9.

10. Atakpa EC, Thorat MA, Cuzick J, et al. Mammographic density, endocrine therapy and breast cancer risk: a prognostic and predictive biomarker review. Cochrane Database Syst Rev 2021;10(10):CD013091.

11. Cuzick J, Warwick J, Pinney E, et al. Tamoxifen-induced reduction in mammographic density and breast cancer risk reduction: a nested case-control study. J Natl Cancer Inst 2011;103(9):744–52.

12. Hartmann LC, Sellers TA, Frost MH, et al. Benign breast disease and the risk of breast cancer. N Engl J Med 2005;353(3):229–37.

13. Wen HY, Brogi E. Lobular Carcinoma in situ. Surg Pathol Clin 2018;11(1):123–45.

14. London SJ, Connolly JL, Schnitt SJ, et al. A prospective study of benign breast disease and the risk of breast cancer. JAMA 1992;267(7):941–4.

15. Graffeo R, Rana HQ, Conforti F, et al. Moderate penetrance genes complicate genetic testing for breast cancer diagnosis: ATM, CHEK2, BARD1 and RAD51D. Breast 2022;65:32–40.

16. National Comprehensive Cancer Network Clinical Practice Guidelines in Oncology: Genetic/Familial High-Risk Assessment: Breast, Ovarian, and Pancreatic Version 2.2023. Available at: https://www.nccn.org/professionals/physician_gls/pdf/genetics_bop.pdf. Accessed January 29, 2023.

17. Lowry KP, Geuzinge HA, Stout NK, et al. Breast cancer screening strategies for women with ATM, CHEK2, and PALB2 pathogenic variants: a comparative modeling analysis. JAMA Oncol 2022;8(4):587–96.

18. Gail MH, Brinton LA, Byar DP, et al. Projecting individualized probabilities of developing breast cancer for white females who are being examined annually. J Natl Cancer Inst 1989;81(24):1879–86.

19. Costantino JP, Gail MH, Pee D, et al. Validation studies for models projecting the risk of invasive and total breast cancer incidence. J Natl Cancer Inst 1999;91(18): 1541–8.

20. National Cancer Institute: Breast Cancer Risk Assessment Tool. Available at: https://bcrisktool.cancer.gov/. Accessed January 29, 2023.

21. Banegas MP, John EM, Slattery ML, et al. Projecting individualized absolute invasive breast cancer risk in US Hispanic Women. J Natl Cancer Inst 2017;109(2). https://doi.org/10.1093/jnci/djw215.

22. Gail MH, Costantino JP, Pee D, et al. Projecting individualized absolute invasive breast cancer risk in African American women. J Natl Cancer Inst 2007;99(23): 1782–92 [published correction appears in J Natl Cancer Inst. 2008 Aug 6;100(15):1118] [published correction appears in J Natl Cancer Inst. 2008 Mar 5;100(5):373].

23. Matsuno RK, Costantino JP, Ziegler RG, et al. Projecting individualized absolute invasive breast cancer risk in Asian and Pacific Islander American women. J Natl Cancer Inst 2011;103(12):951–61.

24. Pankratz VS, Hartmann LC, Degnim AC, et al. Assessment of the accuracy of the Gail model in women with atypical hyperplasia. J Clin Oncol 2008;26(33):5374–9.

25. Wang X, Huang Y, Li L, et al. Assessment of performance of the Gail model for predicting breast cancer risk: a systematic review and meta-analysis with trial sequential analysis. Breast Cancer Res 2018;20(1):18.

26. Tice JA, Cummings SR, Ziv E, et al. Mammographic breast density and the Gail model for breast cancer risk prediction in a screening population. Breast Cancer Res Treat 2005;94(2):115–22.

27. Tice JA, Cummings SR, Smith-Bindman R, et al. Using clinical factors and mammographic breast density to estimate breast cancer risk: development and validation of a new predictive model. Ann Intern Med 2008;148(5):337–47.

28. Tice JA, Miglioretti DL, Li CS, et al. Breast Density and Benign Breast Disease: Risk Assessment to Identify Women at High Risk of Breast Cancer. J Clin Oncol 2015;33(28):3137–43.

29. Tice JA, Bissell MCS, Miglioretti DL, et al. Validation of the breast cancer surveillance consortium model of breast cancer risk. Breast Cancer Res Treat 2019; 175(2):519–23.

30. Breast Cancer Surveillance Consotium Risk Calculator. Available at: https://tools. bcsc-scc.org/BC5yearRisk/calculator.htm. Accessed May 20, 2023.

31. Tyrer J, Duffy SW, Cuzick J. A breast cancer prediction model incorporating familial and personal risk factors. Stat Med 2004;23(7):1111–30. https://doi.org/10. 1002/sim.1668.

32. IBIS Breast Cancer Risk Evaluation Tool, Available at: https://ems-trials.org/ riskevaluator/. Accessed January 29, 2023.

33. Brentnall AR, Cuzick J. Risk models for breast cancer and their validation. Stat Sci 2020;35(1):14–30.

34. Boughey JC, Hartmann LC, Anderson SS, et al. Evaluation of the Tyrer-Cuzick (International Breast Cancer Intervention Study) model for breast cancer risk prediction in women with atypical hyperplasia. J Clin Oncol 2010;28(22):3591–6.

35. Valero MG, Zabor EC, Park A, et al. The Tyrer-Cuzick model inaccurately predicts invasive breast cancer risk in women with LCIS. Ann Surg Oncol 2020;27(3): 736–40.

36. Lo LL, Milne RL, Liao Y, et al. Validation of the IBIS breast cancer risk evaluator for women with lobular carcinoma in-situ. Br J Cancer 2018;119(1):36–9.

37. Cintolo-Gonzalez JA, Braun D, Blackford AL, et al. Breast cancer risk models: a comprehensive overview of existing models, validation, and clinical applications. Breast Cancer Res Treat 2017;164(2):263–84.

38. Kurian AW, Hughes E, Simmons T, et al. Performance of the IBIS/Tyrer-Cuzick model of breast cancer risk by race and ethnicity in the Women's Health Initiative. Cancer 2021;127(20):3742–50.

39. Maas P, Barrdahl M, Joshi AD, et al. Breast cancer risk from modifiable and non-modifiable risk factors among white women in the United States. JAMA Oncol 2016;2(10):1295–302.

40. Antoniou AC, Pharoah PD, McMullan G, et al. A comprehensive model for familial breast cancer incorporating BRCA1, BRCA2 and other genes. Br J Cancer 2002; 86(1):76–83.

41. Antoniou AC, Cunningham AP, Peto J, et al. The BOADICEA model of genetic susceptibility to breast and ovarian cancers: updates and extensions. Br J Cancer 2008;98(8):1457–66.

42. Lee AJ, Cunningham AP, Tischkowitz M, et al. Incorporating truncating variants in PALB2, CHEK2, and ATM into the BOADICEA breast cancer risk model. Genet Med 2016;18(12):1190–8.

43. Mavaddat N, Ficorella L, Carver T, et al. Incorporating alternative Polygenic Risk Scores into the BOADICEA breast cancer risk prediction model. Cancer Epidemiol Biomarkers Prev 2023. https://doi.org/10.1158/1055-9965.EPI-22-0756.

44. CanRisk. Available at: https://www.canrisk.org/. Accessed February 10, 2023.

45. Yang X, Eriksson M, Czene K, et al. Prospective validation of the BOADICEA multifactorial breast cancer risk prediction model in a large prospective cohort study. J Med Genet 2022;59(12):1196–205. https://doi.org/10.1136/jmg-2022-108806.

46. Claus EB, Schildkraut JM, Thompson WD, et al. The genetic attributable risk of breast and ovarian cancer. Cancer 1996;77(11):2318–24.

47. McCarthy AM, Guan Z, Welch M, et al. Performance of breast cancer risk-assessment models in a large mammography cohort. J Natl Cancer Inst 2020;112(5):489–97. https://doi.org/10.1093/jnci/djz177.

48. Parmigiani G, Berry D, Aguilar O. Determining carrier probabilities for breast cancer-susceptibility genes BRCA1 and BRCA2. Am J Hum Genet 1998;62(1):145–58. https://doi.org/10.1086/301670.

49. Mazzola E, Blackford A, Parmigiani G, et al. Recent enhancements to the genetic risk prediction model BRCAPRO. Cancer Inform 2015;14(Suppl 2):147–57. https://doi.org/10.4137/CIN.S17292.

50. Ask2Me: The All Syndromes Known to Man Evaluator, 2023. Available at: https://ask2me.org/. Accessed January 29, 2023.

51. Braun D, Yang J, Griffin M, et al. A Clinical decision support tool to predict cancer risk for commonly tested cancer-related germline mutations. J Genet Couns 2018;27(5):1187–99. https://doi.org/10.1007/s10897-018-0238-4.

52. Gastounioti A, Desai S, Ahluwalia VS, et al. Artificial intelligence in mammographic phenotyping of breast cancer risk: a narrative review. Breast Cancer Re 2022;24(1):14. https://doi.org/10.1186/s13058-022-01509-z.

53. Ho WK, Tai MC, Dennis J, et al. Polygenic risk scores for prediction of breast cancer risk in Asian populations. Genet Med 2022;24(3):586–600. https://doi.org/10.1016/j.gim.2021.11.008.

54. Gao G, Zhao F, Ahearn TU, et al. Polygenic risk scores for prediction of breast cancer risk in women of African ancestry: a cross-ancestry approach. Hum Mol Genet 2022;31(18):3133–43. https://doi.org/10.1093/hmg/ddac102.

55. Kramer I, Hooning MJ, Mavaddat N, et al. Breast cancer polygenic risk score and contralateral breast cancer risk. Am J Hum Genet 2020;107(5):837–48. https://doi.org/10.1016/j.ajhg.2020.09.001.

56. Mavaddat N, Michailidou K, Dennis J, et al. Polygenic risk scores for prediction of breast cancer and breast cancer subtypes. Am J Hum Genet 2019;104(1):21–34. https://doi.org/10.1016/j.ajhg.2018.11.002.

57. Li SX, Milne RL, Nguyen-Dumont T, et al. Prospective evaluation over 15 years of six breast cancer risk models. Cancers 2021;13(20). https://doi.org/10.3390/cancers13205194.

58. Coopey SB, Acar A, Griffin M, et al. The impact of patient age on breast cancer risk prediction models. Breast J 2018;24(4):592–8.

59. McCarthy AM, Liu Y, Ehsan S, et al. Validation of breast cancer risk models by race/ethnicity, family history and molecular subtypes. Cancers 2021;14(1). https://doi.org/10.3390/cancers14010045.

60. National Comprehensive Cancer Network Clinical Practice Guidelines in Oncology: Breast Cancer Screening and Diagnosis version 1.2022. Available at: https://www.nccn.org/professionals/physician_gls/pdf/breast-screening.pdf. Accessed January 29, 2023.

61. National Comprehensive Cancer Network Clinical Practice Guidelines in Oncology: Breast Cancer Risk Reduction Version 1.2023. Available at: https://www.nccn.org/professionals/physician_gls/pdf/breast_risk.pdf. Accessed January 29, 2023.

62. Visvanathan K, Fabian CJ, Bantug E, et al. Use of endocrine therapy for breast cancer risk reduction: ASCO clinical practice guideline update. J Clin Oncol 2019;37(33):3152–65.

63. Howell A, Anderson AS, Clarke RB, et al. Risk determination and prevention of breast cancer. Breast Cancer Res 2014;16(5):446.

64. Korn AR, Reedy J, Brockton NT, et al. The 2018 World Cancer Research Fund/American Institute for Cancer Research Score and Cancer Risk: a longitudinal analysis in the NIH-AARP Diet and Health Study. Cancer Epidemiol Biomarkers Prev 2022;31(10):1983–92.

65. Lynch BM, Neilson HK, Friedenreich CM. Physical activity and breast cancer prevention. Recent Results Cancer Res 2011;186:13–42.

66. Collaborative Group on Hormonal Factors in Breast Cancer. Type and timing of menopausal hormone therapy and breast cancer risk: individual participant meta-analysis of the worldwide epidemiological evidence. Lancet 2019; 394(10204):1159–68.

67. Chen CL, Weiss NS, Newcomb P, et al. Hormone replacement therapy in relation to breast cancer. JAMA 2002;287(6):734–41.

68. Chlebowski RT, Anderson GL, Aragaki AK, et al. Association of menopausal hormone therapy with breast cancer incidence and mortality during long-term follow-up of the Women's Health Initiative randomized clinical trials. JAMA 2020;324(4): 369–80.

69. Million Women Study Collaborators. Breast cancer and hormone-replacement therapy in the Million Women Study. Lancet 2003;362(9382):419–27 [published correction appears in Lancet. 2003 Oct 4;362(9390):1160].

70. Buja A, Pierbon M, Lago L, et al. Breast cancer primary prevention and diet: an umbrella review. Int J Environ Res Public Health 2020;17(13). https://doi.org/10.3390/ijerph17134731.

71. Albuquerque RC, Baltar VT, Marchioni DM. Breast cancer and dietary patterns: a systematic review. Nutr Rev 2014;72(1):1–17.

72. Wei Y, Lv J, Guo Y, et al. Soy intake and breast cancer risk: a prospective study of 300,000 Chinese women and a dose-response meta-analysis. Eur J Epidemiol 2020;35(6):567–78.

73. Messina MJ, Wood CE. Soy isoflavones, estrogen therapy, and breast cancer risk: analysis and commentary. Nutr J 2008;7:17.

74. Dong JY, Zhang L, He K, et al. Dairy consumption and risk of breast cancer: a meta-analysis of prospective cohort studies. Breast Cancer Res Treat 2011; 127(1):23–31.

75. Starek-Świechowicz B, Budziszewska B, Starek A. Alcohol and breast cancer. Pharmacol Rep 2023;75(1):69–84.

76. Chen WY, Rosner B, Hankinson SE, et al. Moderate alcohol consumption during adult life, drinking patterns, and breast cancer risk. JAMA 2011;306(17):1884–90.
77. Suzuki R, Iwasaki M, Inoue M, et al. Body weight at age 20 years, subsequent weight change and breast cancer risk defined by estrogen and progesterone receptor status–the Japan public health center-based prospective study. Int J Cancer 2011;129(5):1214–24.
78. Renehan AG, Pegington M, Harvie MN, et al. Young adulthood body mass index, adult weight gain and breast cancer risk: the PROCAS Study (United Kingdom). Br J Cancer 2020;122(10):1552–61.
79. Teras LR, Patel AV, Wang M, et al. Sustained weight loss and risk of breast cancer in women 50 years and older: a pooled analysis of prospective data. J Natl Cancer Inst 2020;112(9):929–37.
80. Burkbauer L, Goldbach M, Huang C, et al. Awareness of link between obesity and breast cancer risk is associated with willingness to participate in weight loss intervention. Breast Cancer Res Treat 2022;194(3):541–50.
81. Owens DK, Davidson KW, Krist AH, et al. Medication use to reduce risk of breast cancer: US Preventive Services Task Force Recommendation Statement. JAMA 2019;322(9):857–67.
82. Huilgol YS, Keane H, Shieh Y, et al. Elevated risk thresholds predict endocrine risk-reducing medication use in the Athena screening registry. NPJ Breast Cancer 2021;7(1):102.
83. US Preventative Services Task Force. Breast Cancer: Screening, Available at: https://www.uspreventiveservicestaskforce.org/uspstf/recommendation/breast-cancer-screening. Accessed January 29, 2023.
84. American Cancer Society Recommendations for the Early Detection of Breast Cancer. Available at: https://www.cancer.org/cancer/breast-cancer/screening-tests-and-early-detection/american-cancer-society-recommendations-for-the-early-detection-of-breast-cancer.html. Accessed January 29, 2023.
85. Stringer-Reasor EM, Elkhanany A, Khoury K, et al. Disparities in breast cancer associated with African American identity. Am Soc Clin Oncol Educ Book 2021;41:e29–46.
86. Khan A, Rogers CR, Kennedy CD, et al. Genetic evaluation for hereditary cancer syndromes among African Americans: a critical review. Oncol 2022;27(4):285–91.

How to Navigate the Treatment Spectrum from Multimodality Therapy to Observation Alone for ductal carcinoma *in situ*

Sydney M. Record, BA[a], Eun-Sil Shelley Hwang, MD, MPH[a,b], Akiko Chiba, MD[a,b,c],*

KEYWORDS

• DCIS • De-escalation • Active surveillance • Over-treatment

KEY POINTS

- Over 60,000 women in the United States are diagnosed DCIS each year, comprising ~25% of all newly diagnosed breast tumors.
- Based on current guidelines, these women are recommended surgical excision with consideration for radiation therapy and/or endocrine therapy.
- Although there's local control benefit, endocrine therapy, and radiation have not shown breast cancer mortality benefit for DCIS.
- There is a concern for over-treatment of DCIS.

INTRODUCTION

Ductal carcinoma *in situ* (DCIS) represents a unique entity in the spectrum of breast lesions. With the widespread use of screening mammography, the incidence of DCIS has dramatically increased almost 7-fold, now comprising 25% of all newly diagnosed breast cancers.[1] DCIS encompasses a histologically heterogeneous group of neoplastic lesions confined to the breast ducts without invasion into the basement membrane.

Because of DCIS is considered a precursor lesion for invasive breast carcinoma, the goal of management is to prevent the progression to invasive carcinoma, identify

[a] Department of Surgery, Duke University Medical Center, 40 Duke Medicine Circle, 124 Davison Building, Durham, NC 27710, USA; [b] Duke Cancer Institute, 20 Duke Medicine Circle, Durham, NC 27710, USA; [c] Department of Surgery, 508 Fulton Street, Durham, NC 27705, USA
* Corresponding author. DUMC #3513, Durham, NC 27710.
E-mail address: akiko.chiba@duke.edu
Twitter: @sydney_record (S.M.R.); @drshelleyhwang (E.-S.S.H.); @chibaAkiko (A.C.)

Surg Oncol Clin N Am 32 (2023) 663–673
https://doi.org/10.1016/j.soc.2023.05.011
1055-3207/23/Published by Elsevier Inc.
surgonc.theclinics.com

invasive disease which was not identified with core needle biopsy, and prevent breast cancer mortality.[2] It is estimated that 20-30% of DCIS will progress to invasive disease without treatment.[3] However, the current recommended treatment for all patients remains surgical excision with mastectomy or breast-conserving surgery (BCS) with or without radiation therapy and endocrine therapy.

While the progression of DCIS to invasive cancer is well-demonstrated, this may not occur within a patient's lifetime may not cause harm.[2] Current therapeutic approaches likely result in overtreatment those women whose DCIS has limited invasive potential, causing harm from side effects of treatments and promoting unnecessary anxiety in the condition that may not have changed their mortality. The current treatment approach to DCIS has been called into question since mammography has led to a significant increase in DCIS detection, and treatment, without a concomitant reduction in breast cancer incidence and mortality over this same period.

PREVALENCE/INCIDENCE

Prior to the use of mammography, DCIS was rarely diagnosed. It was clinically detected in symptomatic patients as Paget disease of the nipple, nipple discharge, or a palpable mass.[4] DCIS incidence was 1.87 per 100,000 women in the United States in 1973-1975.[5] Between 2007 and 2011, the incidence of DCIS was remarkably higher, at 25.8 per 100,000 women.[6] In contrast, DCIS accounted for 3.8% of new breast cancer diagnoses in 1983.[7] In the United States, over 50,000 women are diagnosed with DCIS each year, over 8,000 in the United Kingdom, and >2500 in the Netherlands.[8]

According to the Surveillance, Epidemiology, and End Results (SEER), invasive breast cancer incidence was 102.13 per 100,000 women in the United States between 1975 and 1979.[9] The U.S. invasive breast cancer incidence per 100,000 women was 131.18 in 2016. Breast cancer mortality has fortunately decreased over this period likely due to the improvement in systemic therapy and earlier diagnosis. Notably however, the incidence of invasive breast cancer has not declined over the same period that DCIS was increasingly treated aggressively by surgical excision.

A comparison can be drawn between the impact of excision of colon polyps on colorectal cancer incidence. Almost all colorectal cancer is adenocarcinoma, which develops from adenoma, a premalignant lesion which presents with varying degrees of dysplasia.[10,11] Based on this understanding, screening for colon cancer with colonoscopy, to detect both adenomas and early colon cancer, was introduced into regular practice in the 1980s.[12] Using SEER data, the incidence of colorectal cancer in the US was 66.30 per 100,000 people in 1985 and 38.02 per 100,000 people in 2016, representing a fairly sharp decline after the adoption of screening colonoscopy.[9] Further, colorectal cancer mortality also declined over this period. This trend has not been observed with the treatment of DCIS.

There is evidence to suggest some cases of DCIS may not progress to invasive cancer during an individual's lifetime. A 1997 systematic review of DCIS detection on autopsy found a median prevalence of DCIS of 8.9%.[13] Interestingly, this review found that the prevalence of DCIS was highest among women who were in the population recommended to undergo screening, women aged 40-70. The detection of DCIS on autopsy shows that these patients died *with* DCIS, rather than *of* DCIS or breast cancer.

PATIENT OVERVIEW

In the current era, the most common presentation of DCIS is in asymptomatic women on routine screening mammography.[4,14] The mammographic finding will be microcalcifications in 62-98% of these patients and other suspicious findings, including masses and parenchymal distortions, in 2–32%.[15–18] Most patients with DCIS are diagnosed via vacuum-assisted breast core needle biopsy.[19] Biopsy allows for the classification of DCIS based on morphological patterns of growth, with five possible designations: comedo-type, cribriform, micropapillary, papillary, and solid.[20] Further, the histologic grade of DCIS can be determined.

Differentiating ADH from low-grade DCIS based on biopsy can be challenging, though the detection of either lesion is commonly followed by wide excision.[18] Because the management after excision will differ, with the management for DCIS typically being more aggressive, a precise diagnosis is required from this larger excision.

TREATMENT OPTIONS
Surgery

According to current NCCN guidelines, surgical resection is recommend for all DCIS.[21] The options of surgical management include breast-conserving surgery (BCS) or mastectomy. The choice to undergo BCS or mastectomy is a personal decision and should involve individualized discussion for shared decision making. Further, patients presenting with extensive DCIS may not be a candidate for BCS.

Another important criterion for patients to undergo BCS is that histologically negative margins are achieved.[22] The excision margins play a critical role in the risk of local recurrence. The meta-analysis of the randomized trials demonstrated that in patients treated with BCS alone, the 10-year risk of IBTR was significantly higher in patients with positive margin compared to those with negative margins. (43.8% vs. 26.0%). The same trend was seen in patients who received adjuvant radiation with a 10-year IBTR of 24.2% in patients with positive margins compared to 12.0% in those with negative margins[15] SSO-ASTRO-ASCO Consensus Guideline recommends margins of at least 2 mm based on the meta-analysis showing reduced risk of IBTR relative to narrower negative margin in patients receiving RT.[23,24] However, clinical judgment should be used in determining whether patients with smaller margin (<2 mm) require re-excision. Patients undergoing BCS should understand the risk of re-excision to obtain negative margins, as well as the rare risk of requiring mastectomy if adequate surgical margins cannot be obtained with BCS.[21]

An important technique in BCS is shaved cavity margins, where surgeons take additional tissue circumferentially around the lumpectomy cavity. This is especially relevant in DCIS, which is associated with a higher risk of positive margins with BCS. A prospective randomized trial showed nearly 65% reduction in the positive-margin rate for pure DCIS (odds ratio 0.366; 95% CI, 0.136 to 0.981; p = 0.046).[25] Other studies have shown to reduce positive margins by up to ~50% with shaved cavity margins for invasive disease and DCIS.[25–27] However, there is some conflicting result showing shaved cavity margins did not show a significant reduction in re-excision rate, in a retrospective review.[28]

Although mastectomy achieves an extremely low recurrence rate, it likely represents an over treatment for many patients. A slightly higher rate of local recurrence has been demonstrated with BCS, but this approach is associated with less morbidity with the same survival.[15,16] In a 2015 observational study of more than 100,000 patients with DCIS in the SEER database, when compared with BCS, mastectomy resulted in a similar 10-year breast cancer-specific mortality (multivariate hazard ratio for mastectomy versus BCS 1.2, 95% CI 0.96–1.50). Studies of early invasive breast cancer demonstrate that both surgeries have low rates of postoperative complications, however, they are more commonly associated with mastectomy.[29]

Another area of discussion in the surgical management of DCIS is sentinel lymph node biopsy (SLNB). NCCN guidelines advise against lymph node resection with BCS.[21] However, these guidelines also state that patients with DCIS undergoing excision in a location that will compromise future SNLB or patients undergoing mastectomy should be considered for SLNB. The justification for this is for the potential for upstage of DCIS to invasive carcinoma at the time of surgery.[30] While SLNB biopsy is generally avoided in the management of DCIS, those patients who are not a candidate for BCS have a larger extent of disease and therefore a higher likelihood of having an invasive cancer and therefore should be considered for SLNB.[5]

Radiation

RT is demonstrated to reduce ipsilateral breast tumor recurrence (IBTR). Meta-analysis of RT compared with no further treatment following lumpectomy showed a reduction in the risk of all ipsilateral breast events (pooled HR 0.49, 95% CI 0.41–0.58).[31] However, most cases of DCIS do not recur when treated with excision alone.[32] RT may be omitted in select low-risk patients.

According to NCCN guidelines, patients with an estrogen-positive lesion who will be undergoing endocrine therapy may be considered for excision alone.[21] Additional criteria presented by NCCN for the consideration of omitting RT are low to intermediate nuclear grade, tumor size $\leq$2.5 cm, and surgical margins >3 mm.

A genomic tool to predict risk of local recurrence has been developed to guide clinical decision marking for DCIS.[33] The Oncotype DX Breast DCIS Score is a 12-gene assay designed to predict the 10-year risk of local recurrence and to predict the benefit of RT. This tool became available in December of 2011. DCISionRT is another predictive tool which uses the assessment of HER2, Ki-67, cycloxxoygenase2(COX2), SIAH2, FOXA1, and p16 expressions by immunohistochemistry as well as clinical factors. This test was validated using samples from the SweDCIS (CORTC 10853) randomized phase II trial comparing BCS alone with BCS + RT.[34] However, neither of the tools has had broad use since these tests are currently not recommended by NCCN guidelines due to lack of prospective validation.

For patients undergoing RT for DCIS, whole breast radiation therapy (WBRT) and accelerated partial breast irradiation (ABPI) may be options. The studies of ABPI are promising. Two single-institution prospective studies of women treated with BCS for DCIS evaluated the recurrence of DCIS after ABPI.[35] Combined analysis found a recurrence rate of 4.1%. This rate was similar to the rate of recurrence following WBRT reported in the NSABP B-17 trial, which showed a DCIS recurrence rate of 2.9% and an invasive cancer recurrence rate of 7.5%.[35] As de-escalation in the treatment of DCIS continues to be evaluated, ABPI may be more appropriate if RT is given.

Of those who experience a local recurrence after BCS, half of those recurrences are found to contain invasive disease.[15,36,37] DCIS has a long clinical course, evidenced by the possibility of recurrence of DCIS after surgical excision over 15 years of follow-up or longer.[36] Previous studies demonstrated that grade is not significantly associated with the risk of local recurrence.[38] The 15-year cumulative incidence of IBRT in NSABP 17 trial of patients with clear margins showed 19.4% in patients who underwent BCS and 8.9% in patients who underwent BCS followed by radiation.[37] Adjuvant radiation decreases the risk of local recurrences by 50%.[15]

Younger age has been associated with higher risk of local recurrence after BCT demonstrated in both randomized clinical trials of RT[36] and retrospective studies.[39] Women <40 years of age were significantly higher risk of invasive breast cancer recurrence of 15.8% compared to 6.5% for those $\geq$40 years of age.[40] These and other clinical variables have been used by investigators at MSKCC to construct a nomogram to predict the risk of recurrence following lumpectomy for DCIS (https://nomograms. mskcc.org/breast/ductalcarcinomainsiturecurrencepage.aspx).

ENDOCRINE THERAPY

Randomized clinical trials have evaluated the role of tamoxifen or aromatase inhibitors (AI) in postmenopausal patients after lumpectomy for DCIS.[36,37] Endocrine therapy has been shown to have local control benefit after surgery in randomized trials. BCS with radiation therapy and tamoxifen reduced ipsilateral invasive recurrence in the NSABP B-17 and B-24. In NSABP B-24 IBTR was reduced by 32% when compared with BCS with radiation + placebo (HR of risk of IBTR = 0.68, 95% CI = 0.49 to 0.95, P = .025). The 15-year cumulative incidence of IBTR was 19.4% for BCS only, 8.9% for BCS + RT, 10% for BCS + RT + placebo (B-24), and 8.5% for BCS + RT + tamoxifen.[37] Adjuvant tamoxifen reduced 10-year risk of any breast cancer event only for ER-positive DCIS. Similarly, the role of tamoxifen was evaluated in the UK, Australia, and New Zealand (UK/ANZ) DCIS trial which demonstrated a reduction in all breast cancer events.[36] Systemic therapy with tamoxifen did not influence overall survival in either trial. Tamoxifen administration appeared to be more effective at reducing the incidence of new breast events in patients who did not receive radiation therapy in the NSABP trials.[36]

   The current NCCN guidelines recommend considering endocrine therapy for 5 years for patients with ER-positive DCIS treated with BCS or unilateral mastectomy to provide risk reduction in the ipsilateral breast treated with BCS and in the contralateral breast in patients treated with mastectomy.[21] Since a survival advantage has not been demonstrated, individual consideration of risks and benefits is important. Tamoxifen is recommended for premenopausal patients and either tamoxifen or AI could be utilized for postmenopausal patients. The standard dose of tamoxifen is 20 mg/day for 5 years; however, the guidelines include the use of low-dose tamoxifen (5 mg/day for 3 year) as an option (as used in the TAM-01 study) if the patient is unwilling or unable to take standard-dose tamoxifen.

ACTIVE SURVEILLANCE/OMISSION OF SURGERY

A study using the data from the SEER registry evaluated the rate of invasive progression in women with DCIS from 1992 to 2014 who did not undergo surgical excision. This study showed 10-year net risk of ipsilateral invasive breast cancer to be 15-28% depending on clinical factors such as age at diagnosis and histologic features.

   Furthermore, some data support selected DCIS may be completely treated with endocrine therapy alone. CALGB 40903 was a phase II prospective trial evaluating neoadjuvant endocrine therapy with letrozole (2.5 mg/day) for 6 months prior to surgery in postmenopausal women with ER + DCIS.[41] 15% of the overall patients achieved pathologic complete response (pCR). Among patients with grade 1 DCIS, 75% achieved pCR, further supporting trials of non-operative management of low-risk DCIS. In patients who had residual disease, the size of DCIS was significantly smaller than initial radiographic measurements.

EVIDENCE FOR ACTIVE SURVEILLANCE

Prostate cancer management provides evidence for AS. The use of AS increased from 22% of cases in 2004–2005 to 50% of cases in 2014–2015 for patients with a Gleason score of 6 or lower.[42]

There is increasing evidence for the efficacy of this management strategy. A 2018 systematic review 13 AS programs for prostate cancer throughout the world found consistent high progression-free and cancer-free survival rates despite significant heterogeneity amongst these large AS cohorts.[43] A 10-year study published in 2023 included 883 men enrolled in 4 differed AS programs in the United Kingdom and found that 106 men (12.0%) of men progressed on AS, no men had distant metastases, and none died of prostate cancer.[44] Given an AS attrition rate of 21.6%, there is now the consideration of even less-intense surveillance strategies for prostate cancer.

Similarly, low-risk well differentiated thyroid cancer can also be effectively managed with AS. The largest prospective series of patients undergoing AS over 22 years in Japan included 2153 patients.[45] 1235 patients underwent AS, compared to immediate surgery, with similar oncologic outcomes. A prospective study of AS for thyroid cancer was also conducted in the United States, with 291 patients undergoing AS.[46] This study also found low rates of tumor growth and no distant or regional metastases during surveillance with only 3.8% of patients experienced tumor growth.

CURRENT ACTIVE SURVEILLANCE TRIALS

There has been broad support for clinical trials to determine whether the de-escalation of treatment for some patients with DCIS may be safe and appropriate. At present, there are four ongoing clinical trials evaluating whether patients with low-risk DCIS can undergo active surveillance rather than surgical treatment with or without adjuvant therapies. These are the COMET trial (NCT02926911) is in the US, LORIS trial (NCT02766881) in the United Kingdom, LORD trial (NCT02492607) in the Netherlands and LORETTA trial in Japan (**Table 1**).

The COMET (Comparison of an Operation to Monitoring with or without Endocrine Therapy) trial is a phase III randomized controlled clinical trial for low-risk DCIS. The primary endpoint is ipsilateral *invasive* breast cancer rate at 2, 5, and 7 years in women undergoing guideline-concordant care compared with active surveillance.[47] The low-risk DCIS (LORD) trial is a randomized international, phase III non-inferiority trial with similar eligibility. The primary outcome is 10-year ipsilateral invasive breast cancer-free survival.[48] The Surgery versus Active Monitoring for Low-Risk DCIS (LORIS) trial is evaluating the safety of observation alone for non-high-grade DCIS. The primary outcome is invasive breast cancer-free survival at five years.[49] The LORETTA trial includes patients with similar eligibility; in addition, endocrine therapy is mandatory for LORETTA whereas in COMET endocrine therapy is optional. Additional outcomes include quality of life between the two treatment arms, as well as biospecimen collections for the discovery of novel markers of invasive progression of DCIS to further individualize treatment plan for optimal treatment.

CONTROVERSIES

Adjuvant radiation and endocrine therapy following BCS have been shown in randomized trials to reduce the risk of invasive and DCIS recurrence, however, neither has improved overall survival. Due to various treatment options available, there has been interest in personalizing treatment to optimize overall outcomes while avoiding overtreatment. Risks and benefits of adjuvant therapies should be discussed with each patient while prioritizing patients' values to make shared treatment decisions.

The role of the physician is to inform the patient with historic as well as modern data and to guide discussions of treatment plan options so that patients can make their best-informed decisions. Although RT has been shown to decrease local recurrence

Table 1
Current international clinical trials of active surveillance for low-risk DCIS

	Study Design	Endocrine Therapy	Age	DCIS Grade	Comedo Necrosis	Imaging	Accrual Target (n)	Accrual End Date
LORIS (UK)	Prospective RCT	Not permitted	≥46	1,2	No	MMG Every 12 months	932	March 31, 2020
COMET (US)	Prospective RCT	Any, optional	≥40	1, 2	Eligible	MMG Every 6 months	1200	Jan 13, 2023
LORD (EU)	Prospective RCT	Not permitted	≥45	1	No	MMG Every 12 months	2500	Dec 31, 2025
LORETTA (Japan)	Prospective single-arm registry	Tamoxifen 20 mg, required	40–75	1, 2	No	MMG, US every 6 months × 2 year, then every 12 months	340	Accrual dependent

Abbreviations: DCIS, ductal carcinoma in situ; MMG, mammogram; RCT, randomized clinical trial.

by 50%, it has no survival benefit. Similarly, ET also shows decreases ipsilateral and contralateral events, again without survival benefit. ET and RT, in particular, may cause side effects that interfere with quality of life. Further, ongoing clinical trials may prove that surgical excision could be omitted in selected low-risk DCIS. Such lines of evidence will help inform how to right-size treatment for DCIS.

DISCUSSION

Due to the adoption of screening mammography, the incidence of DCIS has increased significantly in recent years. Outcomes following current treatment for DCIS are excellent with 10-year breast cancer-specific survival of 98%.[50] There has been increasing concern about the overtreatment of DCIS and treatment de-escalation to decrease toxicity and costs has been considered. It is clear that DCIS is a heterogeneous disease with lack of understanding of its natural history. There is enough evidence to support DCIS is a precursor to invasive disease, however, this progression appears to be non-obligatory, therefore DCIS may remain dormant in some women making current guideline-concordant care result in overtreatment for some patients. At present, we lack evidence to support that equivalent survival could be achieved without surgical treatment, although this question is actively being evaluated in the current clinical trials.

Most importantly, each patient's goals should drive treatment decisions, as patients are increasingly interested in engaging in shared decision making in order to choose a treatment plan that is optimal for them.

CLINICS CARE POINTS

- Radiation therapy results in a ~50% relative risk reduction in local recurrence.
- Endocrine therapy decreases the risk of local recurrence by about 30% after surgical excision and radiation, and also decreases in contralateral events.
- Despite the benefit of adjuvant therapies on local control, neither radiation nor endocrine therapy has shown improved survival.
- The surgical margin width recommended for DCIS is at least 2 mm, and clinical judgment should be utilized to weigh the risk of re-excision with the risk of recurrence for margin <2 mm
- Younger age (<40 years) is associated with higher risk of local recurrence.
- The result of ongoing clinic trials will determine whether active surveillance is non-inferior to surgical excision in patients with low-risk disease.

DISCLOSURE

Dr E.S. Hwang is funded by: R01 CA185138-01 (ESH); U2C CA-17-035 Pre-Cancer Atlas (PCA) Research Centers (ESH); DOD BC132057 (ESH); BCRF 19- 074 (ESH). Dr A. Chiba and S.M. Record have nothing to disclose.

REFERENCES

1. van Seijen M, Lips EH, Thompson AM, et al. Ductal carcinoma in situ: to treat or not to treat, that is the question. Br J Cancer 2019;121(4):285–92.
2. Grimm LJ, Shelley Hwang E. Active surveillance for DCIS: the importance of selection criteria and monitoring. Ann Surg Oncol 2016;23(13):4134–6.

3. Ozanne EM, Shieh Y, Barnes J, et al. Characterizing the impact of 25 years of DCIS treatment. Breast Cancer Res Treat 2011;129(1):165–73.
4. Morrow M, Schnitt SJ, Norton L. Current management of lesions associated with an increased risk of breast cancer. Nat Rev Clin Oncol 2015;12(4):227–38.
5. Virnig BA, Tuttle TM, Shamliyan T, et al. Ductal carcinoma in situ of the breast: a systematic review of incidence, treatment, and outcomes. J Natl Cancer Inst 2010;102(3):170–8.
6. Ward EM, DeSantis CE, Lin CC, et al. Cancer statistics: Breast cancer in situ. CA A Cancer J Clin 2015;65(6):481–95.
7. Ernster VL, Barclay J. Increases in ductal carcinoma in situ (DCIS) of the breast in relation to mammography: a dilemma. JNCI Monographs 1997;1997(22):151–6.
8. Siegel RL, Miller KD, Fuchs HE, et al. Cancer statistics, 2022. CA: A Cancer Journal for Clinicians 2022;72(1):7–33.
9. Surveillance, Epidemiology, and End Results (SEER) Program Populations (1969-2020) (www.seer.cancer.gov/popdata), National Cancer Institute, DCCPS. Surveillance Research Program 2022.
10. Fleming M, Ravula S, Tatishchev SF, et al. Colorectal carcinoma: Pathologic aspects. J Gastrointest Oncol 2012;3(3):153–73.
11. Carvalho B, Sillars-Hardebol AH, Postma C, et al. Colorectal adenoma to carcinoma progression is accompanied by changes in gene expression associated with ageing, chromosomal instability, and fatty acid metabolism. Cell Oncol 2012;35(1):53–63.
12. Brown ML, Potosky AL. The presidential effect: the public health response to media coverage about Ronald Reagan's colon cancer episode. Public Opin Q 1990; 54(3):317–29.
13. Welch HG, Black WC. Using autopsy series to estimate the disease "reservoir" for ductal carcinoma in situ of the breast: how much more breast cancer can we find? Ann Intern Med 1997;127(11):1023–8.
14. Solin LJ. Management of ductal carcinoma in situ (DCIS) of the breast: present approaches and future directions. Curr Oncol Rep 2019;21(4):33.
15. Early Breast Cancer Trialists' Collaborative G. Overview of the randomized trials of radiotherapy in ductal carcinoma in situ of the breast. JNCI Monographs 2010; 2010(41):162–77.
16. Narod SA, Iqbal J, Giannakeas V, et al. Breast cancer mortality after a diagnosis of ductal carcinoma in situ. JAMA Oncol 2015;1(7):888–96.
17. Gunawardena DS, Burrows S, Taylor DB. Non-mass versus mass-like ultrasound patterns in ductal carcinoma in situ: is there an association with high-risk histology? Clin Radiol 2020;75(2):140–7.
18. Farante G, Toesca A, Magnoni F, et al. Advances and controversies in management of breast ductal carcinoma in situ (DCIS). Eur J Surg Oncol 2022;48(4): 736–41.
19. Estévez LG, Álvarez I, Seguí MÁ, et al. Current perspectives of treatment of ductal carcinoma in situ. Cancer Treat Rev 2010/11/01/2010;36(7):507–17.
20. Lester SC, Connolly JL, Amin MB. College of American pathologists protocol for the reporting of ductal carcinoma in situ. Arch Pathol Lab Med 2009;133(1):13–4.
21. NCCN Guidelines Version 4.2022 Ductal Carcinoma in Situ (DCIS). Available at: https://www.nccn.org/guidelines/guidelines-detail?category=1&id=1419.   Accessed January 2023, 08.
22. Morrow M, Van Zee KJ, Solin LJ, et al. Society of surgical oncology-American society for radiation oncology-american society of clinical oncology consensus

guideline on margins for breast-conserving surgery with whole-breast irradiation in ductal carcinoma in situ. Ann Surg Oncol 2016;23(12):3801–10.

23. Marinovich ML, Azizi L, Macaskill P, et al. The association of surgical margins and local recurrence in women with ductal carcinoma in situ treated with breast-conserving therapy: a meta-analysis. Ann Surg Oncol 2016;23(12):3811–21.

24. Morrow M, Van Zee KJ, Solin LJ, et al. Society of surgical oncology-American society for radiation oncology-american society of clinical oncology consensus guideline on margins for breast-conserving surgery with whole-breast irradiation in ductal carcinoma in situ. J Clin Oncol 2016;34(33):4040–6.

25. Howard-McNatt M, Dupont E, Tsangaris T, et al. Impact of cavity shave margins on margin status in patients with pure ductal carcinoma in situ. J Am Coll Surg 2021;232(4):373–8.

26. Unzeitig A, Kobbermann A, Xie X-J, et al. Influence of surgical technique on mastectomy and reexcision rates in breast-conserving therapy for cancer. International Journal of Surgical Oncology 2012;2012:e725121.

27. Chagpar AB, Killelea BK, Tsangaris TN, et al. A randomized, controlled trial of cavity shave margins in breast cancer. N Engl J Med 2015;373(6):503–10.

28. Coopey SB, Buckley JM, Smith BL, et al. Lumpectomy cavity shaved margins do not impact re-excision rates in breast cancer patients. Ann Surg Oncol 2011; 18(11):3036–40.

29. Chatterjee A, Pyfer B, Czerniecki B, et al. Early postoperative outcomes in lumpectomy versus simple mastectomy. J Surg Res 2015;198(1):143–8.

30. Allison KH, Abraham LA, Weaver DL, et al. Trends in breast biopsy pathology diagnoses among women undergoing mammography in the United States: A report from the Breast Cancer Surveillance Consortium. Cancer 2015;121(9):1369–78.

31. Goodwin A, Parker S, Ghersi D, et al. Post-operative radiotherapy for ductal carcinoma in situ of the breast–a systematic review of the randomised trials. Breast 2009;18(3):143–9.

32. Silverstein MJ, Lagios MD. Should all patients undergoing breast conserving therapy for DCIS receive radiation therapy? No. One size does not fit all: an argument against the routine use of radiation therapy for all patients with ductal carcinoma in situ of the breast who elect breast conservation. J Surg Oncol 2007;95(8): 605–9.

33. Coates AS, Winer EP, Goldhirsch A, et al. Tailoring therapies–improving the management of early breast cancer: St Gallen international expert consensus on the primary therapy of early breast cancer 2015. Ann Oncol 2015;26(8):1533–46.

34. Bremer T, Whitworth PW, Patel R, et al. a biological signature for breast ductal carcinoma in situ to predict radiotherapy benefit and assess recurrence risk. Clin Cancer Res 2018;24(23):5895–901.

35. Ciervide R, Dhage S, Guth A, et al. Five year outcome of 145 patients with ductal carcinoma in situ (DCIS) after accelerated breast radiotherapy. Int J Radiat Oncol Biol Phys 2012;83(2):e159–64.

36. Cuzick J, Sestak I, Pinder SE, et al. Effect of tamoxifen and radiotherapy in women with locally excised ductal carcinoma in situ: long-term results from the UK/ANZ DCIS trial. Lancet Oncol 2011;12(1):21–9.

37. Wapnir IL, Dignam JJ, Fisher B, et al. Long-term outcomes of invasive ipsilateral breast tumor recurrences after lumpectomy in NSABP B-17 and B-24 randomized clinical trials for DCIS. J Natl Cancer Inst 2011;103(6):478–88.

38. Bijker N, Peterse JL, Duchateau L, et al. Risk factors for recurrence and metastasis after breast-conserving therapy for ductal carcinoma-in-situ: analysis of

European Organization for Research and Treatment of Cancer Trial 10853. J Clin Oncol 2001;19(8):2263–71.

39. Van Zee KJ, Liberman L, Samli B, et al. Long term follow-up of women with ductal carcinoma in situ treated with breast-conserving surgery: the effect of age. Cancer 1999;86(9):1757–67.

40. Cronin PA, Olcese C, Patil S, et al. Impact of age on risk of recurrence of ductal carcinoma in situ: outcomes of 2996 women treated with breast-conserving surgery over 30 years. Ann Surg Oncol 2016;23(9):2816–24.

41. Hwang ES, Hyslop T, Hendrix LH, et al. Phase II single-arm study of preoperative letrozole for estrogen receptor-positive postmenopausal ductal carcinoma in situ: CALGB 40903 (Alliance). J Clin Oncol 2020;38(12):1284–92.

42. Liu Y, Hall IJ, Filson C, et al. Trends in the use of active surveillance and treatments in Medicare beneficiaries diagnosed with localized prostate cancer. Urol Oncol: Seminars and Original Investigations 2021;39(7):432.e1–10.

43. Kinsella N, Helleman J, Bruinsma S, et al. Active surveillance for prostate cancer: a systematic review of contemporary worldwide practices. Transl Androl Urol 2018;7(1):83–97.

44. Light A, Lophatananon A, Keates A, et al. Development and External Validation of the STRATified CANcer Surveillance (STRATCANS) Multivariable model for predicting progression in men with newly diagnosed prostate cancer starting active surveillance. J Clin Med 2023;12(1):216.

45. Ito Y, Miyauchi A, Kihara M, et al. Patient age is significantly related to the progression of papillary microcarcinoma of the thyroid under observation. Thyroid 2014;24(1):27–34.

46. Tuttle RM, Fagin JA, Minkowitz G, et al. Natural history and tumor volume kinetics of papillary thyroid cancers during active surveillance. JAMA Otolaryngol Head Neck Surg 2017;143(10):1015–20.

47. Hwang ES, Hyslop T, Lynch T, et al. The COMET (Comparison of Operative versus Monitoring and Endocrine Therapy) trial: a phase III randomised controlled clinical trial for low-risk ductal carcinoma in situ (DCIS). BMJ Open 2019;9(3):e026797.

48. Elshof LE, Tryfonidis K, Slaets L, et al. Feasibility of a prospective, randomised, open-label, international multicentre, phase III, non-inferiority trial to assess the safety of active surveillance for low risk ductal carcinoma in situ - The LORD study. Eur J Cancer 2015;51(12):1497–510.

49. Francis A, Thomas J, Fallowfield L, et al. Addressing overtreatment of screen detected DCIS; the LORIS trial. Eur J Cancer 2015;51(16):2296–303.

50. Worni M, Akushevich I, Greenup R, et al. Trends in treatment patterns and outcomes for ductal carcinoma in situ. J Natl Cancer Inst 2015;107(12):djv263.

Is Axillary Staging Obsolete in Early Breast Cancer?

Monica Morrow, MD

KEYWORDS

- Axillary staging • Early breast cancer • Sentinel lymph node biopsy • Axilla
- Local control

KEY POINTS

- Extensive nodal metastases (N2–3) are present in less than 4% of patients with a negative clinical examination of the axilla, and do not constitute a reason for axillary staging in clinical stage 1 and 2 breast cancer.
- Sentinel lymph node biopsy results in paresthesia, pain, and lymphedema in 3% to 15% of patients.
- In prospective trials of no axillary surgery, axillary recurrence occurred in 3% to 6% of patients treated without surgery.
- In postmenopausal women with HR+/HER2− stage 1 and 2 breast cancer, results of genomic assays, not nodal status, determine the need for systemic therapy.
- At present, axillary staging is not indicated for staging, local control, or determining the need for systemic therapy in women age ≥70 years with cT1–2 N0 HR+/HER2− breast cancer.

INTRODUCTION

Historically, axillary lymph node dissection (ALND) was regarded as part of the curative management of breast cancer. However, after clinical trials made it clear that ALND did not contribute to survival,[1] ALND came to be regarded as a staging procedure as well as a means of maintaining local control in the axilla. Subsequently, ALND was replaced by the less-morbid sentinel lymph node biopsy (SLNB) for staging, and for therapy in those with limited nodal disease burdens. The impetus to eliminate SLNB arises from recognition that in the current era of molecular medicine, decisions regarding adjuvant systemic therapy are frequently made based on estrogen receptor (ER), progesterone receptor (PR), and human epidermal growth factor receptor 2 (HER2) status as well as genomic tests, rather than nodal status, raising the question of whether any form of axillary surgery is necessary in early-stage breast cancer. In addition, the widespread adoption of screening mammography has resulted in the

Breast Service, Department of Surgery, Memorial Sloan Kettering Cancer Center, 300 East 66th Street, New York, NY 10065, USA
E-mail address: morrowm@mskcc.org

Surg Oncol Clin N Am 32 (2023) 675–691
https://doi.org/10.1016/j.soc.2023.05.002
1055-3207/23/© 2023 Elsevier Inc. All rights reserved.
surgonc.theclinics.com

diagnosis of smaller breast cancers, which are less likely to have nodal metastases, and, in those with nodal metastases, lower disease burdens, suggesting a decreased need for axillary surgery for local control. Additionally, there is an increasing awareness of the morbidity of SLNB.

SLNB has been shown in randomized trials to have a lower risk of lymphedema and sensory loss when compared with ALND,[2] but adverse outcomes from the procedure still occur in a substantial minority of patients. Although perioperative complications, such as wound infection or hematoma, are uncommon,[3] long-term sequelae are more frequent.

At the 6-month timepoint in the American College of Surgeons Oncology Group (ACOSOG) Z0010 trial of 4069 patients undergoing SLNB alone, 8.6% of patients had axillary paresthesias, 3.8% had decreased range of motion in the upper extremity, and 6.9% had lymphedema.[3] Other early studies reported axillary paresthesias in 16% to 30% of patients undergoing SLNB.[4,5] In a detailed evaluation of arm function and quality of life performed 18 months postoperatively in the randomized ALMANAC (Axillary Lymphatic Mapping Against Nodal Axillary Clearance) trial, 17% of patients undergoing SLNB alone reported at least 1 arm problem: numbness in 8.7%, and lymphedema in 7%.[2] In studies examining the effect of age on symptoms, symptoms were noted to be more severe in younger patients.[2,6] In a meta-analysis of 17 studies conducted between 2001-2008 reporting arm symptoms after SLNB alone, rates of pain varied from 7.5-36.0%, decreased range of motion varied from 0-31%, decreased strength varied from 11-19%, and sensory disorders varied from 1-66%. Lymphedema rates ranged from 0% to 14%.[7] Although the relatively high rate of sequelae of SLNB in these early studies might be attributed to lack of familiarity with the procedure, similar results have been reported in more recent studies. Kootstra and colleagues[8] observed limitations in anteflexion and abduction-exrotation of the shoulder 2 years postoperatively in a longitudinal follow-up study of the effects of axillary surgery on arm function, which included 61 women undergoing SLNB alone, and in a retrospective study including 600 patients treated between 2014 and 2021, paresthesias were seen in 14%, lymphedema in 4%, and decreased range of motion in 3.5%.[9] In the initial 176 patients enrolled in the SOUND (Sentinel node vs Observation after Axillary Ultrasound) trial , a randomized comparison of outcomes after SLNB and no axillary surgery, significant differences favoring the no-axillary-surgery group were observed in the Disability Arm and Shoulder questionnaire at 1 week postoperatively, but did not persist at 6 months' follow-up.[10] Although SLNB clearly decreases the morbidity of axillary staging compared with ALND, short- and long-term sequelae are seen even after years of experience with the procedure, providing the impetus to critically examine the need for axillary staging in early breast cancer today.

AXILLARY STAGING TO MAINTAIN LOCAL CONTROL

The need for axillary staging to maintain local control is dependent on the likelihood of nodal metastases in patients deemed node negative by physical examination with or without imaging studies, and the risk of nodal recurrence in patients treated without axillary surgery or node field radiotherapy (RT). A substantial body of literature is available to address both questions.

Axillary Tumor Burden

The likelihood of nodal metastases varies with tumor size, histology, ER, PR, and HER2 status, multicentricity, and the presence of lymphovascular invasion, as well as other patient and tumor features. In a large SEER (Surveillance, Epidemiology and End Results) data set, the incidence of nodal metastases was under 20% for tumors up to 1.5 cm in size, and ranged from 20% to 60% for T2 tumors,[11] but the data set was not restricted to those without palpable adenopathy and included patients diagnosed before the widespread uptake of screening mammography. McCartan and colleagues[12] examined the incidence of nodal metastases in a consecutive series of 5142 clinically node-negative patients who had an SLNB between 2006 and 2011. Median age was 58 years; median tumor size was 1.3 cm (range, 0.1–12.4 cm), and 85% had hormone receptor–positive (HR+) disease. Nodal metastases were present in 19%, and younger age, larger tumor size, high nuclear grade, multifocality/centricity, and lymphovascular invasion were all significantly associated with nodal metastases. Somewhat surprisingly, increased body mass index did not correlate with a higher incidence of nodal positivity, although 28% of the population was obese.

It is now recognized that receptor status is also associated with the risk of nodal metastases. In 11,496 women having surgery at Memorial Sloan Kettering Cancer Center between 1998 and 2010, nodal macrometastases were present in 25% of HR+/HER2− patients, 32% of HR+/HER+ patients, 36% of HR−/HER+ patients, and 28% of those with triple-negative cancers. Metastases in $\geq$4 nodes were present in 9%, 16%, 22%, and 13% of these groups, respectively.[13] On multivariable analysis after controlling for tumor size, grade, lymphovascular invasion, and age, receptor status was significantly associated with the presence of nodal metastases and involvement of $\geq$4 nodes ($P<.0001$ for both). Patients with triple-negative tumors were the least likely to have any nodal involvement, whereas those with HR−/HER2+ tumors were most likely to have nodal involvement and to have $\geq$4 involved nodes. Others have demonstrated a relationship between receptor status and nodal involvement, with the lowest likelihood of nodal disease in those with triple-negative cancers.[14,15] Particular attention has been given to the incidence of nodal metastases in postmenopausal women because it is in this group that axillary staging is thought to be least likely to change clinical management. Amlicke and colleagues[16] examined the incidence of nodal metastases in 325,692 women with cN0 ER+/HER2− breast cancer reported to the National Cancer Database. In those with T1 tumors, 87% were node negative, whereas 67% of T2 tumors and 31% of T3 tumors were node negative. Pathologic N2/3 disease was present in 1.2% of T1 tumors, 5.9% of T2 tumors, and 17.3% of T3 tumors. In a multivariable model, higher T stage, lobular histology, and high histologic grade were significantly associated with pN2/3 disease. Lee and colleagues[17] reported a series of 3363 consecutive postmenopausal women with cT1–2N0 breast cancers and found that 19% had pN1 disease, and only 3.6% had pN2/3 disease. In the subset of 2639 women with HR+/HER2− disease, 3.5% had pN2/3 disease. On multivariable analysis, age less than 65 years, T2 tumors, lymphovascular invasion, and multifocality/centricity were significantly associated with pN2/3 disease. Rates of pN2/3 disease were 4.1% among patients less than 65 years of age, 7.7% in those with multifocal/centric tumors, and 12.6% among patients with tumors greater than 2 cm.

In aggregate, these studies demonstrate that although nodal metastases are not uncommon with a normal physical examination, a heavy nodal disease burden is rare in more recent studies (**Table 1**).[12,16–19] The accuracy of clinical evaluation of the axilla can be improved with the addition of axillary ultrasound and axillary node biopsy. The identification of abnormal nodes on axillary ultrasound is dependent on nodal enlargement and abnormal morphology with cortical thickening. In an early systematic review of the accuracy of ultrasound-guided biopsy of axillary nodes for staging,

Table 1
Nodal metastasis in clinically node-negative patients

Author	Number of Patients	Population	Nodal Macrometastases Any (%)	N2-N3 (%)
Majid et al,[18] 2013	1435	All, population based	33	NS
Voogd et al,[19] 2000	5125	All, population based	34	NS
McCartan et al,[12] 2016	5142	T1-T3, any receptor status	19	4.1
Amlicke et al,[16] 2022	325,692	T1-T4, postmenopausal ER+/HER2−		2.2
		T1	13	
		T2	33	
		T3	48	
		T4	51	
Lee et al,[17] 2023	3363	cT 1–2, postmenopausal, any receptor status	23	3.6
	2639	HR+/HER2−		3.5

Abbreviation: NS, not significant.

Houssami and colleagues[20] showed that the procedure is accurate with sensitivity of 79.6% (95% confidence interval [CI], 74.1 to 84.2) for the detection of metastases and a false-negative rate of 20.4%. In another meta-analysis published in 2021, which included 10,374 patients, the sensitivity of axillary ultrasound for the detection of nodal metastases was 51% (95% CI, 43%–59%),[21] and the false-negative rate for the identification of patients with metastases in $\geq$3 nodes was 28%.

Other studies have examined the ability of axillary ultrasound to exclude a heavy nodal disease burden. In retrospective studies, 3% to 7% of patients with negative axillary ultrasounds are found to have metastases in $\geq$3 nodes.[22–26] In these studies, features associated with the presence of nodal metastases in general, such as larger tumor size, high grade, lymphovascular invasion, and younger age, as well as lobular histology, tended to be associated with higher false-negative rates for axillary ultrasound and heavier disease burdens. Studies examining the ability of axillary ultrasound to identify patients with heavy axillary tumor burdens are summarized in **Table 2**.[7,22,23,25–28] All studies demonstrate a negative predictive value of 90% or

Table 2
Accuracy of ultrasound ± biopsy in identifying extensive (N2-N3) nodal disease

Author	Number of Patients	Clinical Stage	NPV (%)	FNR (%)
Abe et al,[22] 2013	539	T1–4, cN0	97	17
Amonkar et al,[27] 2013	439	T1–4, cN0, N+	97	23
Jackson et al,[23] 2015	494	T1–4, cN0	96	29
Neal et al,[26] 2010	208	T1–4, cN0, N+	93	4
Liu et al,[7] 2009	3944	T1–4, cN0	97	10
Moorman et al,[25] 2014[a]	1060	T < 5 cm, cN0	96	36
Kramer et al,[28] 2016[a]	2130	T1–3	93	7

Abbreviations: FNR, false-negative rate; NPV, negative predictive value.
[a] Extensive nodal disease defined as involvement of $\geq$3 nodes.

better, with variable false-negative rates, which are likely due to differences in the clinical stages of patients included in the studies.

Several ongoing clinical trials have provided information on the accuracy of physical examination, tumor characteristics, and axillary ultrasound in identifying patients with low-volume axillary disease. The SOUND trial included 1560 patients with T1 tumors and a clinically negative axilla, and a negative axillary ultrasound with or without fine-needle aspiration, who were undergoing breast-conserving surgery (BCS) and were randomized to SLNB or no axillary staging.[29] The INSEMA (Intergroup-Sentinel-Mamma) trial had a similar design but included T1 and T2 patients. More than 90% of patients in both studies had HR+ disease, and the median patient age was 61 years. Although the primary endpoints have not been reported, information on tumor burden in the patients randomized to the axillary surgery arms is available. Macrometastases were seen in 14% of patients in both studies, but pN2/3 disease was present in only 0.5% of the patients in SOUND, and metastases to 3 or more nodes in 1.3% of those in the INSEMA trial, indicating that the combination of low T stage, normal physical examination, and a normal axillary ultrasound excludes the presence of a high-nodal disease burden with a high degree of reliability (Gentilini O, presented at the St. Gallen International Consensus Conference, Vienna, Austria, March 2023).[30]

RELATIONSHIP BETWEEN AXILLARY TUMOR BURDEN AND NODAL RECURRENCE

In considering the potential for axillary recurrence if axillary staging is omitted, it is important to remember that the presence of axillary node metastases, which are not treated with surgery or RT, does not translate to local failure in the majority of cases. This was demonstrated in the landmark NSABP (National Surgical Adjuvant Breast and Bowel Project) B04 trial, a study that recruited patients with primary operable breast cancer confined to the breast, or breast and axilla, in the prescreening mammography era and at a time when adjuvant systemic therapy was not in routine use.[1] Clinically node-negative patients (n = 1079) were randomized to radical mastectomy, total mastectomy, or total mastectomy with RT. Despite 39% of patients in the radical mastectomy arm having nodal metastases, only 12% of those who did not undergo axillary surgery developed axillary first failure even in the absence of systemic therapy.

Although this study did not lead to the abandonment of ALND, it provided an important proof of principle, which has been redemonstrated in multiple more recent studies. Additional evidence that residual nodal disease does not translate into regional recurrence in women of all ages comes from the early experience with SLNB in which false-negative rates for the procedure were reported to range from 2.7% to 9.8%,[31–33] yet less than 1% of those with negative sentinel lymph nodes (SLNs) experienced an axillary recurrence within the initial 5 postoperative years.[32,34] Addressing concerns that the use of adjuvant systemic therapy might result in a delay in axillary recurrence, particularly in patients with HR+ cancers receiving 5 years of endocrine therapy, Galimberti and colleagues[35] reported a 1.7% rate of axillary recurrence in 5262 consecutive SLN-negative patients after a median follow-up of 7 years. Similar findings were reported from Memorial Sloan Kettering Cancer Center in 1529 SLN-negative patients followed a median of 10.8 years in which the cumulative incidence of recurrence was 0.6% at 10 years and 0.9% at 15 years.[36]

In the ACOSOG Z0011 trial of patients with metastases in 1 to 2 sentinel nodes treated with BCS and whole-breast irradiation, 27.3% of those randomized to ALND had macrometastases in non-sentinel nodes, yet only 1.5% of those in the no-additional-axillary-treatment group had a regional recurrence.[37,38]

Outcome data on the incidence of nodal recurrence in HR+ patients age ≥65 years who did not have axillary surgery are also available. The CALGB 9343 trial randomized women age ≥70 years with T1N0, HR+ breast cancer undergoing lumpectomy and treatment with tamoxifen to RT versus no RT. Initially, ALND was required for staging, but this requirement was subsequently dropped, providing outcome information for 3 patient groups. In the 244 patients who had ALND, no axillary recurrences were observed. In the group that did not have axillary surgery, no recurrences were seen in the patients receiving RT, whereas 6 of the 200 who had tamoxifen and no RT had an axillary recurrence at a median follow-up of 12.6 years.[39]

The IBCSG 10-93 trial randomized women age ≥60 years with clinically node-negative breast cancer who received tamoxifen to undergo ALND or no axillary surgery.[40] At 6 years' follow-up, the nodal recurrence rate was 1% in the ALND arm, and 3% in the no-axillary-surgery arm. No differences in overall survival (OS) were noted, and patients in the no-axillary-surgery arm had a better quality of life at the first postoperative assessment ($P = .01$); however, there was a return to baseline quality of life for both groups at later time points. A third trial conducted by Martelli and colleagues[41] randomized women age 65 to 80 years with cT1N0 cancer undergoing BCT to ALND or no ALND. No survival difference was seen between groups, and at a median follow-up of 15 years, only 6% of the patients in the no-axillary-surgery group had an axillary recurrence.

These findings, coupled with the remarkable decrease in the rates of in-breast recurrence seen in patients receiving systemic therapy,[42] emphasize the opportunity for further de-escalation of axillary surgery in an era when the majority of women with invasive breast cancer receive systemic therapy, and that therapy is increasingly effective.

AXILLARY STAGING TO GUIDE ADJUVANT SYSTEMIC THERAPY

In addition to the need for axillary staging to maintain local control, the presence of axillary node metastases has been an important determinant of the need for adjuvant systemic therapy. Historically, the use of adjuvant systemic therapy was limited to women with nodal metastases, but currently, most patients with breast cancer receive adjuvant endocrine therapy and/or chemotherapy, and the importance of nodal status in determining the need for systemic therapy and the type of systemic therapy varies with HR and HER2 status. This is an important consideration when discussing the possibility of eliminating axillary staging, because although, as discussed previously, metastases to ≥3 axillary nodes can be reliably excluded with a normal physical examination and a negative axillary ultrasound, nodal metastases were present in 14% of the patients enrolled in the SOUND and INSEMA trials who met these criteria (Gentilini O, presented at the St. Gallen International Consensus Conference, Vienna, Austria, March 2023).[30]

Axillary staging remains important for patients with HER2+ and triple-negative breast cancers where the presence of nodal metastases is usually considered an indication for neoadjuvant chemotherapy (NAC), allowing the use of dual HER2 blockade in patients with HER2 overexpressing tumors, and trastuzumab emtansine (TDM-1) for those who do not have a pathologic complete response (pCR) to NAC.[43] Conversely, in patients with stage 1 HER2+ breast cancers, treatment can be de-escalated to paclitaxel and trastuzumab with excellent outcomes, as demonstrated in the APT trial.[44] In node-positive patients with triple-negative breast cancer, pembrolizumab is used in combination with NAC, and capecitabine is given to those who do not have a pCR, whereas for those with tumors less than 5 mm in size and negative lymph nodes, systemic therapy can be avoided.[43]

Axillary staging is the least likely to alter the selection of systemic therapy for postmenopausal HR+/HER2− patients with breast cancer. The TAILORx trial showed that the Oncotype DX 21-gene recurrence score (Exact Sciences, Redwood City, CA, USA) was both prognostic and predictive of the benefit of chemotherapy in both premenopausal and postmenopausal women with node-negative breast cancer, with no chemotherapy benefit seen in those with recurrence scores less than 25.[45] The RxPONDER trial enrolled women with metastases in 1 to 3 axillary nodes and randomized those with recurrence scores of less than 25 to endocrine therapy alone or endocrine therapy plus chemotherapy. A subset of premenopausal women not deriving a benefit from chemotherapy was not identified, but in the postmenopausal women, no improvement in invasive disease-free survival (IDFS) was seen with the addition of chemotherapy to endocrine therapy.[46] A chemotherapy benefit was absent among postmenopausal women regardless of tumor size, number of involved axillary nodes (range 1–3), histologic grade, and age. Thus, for postmenopausal women with HR+/HER2− breast cancers and involvement of 0, 1, 2, or 3 lymph nodes, the Oncotype DX 21-gene recurrence score, not nodal status, is the determinant of chemotherapy benefit. Concerns have been raised that in the absence of axillary staging, women with metastases in ≥4 nodes who were not eligible for RxPONDER might not be identified, leading to undertreatment. It is worth noting that 37.4% of patients enrolled in RxPONDER had axillary metastases identified with SLNB alone and did not undergo ALND to determine if ≥4 nodes were involved. Despite this, no difference in outcome was observed between patients with nodal involvement identified by SLNB alone or by ALND. As discussed previously, metastases in ≥3 nodes were present in only 3.6% of 3363 postmenopausal women with T1–2 tumors and a normal physical examination reported by Lee and colleagues,[17] and in fewer than 1.5% of patients enrolled in SOUND and INSEMA who also had a normal axillary ultrasound (Gentilini O, presented at the St. Gallen International Consensus Conference, Vienna, Austria, March 2023).[30] Pilewskie and colleagues[47] retrospectively examined the impact of SLNB on the use of chemotherapy in a group of 1786 postmenopausal women with T1–2, cN0 HR+/HER2− breast cancers and found that even in the absence of the routine use of axillary ultrasound, only 17 patients (1%) were found to have pathologic N2 or N3 disease and received chemotherapy, and that 20 required ALND owing to identification of ≥3 positive SLNs.

Concern has also been raised that elimination of axillary staging in postmenopausal HR+/HER2− women might result in failure to identify high-risk women who would benefit from treatment with abemaciclib. The monarchE trial randomized HR+/HER2− patients defined as high risk on the basis of metastases to ≥4 axillary nodes, or involvement of 1 to 3 nodes and a tumor size of ≥5 cm, or histologic grade 3, or a Ki67 greater than 20% to endocrine therapy alone, or with abemaciclib.[48] At a median follow-up of 24 months, a significant improvement in IDFS was seen for the abemaciclib arm. As noted above, N2/3 disease is uncommon in clinically node-negative women with T1 and T2 tumors. Concerns regarding undertreatment in the absence of axillary staging would be limited to those with grade 3 tumors or an elevated Ki67, in which cases the identification of any nodal metastases might be sufficient to justify abemaciclib treatment. Individual patient characteristics must be considered in the decision to forgo SLNB, and in those with larger T2 tumors and unfavorable characteristics on core biopsy, such as grade 3 and lymphovascular invasion, axillary staging with SLNB would be a reasonable approach. Such a policy would still allow elimination of axillary staging for the majority of HR+/HER2−postmenopausal women with T1 and T2 tumors.

AXILLARY STAGING TO GUIDE POSTMASTECTOMY RADIOTHERAPY AND REGIONAL NODAL IRRADIATION

The most compelling argument for axillary staging in postmenopausal HR+/HER2− patients with breast cancer is the central role that nodal staging plays in determining the need for postmastectomy radiotherapy (PMRT) and regional nodal irradiation (RNI). The use of PMRT and RNI in patients with metastases to ≥4 axillary nodes has been standard for many years because of the high risk of locoregional recurrence in this group. The finding in the 2014 EBCTCG (Early Breast Cancer Trialists' Collaborative Group) Overview analysis that after 15 years follow-up, breast cancer-specific survival was improved with the use of RT, and that the relative survival benefit was comparable for women with metastases in 1 to 3 nodes and those with involvement of ≥4 nodes,[49] coupled with the subsequent publication of 2 prospective randomized trials and 1 population-based cohort study demonstrating a benefit of RNI in more modern groups of patients with breast cancer, further enhanced this trend.[50–52] However, the very modest magnitude of the DFS and distant disease-free survival (DDFS) benefits, coupled with the limited but real toxicity of RNI and PMRT (particularly in patients with breast reconstruction), has led to variable adoption of the use of PMRT/RNI in patients with 1 to 3 nodal metastases, and to attempts to identify low-risk subgroups who can be spared the toxicity of RT. Current National Comprehensive Cancer Network (NCCN) guidelines recommend "strongly considering" comprehensive nodal irradiation in patients with metastases to 1 to 3 axillary nodes.[43] Retrospective studies have shown low rates of locoregional recurrence when patients were selected for PMRT based on clinico-pathologic risk factors,[53,54] and a prediction model has been developed using data from 3532 patients treated at 5 institutions in North America to try and individualize risk.[55] The impact of eliminating nodal staging on the use of RNI/PMRT will depend on the thresholds used for treatment. If the presence of a single nodal metastasis is thought to warrant irradiation regardless of other tumor characteristics, axillary staging will remain essential.

More definitive information upon which to base decisions regarding PMRT/RNI in HR+ patients will be provided by the results of the TAILOR RT trial, in which 2140 women with pT1–2 N1a, HR+/HER2− breast cancer and an Oncotype DX 21-gene recurrence score less than 18 undergoing BCS or mastectomy are randomized to whole-breast irradiation with or without RNI if treated with BCS, or to PMRT and RNI versus no RT if treated with mastectomy. The primary endpoint is breast cancer recurrence-free interval. This study will determine if RNI is beneficial in patients with a limited nodal disease burden and a favorable genomic risk profile, an important question when considering eliminating nodal staging.

OMISSION OF SENTINEL LYMPH NODE BIOPSY IN WOMEN GREATER THAN 70 YEARS OF AGE WITH HORMONE RECEPTOR POSITIVE/HUMAN EPIDERMAL GROWTH FACTOR RECEPTOR 2 NEGATIVE BREAST CANCERS: A TEST CASE

The data discussed previously, demonstrating low rates of local recurrence in women age ≥70 years with early-stage HR+ breast cancer not undergoing axillary surgery, coupled with acceptance of the idea that axillary surgery is a staging rather than a therapeutic procedure, and with the relatively infrequent use of chemotherapy in this patient population, led the Society of Surgical Oncology, in conjunction with the Choosing Wisely campaign, to recommend avoiding SLNB in women age ≥70 years with HR+/HER2− early-stage breast cancers who will receive endocrine therapy for 5 years[56]; NCCN guidelines also consider SLNB optional in this population.[57] Despite a fairly large body of high-quality evidence supporting the safety of SLNB omission, including the CALGB 9343 trial, the IBCSG 1-93 trial, and the study of Martelli and colleagues discussed previously,[39–41] the surgical procedure continues to be performed in a large number of patients. A National Cancer Database study examining time trends in the use of axillary surgery from 2013 to 2016 in women age ≥70 years found that more than 75% of those age 70 to 84 years with cT1–2N0 cancers had an SLNB, and that, remarkably, approximately 50% of those age ≥85 years had the procedure.[58] Other studies examining the use of SLNB in this population in the United States and Canada document rates of SLNB that exceed 80%.[59,60]

In an effort to understand patient attitudes about de-escalation of axillary surgery in women age ≥70 years with HR+ breast cancer, Wang and colleagues[61] classified women as high or low users of breast cancer treatment based on use of SLNB and breast RT. Semistructured interviews were conducted with a total of 12 women—8 high users and 4 low users of treatment—with similar themes regarding treatment selection identified in both groups. Understanding of the role of SLNB was poor, and most patients did not recall a discussion of the possibility of omitting the procedure. In contrast, most did recall a discussion about omitting RT. The most significant factor influencing decisions about SLNB and RT was a physician's recommendation about the procedure. Peace of mind was also given as a reason for pursuing more treatment, and some patients thought that age-based guidelines might be discriminatory. The importance of physician recommendation and the desire to pursue more treatment for peace of mind in the absence of evidence of clear benefit echo the findings of larger studies examining factors influencing the breast cancer surgical decision.[62] Minami and colleagues[63] examined the perspectives of surgical oncologists (n = 16), medical oncologists (n = 6), and radiation oncologists (n = 7) in both academic and community practice on this issue using semistructured interviews conducted in 2020. The interviews revealed poor knowledge of the randomized trial evidence supporting omission of SLNB, the feeling that patient preference was an important consideration, and the difficulty of avoiding giving mixed messages to patients when providers from different specialties have different perspectives on the issue. The failure to abandon SLNB in women age ≥70 years with early HR+/HER2− breast cancers illustrates the difficulties inherent in elimination of axillary staging in broader patient groups.

FUTURE DIRECTIONS

Another group for whom elimination of axillary staging is being considered consists of patients, sometimes known as "exceptional responders," who appear to have a pCR to neoadjuvant therapy. Although clinical trials to date examining the ability of imaging and image-guided biopsy to identify pCR in the breast have had unacceptably high false-negative rates,[64,65] rates of pCR in the nodes are known to be higher than those seen in the breast, even when ductal carcinoma in situ is not included in the definition of pCR.[66] In patients who are clinically node negative at presentation and have a breast pCR, nodal metastases are uncommon. In a

National Cancer Database study of HER2+ (n = 3062) and triple negative patients (n = 2315) receiving NAC, those who were cN0 and had a breast pCR had a 1.6% incidence of nodal metastases, which did not differ by subtype.[67] Similar findings were reported from the Netherlands Cancer Registry.[68] In light of these observations, EUBREAST-01, a multi-institutional single-arm trial of no axillary surgery for patients with cT1–3N0 triple-negative or HER2+ breast cancer who have a radiologic complete response to NAC and pCR confirmed with lumpectomy, will be performed. The primary endpoint is 3-year axillary recurrence-free survival, and 267 patients will be recruited.[69]

As summarized in **Table 3**,[10,30,70] 5 prospective randomized trials are evaluating the need for SLNB in patients with cT1–2N0 disease undergoing initial surgery. The SOUND and INSEMA trials have completed recruitment, and reports of the characteristics of trial participants indicate that although these studies were open to women of all ages and receptor subtypes, the vast majority of study participants were postmenopausal women with HR+/HER2− tumors, likely reflecting greater physician comfort with the idea that nodal status is unlikely to change treatment for this patient subgroup. In contrast to the other studies, the SOAPET study uses a PET scan rather than axillary ultrasound to exclude the presence of significant nodal disease, and the initial phase of this study will establish the negative predictive value of PET scanning before proceeding to a second study phase examining elimination of SLNB. Although it is possible that PET scanning will have a greater sensitivity than axillary ultrasound for the detection of small tumor deposits in the SLN, the cost-effectiveness of this approach is unclear, because a metastatic workup is not indicated in patients with cT1–2N0 disease. In addition, the high cost of PET scanning and more limited availability will limit the generalizability of this approach on a worldwide basis.

The outlook for eliminating SLN biopsy for premenopausal women with HR+/HER2− tumors and for all patients with HER2+ or triple-negative cancers is less clear. Although great strides have been made in refining prognosis in HR+ breast cancer using genomic markers,[71,72] nodal metastases remain prognostic, as illustrated in studies of the Oncotype DX 21-gene recurrence score whereby nodal status is an independent prognostic factor for recurrence even when the Oncotype DX 21-gene recurrence score is included in the model.[73] However, nodal status is not predictive of the benefit of chemotherapy in postmenopausal women as demonstrated in the RxPONDER trial,[46] opening the door to omitting axillary staging for this subgroup. In contrast, for triple-negative and HER2+ patients, specific markers predicting the benefit of particular anti-HER therapies, specific chemotherapy agents, and immunotherapy are lacking, so the prognostic information provided by nodal status is critical in weighing the risks and benefits of treatment. Similarly, the importance of nodal status in assessing prognosis in HR+ patients could increase if the use of cyclin-dependent kinase (CDK) 4/6 inhibitors is expanded to lower-risk patient subsets. At present, nodal staging remains the standard of care for women less than 70 years of age regardless of receptor status, but this is something that is likely to change as results of ongoing trials become available, and indications for systemic therapy and RNI continue to evolve. A cost-effectiveness analysis has demonstrated both cost savings and improved quality of life for observation versus SLNB in postmenopausal women with cT1–2N0, HR+/HER2− cancers,[74] but the experience with omission of SLNB in women age ≥70 years with these tumors suggests that educational interventions targeting both providers and patients, as well as multidisciplinary acceptance of this approach, will be necessary for implementation.

Table 3
Omission of sentinel lymph node biopsy: ongoing randomized trials

Trial	Country	Number of Patients	Inclusion	Randomization Arms	Endpoints
SOUND (2012–2021)[10] Active, not recruiting	Italy	1560	BCS + XRT, cT1N0	Observation SLNB	DDFS (6 mo)
INSEMA (2015–2024)[30] Active, not recruiting	Germany	5505	BCS + XRT, cT1–2N0	Observation SLNB ↓ 1–3 SLNs macromet ALND vs no ALND	IDFS (5 y)
BOOG 2013–08 (2015–2027)[70] Active, recruiting	Netherlands	1644	BCS + XRT, cT1–2N0	Observation SLNB	Regional recurrence (up to 10 y)
NAUTILUS (2020–2027)[70] Active, recruiting	Korea	1734	BCS + XRT, cT1–2N0	Observation SLNB	IDFS (5 y)
SOAPET (2019–2027)[70]	China	1528	cT1–2N0	PET Stage 1: assess NPV Stage 2: SLNB omitted	Stage 1: NPV Stage 2: RFS/DDFS (5 y)

Abbreviations: BCS, breast-conserving surgery; XRT, radiotherapy; SLNB, sentinel lymph node biopsy; DDFS, distant disease-free survival; SLNs, sentinel lymph nodes; macromet, macrometastases; ALND, axillary lymph node dissection; IDFS, invasive disease-free survival; PET, positron emission tomography; NPV, negative predictive value; RFS, recurrence-free survival.

CLINICS CARE POINTS

- Extensive nodal metastases (N2–3) are present in less than 4% of patients with a negative clinical examination of the axilla and do not constitute a reason for axillary staging in clinical stage 1 and 2 breast cancer.
- Sentinel lymph node biopsy results in paresthesia, pain, and lymphedema in 3% to 15% of patients.
- In prospective trials of no axillary surgery, axillary recurrence occurred in 3% to 6% of patients treated without surgery.
- In postmenopausal women with HR+/HER2– stage 1 and 2 breast cancer, results of genomic assays, not nodal status, determine the need for systemic therapy.
- At present, axillary staging is not indicated for staging, local control, or determining the need for systemic therapy in women age ≥70 years with cT1–2N0 HR+/HER2– breast cancer

DISCLOSURE

The author has no disclosures to report.

ACKNOWLEDGMENTS

The author acknowledges V. Morgan Jones, MD for assistance in literature review.

REFERENCES

1. Fisher B, Jeong JH, Anderson S, et al. Twenty-five-year follow-up of a randomized trial comparing radical mastectomy, total mastectomy, and total mastectomy followed by irradiation. N Engl J Med 2002;347(8):567–75.
2. Fleissig A, Fallowfield LJ, Langridge CI, et al. Post-operative arm morbidity and quality of life. Results of the ALMANAC randomised trial comparing sentinel node biopsy with standard axillary treatment in the management of patients with early breast cancer. Breast Cancer Res Treat 2006;95(3):279–93.
3. Wilke LG, McCall LM, Posther KE, et al. Surgical complications associated with sentinel lymph node biopsy: results from a prospective international cooperative group trial. Ann Surg Oncol 2006;13(4):491–500.
4. Burak WE, Hollenbeck ST, Zervos EE, et al. Sentinel lymph node biopsy results in less postoperative morbidity compared with axillary lymph node dissection for breast cancer. Am J Surg 2002;183(1):23–7.
5. Swenson KK, Nissen MJ, Ceronsky C, et al. Comparison of side effects between sentinel lymph node and axillary lymph node dissection for breast cancer. Ann Surg Oncol 2002;9(8):745–53.
6. Temple LK, Baron R, Cody HS 3rd, et al. Sensory morbidity after sentinel lymph node biopsy and axillary dissection: a prospective study of 233 women. Ann Surg Oncol 2002;9(7):654–62.
7. Liu CQ, Guo Y, Shi JY, et al. Late morbidity associated with a tumour-negative sentinel lymph node biopsy in primary breast cancer patients: a systematic review. Eur J Cancer 2009;45(9):1560–8.
8. Kootstra JJ, Hoekstra-Weebers JE, Rietman JS, et al. A longitudinal comparison of arm morbidity in stage I-II breast cancer patients treated with sentinel lymph node biopsy, sentinel lymph node biopsy followed by completion lymph node

dissection, or axillary lymph node dissection. Ann Surg Oncol 2010;17(9): 2384–94.

9. Lorek A, Steinhof-Radwańska K, Zarębski W, et al. Comparative Analysis of Post-operative Complications of Sentinel Node Identification Using the SentiMag(®) Method and the Use of a Radiotracer in Patients with Breast Cancer. Curr Oncol 2022;29(5):2887–94.

10. Gentilini O, Botteri E, Dadda P, et al. Physical function of the upper limb after breast cancer surgery. Results from the SOUND (Sentinel node vs. Observation after axillary Ultra-souND) trial. Eur J Surg Oncol 2016;42(5):685–9.

11. Paramanandam VS, Dylke E, Clark GM, et al. Prophylactic Use of Compression Sleeves Reduces the Incidence of Arm Swelling in Women at High Risk of Breast Cancer-Related Lymphedema: A Randomized Controlled Trial. J Clin Oncol 2022; 40(18):2004–12.

12. McCartan D, Stempel M, Eaton A, et al. Impact of Body Mass Index on Clinical Axillary Nodal Assessment in Breast Cancer Patients. Ann Surg Oncol 2016; 23(10):3324–9.

13. Ugras S, Stempel M, Patil S, et al. Estrogen receptor, progesterone receptor, and HER2 status predict lymphovascular invasion and lymph node involvement. Ann Surg Oncol 2014;21(12):3780–6.

14. Crabb SJ, Cheang MC, Leung S, et al. Basal breast cancer molecular subtype predicts for lower incidence of axillary lymph node metastases in primary breast cancer. Clin Breast Cancer 2008;8(3):249–56.

15. Voduc KD, Cheang MC, Tyldesley S, et al. Breast cancer subtypes and the risk of local and regional relapse. J Clin Oncol 2010;28(10):1684–91.

16. Amlicke MJ, Park J, Agala CB, et al. Prevalence of Pathologic N2/N3 Disease in Postmenopausal Women with Clinical N0 ER+/HER2- Breast Cancer. Ann Surg Oncol 2022;29(12):7662–9.

17. Lee MK, Montagna G, Pilewskie ML, et al. Axillary Staging Is Not Justified in Post-menopausal Clinically Node-Negative Women Based on Nodal Disease Burden. Ann Surg Oncol 2023;30(1):92–7.

18. Majid S, Tengrup I, Manjer J. Clinical assessment of axillary lymph nodes and tumor size in breast cancer compared with histopathological examination: a population-based analysis of 2,537 women. World J Surg 2013;37(1):67–71.

19. Voogd AC, Coebergh JW, Repelaer van Driel OJ, et al. The risk of nodal metastases in breast cancer patients with clinically negative lymph nodes: a population-based analysis. Breast Cancer Res Treat 2000;62(1):63–9.

20. Houssami N, Ciatto S, Turner RM, et al. Preoperative ultrasound-guided needle biopsy of axillary nodes in invasive breast cancer: meta-analysis of its accuracy and utility in staging the axilla. Ann Surg 2011;254(2):243–51.

21. Le Boulc'h M, Gilhodes J, Steinmeyer Z, et al. Pretherapeutic Imaging for Axillary Staging in Breast Cancer: A Systematic Review and Meta-Analysis of Ultrasound, MRI and FDG PET. J Clin Med 2021;10(7):1543.

22. Abe H, Schacht D, Sennett CA, et al. Utility of preoperative ultrasound for predicting pN2 or higher stage axillary lymph node involvement in patients with newly diagnosed breast cancer. AJR Am J Roentgenol 2013;200(3):696–702.

23. Jackson RS, Mylander C, Rosman M, et al. Normal Axillary Ultrasound Excludes Heavy Nodal Disease Burden in Patients with Breast Cancer. Ann Surg Oncol 2015;22(10):3289–95.

24. Keelan S, Heeney A, Downey E, et al. Breast cancer patients with a negative axillary ultrasound may have clinically significant nodal metastasis. Breast Cancer Res Treat 2021;187(2):303–10.

25. Moorman AM, Bourez RL, Heijmans HJ, et al. Axillary ultrasonography in breast cancer patients helps in identifying patients preoperatively with limited disease of the axilla. Ann Surg Oncol 2014;21(9):2904–10.

26. Neal CH, Daly CP, Nees AV, et al. Can preoperative axillary US help exclude N2 and N3 metastatic breast cancer? Radiology 2010;257(2):335–41.

27. Amonkar SJ, Oates E, McLean L, et al. Pre-operative staging of the axilla in primary breast cancer. By redefining the abnormal appearing node can we reduce investigations without affecting overall treatment? Breast 2013;22(6):1114–8.

28. Kramer GM, Leenders MW, Schijf LJ, et al. Is ultrasound-guided fine-needle aspiration cytology of adequate value in detecting breast cancer patients with three or more positive axillary lymph nodes? Breast Cancer Res Treat 2016;156(2): 271–8.

29. Gentilini O, Veronesi U. Abandoning sentinel lymph node biopsy in early breast cancer? A new trial in progress at the European Institute of Oncology of Milan (SOUND: Sentinel node vs Observation after axillary UltraSouND). Breast 2012; 21(5):678–81.

30. Reimer T, Stachs A, Nekljudova V, et al. Restricted Axillary Staging in Clinically and Sonographically Node-Negative Early Invasive Breast Cancer (c/iT1-2) in the Context of Breast Conserving Therapy: First Results Following Commencement of the Intergroup-Sentinel-Mamma (INSEMA) Trial. Geburtshilfe Frauenheilkd 2017;77(2):149–57.

31. Ahlgren J, Holmberg L, Bergh J, et al. Five-node biopsy of the axilla: an alternative to axillary dissection of levels I-II in operable breast cancer. Eur J Surg Oncol 2002;28(2):97–102.

32. Krag DN, Anderson SJ, Julian TB, et al. Sentinel-lymph-node resection compared with conventional axillary-lymph-node dissection in clinically node-negative patients with breast cancer: overall survival findings from the NSABP B-32 randomised phase 3 trial. Lancet Oncol 2010;11(10):927–33.

33. McMasters KM, Wong SL, Chao C, et al. Defining the optimal surgeon experience for breast cancer sentinel lymph node biopsy: a model for implementation of new surgical techniques. Ann Surg 2001;234(3):292–9 [discussion: 299–300].

34. van der Ploeg IM, Nieweg OE, van Rijk MC, et al. Axillary recurrence after a tumour-negative sentinel node biopsy in breast cancer patients: A systematic review and meta-analysis of the literature. Eur J Surg Oncol 2008;34(12):1277–84.

35. Galimberti V, Manika A, Maisonneuve P, et al. Long-term follow-up of 5262 breast cancer patients with negative sentinel node and no axillary dissection confirms low rate of axillary disease. Eur J Surg Oncol 2014;40(10):1203–8.

36. Matsen C, Villegas K, Eaton A, et al. Late Axillary Recurrence After Negative Sentinel Lymph Node Biopsy is Uncommon. Ann Surg Oncol 2016;23(8): 2456–61.

37. Giuliano AE, Ballman K, McCall L, et al. Locoregional Recurrence After Sentinel Lymph Node Dissection With or Without Axillary Dissection in Patients With Sentinel Lymph Node Metastases: Long-term Follow-up From the American College of Surgeons Oncology Group (Alliance) ACOSOG Z0011 Randomized Trial. Ann Surg 2016;264(3):413–20.

38. Giuliano AE, Ballman KV, McCall L, et al. Effect of Axillary Dissection vs No Axillary Dissection on 10-Year Overall Survival Among Women With Invasive Breast Cancer and Sentinel Node Metastasis: The ACOSOG Z0011 (Alliance) Randomized Clinical Trial. JAMA 2017;318(10):918–26.

39. Hughes KS, Schnaper LA, Bellon JR, et al. Lumpectomy plus tamoxifen with or without irradiation in women age 70 years or older with early breast cancer: long-term follow-up of CALGB 9343. J Clin Oncol 2013;31(19):2382–7.
40. Rudenstam CM, Zahrieh D, Forbes JF, et al. Randomized trial comparing axillary clearance versus no axillary clearance in older patients with breast cancer: first results of International Breast Cancer Study Group Trial 10-93. J Clin Oncol 2006;24(3):337–44.
41. Martelli G, Boracchi P, Ardoino I, et al. Axillary dissection versus no axillary dissection in older patients with T1N0 breast cancer: 15-year results of a randomized controlled trial. Ann Surg 2012;256(6):920–4.
42. Bouganim N, Tsvetkova E, Clemons M, et al. Evolution of sites of recurrence after early breast cancer over the last 20 years: implications for patient care and future research. Breast Cancer Res Treat 2013;139(2):603–6.
43. National Comprehensive Cancer Network (NCCN). NCCN Clinical Practice Guidelines in Oncology. Breast Cancer V4 2002. Available at: https://www.nccn.org/guidelines/guidelines-detail?category=1&id=1419. Accessed January 19, 2023.
44. Tolaney SM, Barry WT, Dang CT, et al. Adjuvant paclitaxel and trastuzumab for node-negative, HER2-positive breast cancer. N Engl J Med 2015;372(2):134–41.
45. Sparano JA, Gray RJ, Makower DF, et al. Prospective Validation of a 21-Gene Expression Assay in Breast Cancer. N Engl J Med 2015;373(21):2005–14.
46. Kalinsky K, Barlow WE, Gralow JR, et al. 21-Gene Assay to Inform Chemotherapy Benefit in Node-Positive Breast Cancer. N Engl J Med 2021;385(25):2336–47.
47. Pilewskie M, Sevilimedu V, Eroglu I, et al. How Often Do Sentinel Lymph Node Biopsy Results Affect Adjuvant Therapy Decisions Among Postmenopausal Women with Early-Stage HR(+)/HER2(-) Breast Cancer in the Post-RxPONDER Era? Ann Surg Oncol 2022;29(10):6267–73.
48. Johnston SRD, Harbeck N, Hegg R, et al. Abemaciclib Combined With Endocrine Therapy for the Adjuvant Treatment of HR+, HER2-, Node-Positive, High-Risk, Early Breast Cancer (monarchE). J Clin Oncol 2020;38(34):3987–98.
49. McGale P, Taylor C, Correa C, et al. Effect of radiotherapy after mastectomy and axillary surgery on 10-year recurrence and 20-year breast cancer mortality: meta-analysis of individual patient data for 8135 women in 22 randomised trials. Lancet 2014;383(9935):2127–35.
50. Poortmans PM, Collette S, Kirkove C, et al. Internal Mammary and Medial Supraclavicular Irradiation in Breast Cancer. N Engl J Med 2015;373(4):317–27.
51. Thorsen LB, Offersen BV, Danø H, et al. DBCG-IMN: A Population-Based Cohort Study on the Effect of Internal Mammary Node Irradiation in Early Node-Positive Breast Cancer. J Clin Oncol 2016;34(4):314–20.
52. Whelan TJ, Olivotto IA, Parulekar WR, et al. Regional Nodal Irradiation in Early-Stage Breast Cancer. N Engl J Med 2015;373(4):307–16.
53. Muhsen S, Moo TA, Patil S, et al. Most Breast Cancer Patients with T1-2 Tumors and One to Three Positive Lymph Nodes Do Not Need Postmastectomy Radiotherapy. Ann Surg Oncol 2018;25(7):1912–20.
54. Tendulkar RD, Rehman S, Shukla ME, et al. Impact of postmastectomy radiation on locoregional recurrence in breast cancer patients with 1-3 positive lymph nodes treated with modern systemic therapy. Int J Radiat Oncol Biol Phys 2012;83(5):e577–81.
55. Sittenfeld SMC, Zabor EC, Hamilton SN, et al. A multi-institutional prediction model to estimate the risk of recurrence and mortality after mastectomy for T1-2N1 breast cancer. Cancer 2022;128(16):3057–66.

56. Society of Surgical Oncology, Choosing Wisely. Five Things Physicians and Patients Should Question, Available at: https://www.choosingwisely.org/societies/society-of-surgical-oncology/July 2016 (Accessed January 19, 2023).
57. Gradishar WJ, Anderson BO, Balassanian R, et al. NCCN Guidelines Insights: Breast Cancer, Version 1.2017. J Natl Compr Canc Netw 2017;15(4):433–51.
58. Minami CA, Jin G, Schonberg MA, et al. Variation in Deescalated Axillary Surgical Practices in Older Women with Early-Stage Breast Cancer. Ann Surg Oncol 2022. https://doi.org/10.1245/s10434-022-11677-z.
59. Louie RJ, Gaber CE, Strassle PD, et al. Trends in Surgical Axillary Management in Early Stage Breast Cancer in Elderly Women: Continued Over-Treatment. Ann Surg Oncol 2020;27(9):3426–33.
60. Thompson J, Le J, Hop A, et al. Impact of Choosing Wisely Recommendations on Sentinel Lymph Node Biopsy and Postoperative Radiation Rates in Women Over Age 70 Years with Hormone-Positive Breast Cancer. Ann Surg Oncol 2021;28(10):5716–22.
61. Wang T, Baskin A, Miller J, et al. Trends in Breast Cancer Treatment De-Implementation in Older Patients with Hormone Receptor-Positive Breast Cancer: A Mixed Methods Study. Ann Surg Oncol 2021;28(2):902–13.
62. Jagsi R, Hawley ST, Griffith KA, et al. Contralateral Prophylactic Mastectomy Decisions in a Population-Based Sample of Patients With Early-Stage Breast Cancer. JAMA Surg 2017;152(3):274–82.
63. Minami CA, Bryan AF, Freedman RA, et al. Assessment of Oncologists' Perspectives on Omission of Sentinel Lymph Node Biopsy in Women 70 Years and Older With Early-Stage Hormone Receptor-Positive Breast Cancer. JAMA Netw Open 2022;5(8):e2228524.
64. Basik M, Cecchini RS, De Los Santos JF, et al. Abstract no. GS5-05. Primary analysis of NRG-BR005, a phase II trial assessing accuracy of tumor bed biopsies in predicting pathologic complete response (pCR) in patients with clinical/radiological complete response after neoadjuvant chemotherapy (NCT) to explore the feasibility of breast-conserving treatment without surgery. Presented at the 42nd Annual San Antonio Breast Cancer Symposium, December 10-14, 2019, San Antonio, Texas. Cancer Res 2020;80(4_Supplement). GS5-05.
65. van Loevezijn AA, van der Noordaa MEM, van Werkhoven ED, et al. Minimally Invasive Complete Response Assessment of the Breast After Neoadjuvant Systemic Therapy for Early Breast Cancer (MICRA trial): Interim Analysis of a Multicenter Observational Cohort Study. Ann Surg Oncol 2021;28(6):3243–53.
66. Mamtani A, Barrio AV, King TA, et al. How Often Does Neoadjuvant Chemotherapy Avoid Axillary Dissection in Patients With Histologically Confirmed Nodal Metastases? Results of a Prospective Study. Ann Surg Oncol 2016;23(11):3467–74.
67. Barron AU, Hoskin TL, Day CN, et al. Association of Low Nodal Positivity Rate Among Patients With ERBB2-Positive or Triple-Negative Breast Cancer and Breast Pathologic Complete Response to Neoadjuvant Chemotherapy. JAMA Surg 2018;153(12):1120–6.
68. Samiei S, van Nijnatten TJA, de Munck L, et al. Correlation Between Pathologic Complete Response in the Breast and Absence of Axillary Lymph Node Metastases After Neoadjuvant Systemic Therapy. Ann Surg 2020;271(3):574–80.
69. Reimer T, Glass A, Botteri E, et al. Avoiding Axillary Sentinel Lymph Node Biopsy after Neoadjuvant Systemic Therapy in Breast Cancer: Rationale for the Prospective, Multicentric EUBREAST-01 Trial. Cancers (Basel) 2020;12(12).

70. U.S. National Library of Medicine. Available at: ClinicalTrials.giv. Accessed January 26, 2023.
71. Cardoso F, van't Veer LJ, Bogaerts J, et al. 70-Gene Signature as an Aid to Treatment Decisions in Early-Stage Breast Cancer. N Engl J Med 2016;375(8):717–29.
72. Sparano JA, Gray RJ, Makower DF, et al. Adjuvant Chemotherapy Guided by a 21-Gene Expression Assay in Breast Cancer. N Engl J Med 2018;379(2):111–21.
73. Dowsett M, Cuzick J, Wale C, et al. Prediction of risk of distant recurrence using the 21-gene recurrence score in node-negative and node-positive postmenopausal patients with breast cancer treated with anastrozole or tamoxifen: a Trans-ATAC study. J Clin Oncol 2010;28(11):1829–34.
74. McEvoy AM, Poplack S, Nickel K, et al. Cost-effectiveness analyses demonstrate that observation is superior to sentinel lymph node biopsy for postmenopausal women with HR + breast cancer and negative axillary ultrasound. Breast Cancer Res Treat 2020;183(2):251–62.

Evidence-Based Strategies to Minimize the Likelihood of Axillary Lymph Node Dissection in Clinically Node-Positive Patients Following Neoadjuvant Chemotherapy

Ashley A. Woodfin, MD[a], Abigail S. Caudle, MD[b],*

KEYWORDS

- Breast cancer • Axillary management • Neoadjuvant chemotherapy • Node positive
- Sentinel lymph node biopsy • Target axillary dissection

KEY POINTS

- Sentinel lymph node biopsy (SLNB) is feasible in cN + after neoadjuvant chemotherapy (NAC), if done with dual tracer technique, removal of 2 or more nodes, and the use of immunohistochemistry.
- Performing targeted axillary dissection in cN + patients after NAC has consistently demonstrated a false-negative rate below that of SLNB alone.
- Patient selection is important for axillary de-escalation. Long-term outcomes on minimal axillary surgery are limited but even low-volume residual axillary disease portends poorer prognosis than ypN0.

INTRODUCTION

The morbidity of axillary lymph node dissection (ALND) has been well studied, with lymphedema as the most concerning complication that can affect quality of life. Current literature quotes rates of lymphedema that range from 20% to 30% following ALND that can double with the addition of adjuvant nodal radiation.[1–3] Although there are surgical techniques in development that may treat or prevent lymphedema in the future, understanding when extensive axillary surgery improves oncologic outcomes, and is thus necessary, is critical.[1,4]

---

[a] MD Anderson Cancer Center, Breast Surgical Oncology, 1515 Holcombe Boulevard, Houston TX 77030, USA; [b] MD Anderson Cancer Center, 1515 Holcombe Boulevard, Unit 1484, Houston TX 77030-4009, USA
* Corresponding author.
E-mail address: ascaudle@mdanderson.org

Surg Oncol Clin N Am 32 (2023) 693–703
https://doi.org/10.1016/j.soc.2023.05.003
surgonc.theclinics.com

ALND has historically been the standard of care for patients who present with clinically node-positive (cN+) breast cancer after neoadjuvant chemotherapy (NAC) despite the fact that many convert to pathologically node negative. As systemic therapy regimens have advanced in the neoadjuvant setting, we are now seeing higher rates of achieving pathologic complete response (pCR). For triple negative and Human Growth Factor Receptor 2 (HER2+) cancers, this has been more significant with the addition of immunotherapy and HER2-targeted therapy achieving overall pCR rates of 45% to 65%,[5–7] with an axillary pCR in up to 75% in these populations.[8–10] Identifying the patients who have eradication of nodal disease is difficult without complete axillary clearance, so all patients were committed to this operation. However, there are multiple recent trials that have evaluated the accuracy of minimally invasive techniques to assess axillary response to chemotherapy. In the following article, we will discuss the current evidence on safely minimizing axillary surgery in cN + patients following NAC.

BACKGROUND
Sentinel Lymph Node Biopsy

Feasibility
Sentinel lymph node biopsy (SLNB) has been well established as technically feasible after NAC despite initial concerns that systemic therapy may lead to fibrosis in lymphatic channels that could affect drainage patterns. In upfront surgery, sentinel lymph node (SLN) detection rates now approach 100%,[11–13] with similar rates seen in those patients who are clinically N0 (cN0) that undergo NAC when using dual tracer for the identification at the time of surgery. A single-center retrospective study out of MD Anderson Cancer Center (MDACC) demonstrated no significant difference in the detection rate when looking at patients with cN0 disease that underwent surgery first (99%) compared with those undergoing NAC followed by SLNB (97%) in a study population of more than 3700 patients.[14] GANEA, a French multicenter prospective trial, demonstrated a similar SLN detection rate of 94.6% after NAC in those initially cN0, however, found that the detection dropped significantly in patients with initial cN1 disease (81.5%).[15]

More recent studies including the SENTinel NeoAdjuvant (SENTINA), American College of Surgeons Oncology Group Z1071 (ACOSOG Z1071), and the Sentinel Node Biopsy After NeoAdjuvant Chemotherapy (SN FNAC) trials have included patient populations with cN1-N2 disease before NAC and reported identification rates between 80% and 93%.[16–18] A variety of techniques for sentinel lymph node mapping was used in these studies, which may have affected the identification rates. The SENTINA study used radiocolloid alone in 61% of its population, and radiocolloid plus blue dye in 34%, and had the lowest reported SLN detection rate at 80%.[16] Whereas the ACOSOG Z1071 trial used dual tracer in 79.1% of the population (4.1% using blue dye only, 16.8% with radiocolloid only) and found that detection rates of at least one SLN was slightly lower in those patients with cN2 disease versus cN1 disease (89.5% vs 92.9%, respectively).[17] The SN FNAC trial also had a mix of single versus dual tracer use in their study population and reported a detection rate of 88%.[18]

Accuracy
In the setting of SLNB, the false-negative rate (FNR) is defined as the proportion of patients with residual nodal disease who had no metastases seen in sentinel nodes. Thus, relying on sentinel node pathologic condition alone would have understaged the extent of residual disease. Although there has been interest in minimally invasive techniques to assess axillary response to NAC, early studies showed an unacceptable FNR although they were primarily single-institutional, retrospective studies.

Three multiinstitutional, prospective registry trials were established to better evaluate the use of SLNB in cN + patients after completion of NAC. All 3 trials enrolled cN + patients who underwent NAC. At the time of surgery, enrolled patients underwent SLNB followed by completion ALND so that the pathologic condition of the sentinel nodes could be compared with that of the remaining nodes in order to determine the FNR. These 3 trials, SENTINA, ACOSOG Z1071, and the SN FNAC had striking similarities between the trials' results both as to the accuracy of SLNB as well as technical factors that affect FNR. However, there were some key differences in study design.

SENTINA was a 4-armed study including patients with cN0, cN + that converted to cN0 after NAC, and those cN + that remained cN + after NAC. A unique aspect of this study included performing upfront SLNB on patients in the cN0 arm, with repeat SLNB following NAC in those with initial positive SLNB (arm B). This demonstrated repeat SLNB after NAC was not feasible (detection rate of only 60.8%) nor accurate (FNR 51.6%). When investigating initial SLNB accuracy after NAC, Arm C of the study contained 592 patients that converted from cN + to cN0 after NAC. SLNB after NAC performed had an FNR of 14.2%. However, it is notable that only 25% of those in Arm C underwent biopsy to verify nodal status before NAC,[16] meaning a quarter of the patients in this cohort could have been cN0.

The ACOSOG Z1071 enrolled 756 patients with cT0-4, cN1-2, M0 breast cancer that underwent NAC, 663 of which were cN1 with ultimately evaluable disease receiving SLNB followed by completion ALND. After data analysis, the FNR of SLNB was calculated at 12.6%, similar to that up the SENTINA trial, and above the prespecified cutoff of 10%.[17]

SN FNAC included cT0-3, cN1-2, and M0-X receiving NAC. However, this study underwent unplanned interim analysis after the presentation of ACOSOG Z1071, at which point the trial was only at approximately 50% accrual. Considering the similar trial design and goals to ACOSOG Z1071, the study was ended early. The calculated SLNB FNR in this study with n = 153 was 8.4%, furthermore an axillary PCR of 34.5% was reported.[18]

Dual tracer

The use of dual tracer refers to using 2 different techniques for sentinel lymph node mapping and identification, including use of a radiotracer such as Tc99 in addition to dye such as isosulfan or methylene blue. Single tracer technique has been shown effective in accurately identifying SLNs in cN0; however, multiple studies have shown that dual tracer technique is superior in cN + pts after NAC.[14,16–18] All 3 large trials above demonstrated a decrease in the FNR when dual tracers were used: SENTINA 16% versus 9%.[16] ACOSOG Z1071 20% versus 11%.[17] SN FNAC 16% versus 5.2%.[18]

Number of sentinel lymph node resected

All 3 trials also demonstrated an inverse correlation between the number of SLN resected and FNR on subgroup analysis. In the SENTINA and ACOSOG Z1071 trials, resection of 3 or more nodes decreased the FNR to less than 10% (FNRs of 7% and 9%, respectively).[16,17] Whereas in the SN FNAC trial, a resection of 2 or more nodes lowered the FNR to 4.9%.[18]

Immunohistochemistry

Use of immunohistochemistry (IHC) plays a significant role in the accuracy of SLNB in this patient population. In the SN FNAC study, all SLNs negative for metastases on hematoxylin-eosin stain (H&E) staining underwent IHC, and all nodal disease was considered positive including isolated tumor cells (ITCs) and micrometastases (<2 mm). Using H&E evaluation alone, the FNR would have been 13%. The addition of IHC reduced this to less than 10%.[18] Once this data was published, the *ACOSOG Z1071* did a central analysis of their nodal pathologic condition with IHC and also found a reduced FNR.[19]

Assessment of the clipped node
Finally, a subgroup of 170 patients in the *ACOSOG Z1071* study had a clip placed in their biopsied positive node, even though this was not a mandatory part of the trial. The authors found analysis of the clipped node significant to the accuracy of the SLNB after NAC. It was reported that when the clipped node was retrieved as an SLN, the FNR dropped to 6.8% (CI: 1.9%–16.5%).[20] See **Table 1**.

Techniques to improve the false negative rate of sentinel lymph node biopsy
After review of the 3 large studies above, there are some take away points from subgroup analysis that suggest techniques to reduce the FNR.

1. Use of dual tracer for SLN mapping
2. Resecting 2 or more SLN
3. Confirmatory testing with IHC on negative SLN
4. Resection of previously biopsied node (clipped node)

Targeted axillary dissection
The data from the *ACOSOG Z1071* trial showing an advantage to marking nodes after biopsy confirms the presence of metastatic disease led to the development of targeted axillary dissection (TAD). TAD consists of selectively localizing and removing the marked in node in addition to removing the sentinel nodes. The clipped node can be localized by a variety of techniques similar to localization techniques for the breast (ie, wire placement, magnetic localizer, radioactive seed, and reflector seed). This technique was demonstrated as feasible after NAC[21] and shown to be beneficial in increasing the accuracy of axillary staging in patients with cN + disease after NAC.[22]

It is worth noting that the clipped node is not always a sentinel node, explaining why it needs to be localized to ensure resection. In the 141 patients that had a clipped node in the *ACOSOG Z1071* trial with documented location at time of resection (either in SLNB specimen or in completion ALND [cALND] specimen), the clipped node was in the SLN in 107, and in the cALND specimen in 34, or approximately 24% of the

Table 1
Feasibility and accuracy of sentinel lymph node biopsy after neoadjuvant chemotherapy

	ACOSOG Z1071[17,19]	SENTINA[16]	SN FNAC[18]
SLN Identification Rate	92.7%	80%	88%
False-negative rates:			
Overall	12.6%	14.2%	13.4%
Single tracer	20.3%	16.0%	16%
Dual tracer	10.8%	8.6%	5.2%
Remove 1 SLN	31%	24.3%	18.2%
Remove 2 SLN	21.1%	18.5%	>1 SLN – 4.9%
Remove 3 SLN	9.1%	7.3%	
Immunohistochemistry	8.7%	Not reported	8.4%

time, which is consistent with current literature quoting rates 23% to 37%.[20,22–24] This means that if relying only on lymphatic mapping and resection of the SLNs, the clipped node will be missed in approximately a quarter of patients.

The first study evaluating TAD as a surgical technique aimed to evaluate whether pathologic changes in the clipped node after NAC are reflective of the entire nodal basin and whether ensuring the removal of the clipped node in addition to SLNs improves the accuracy of axillary staging. They found that the evaluation of the clipped node alone resulted in an FNR of 4.2%, advocating that the clipped node is a valuable staging element. Evaluation of SLNB alone resulted in an FNR of 10.1%, whereas adding the evaluation of clipped node reduced the FNR to 1.4%. After an initial trial to establish the safety of TAD,[21] they reported on 85 patients undergoing TAD showing an FNR of 2% (95% CI 0.05–10.7).[22]

SenTa
This was a German prospective, multicenter registry that included patients cT1-4, cN+, M0 who underwent NAC. The primary aim of this study was to explore the detection rate of SLNs, the clipped node, as well as TAD, and determine the FNR and negative predictive value (NPV) for each. With examination of the clipped node alone, the detection rate was 77.8% with an FNR of 7.2% and NPV of 92%. With TAD, the detection rate was 86.9%, FNR was 4.2%, and NPV was 93.9%.[23] However, the successful replication of TAD in a nonselected multicenter trial validates the clinical feasibility and accuracy of TAD. Furthermore, SenTa 2 is a future study that is currently enrolling and investigating the accuracy of TAD in those patients presenting with 3 or more initially suspicious lymph nodes that convert to cN0 following NAC.

Radioactive iodine seed localization in the axilla combined with sentinel node
This was prospective, multicenter validation trial in cN + patients treated with NAC that demonstrates the replicability of TAD. Of note, in order to perform TAD in this study, they used their original *MARI* (Marking Axillary Lymph Nodes with Radioactive Iodine Seeds) technique placing I^{125} radioactive seeds in the positive node before NAC to guide resection of the biopsied node,[25] at the time of definitive surgery. They reported a detection rate of the targeted node in 98% and FNR of 3.47% in a population of more than 200 patients.[24] This is consistent with the findings of *SenTa* and the MDACC study, with future studies ongoing to examine outcomes and patient selection for TAD (**Table 2**).

Future trials
The AXSANA (Axillary Surgery After NeoAdjuvant Treatment) European prospective multicenter cohort study from the European Breast Cancer Research Association of Surgical Trialists (EUBREAST) network is evaluating different surgical methods of axillary staging in cN + patients treated with NAC. Surgical management after NAC will be up to institutional/national standards and will evaluate SLNB, TAD, and ALND. The aim is to analyze the clinical landscape of axillary surgery in this patient population

Table 2
Feasibility and accuracy of removing SLNs and marked nodes after neoadjuvant chemotherapy

	Identification Rate	False-Negative Rate
MD Anderson (TAD)[22]	Not reported	2%
SenTa (TAD)[23]	87%	4.2%
Netherlands (RISAS)[24]	98%	3.5%

because there are currently discrepancies in technique and findings. Primary endpoints are invasive disease-free survival (DFS), axillary recurrence, health-related quality of life, and arm morbidity.[26] The study is still accruing and has enrolled more than 300 patients. Similarly, GANEA-3, a French prospective, multicenter diagnostic study that will be assessing TAD, as well as breast tumor characteristics to predict axillary response after NAC. All enrolled patients will undergo TAD and completion ALND, with primary aim to help identify patients in whom ALND could be avoided.[27]

DISCUSSION
Oncologic Safety

Despite current literature on feasibility and accuracy of SLNB and TAD in cN + after NAC, we still do not have data on the oncologic outcomes. The hypothetical risk in leaving it behind chemoresistant disease is an area of concern when considering de-escalation of axillary surgery.

Residual Axillary Disease

Prognostically, low-volume axillary disease in the form of ITCs and micrometastases has been shown as similar to pN0 disease in upfront surgery.[28,29] However, Wong and coauthors indicate that DFS and overall survival (OS) worsens with even low-volume residual axillary disease after NAC. They performed a single-institution retrospective review with median follow-up of 5.3 years to assess locoregional recurrence (LRR), DFS, and OS in cT1-4, N0-1 patients undergoing NAC. In addition, they reported an National Cancer Database (NCDB) query for cT1-3, N0-1 patients undergoing NAC with a mean follow-up of 3.7 years to assess OS. The population with ITCs after NAC had significantly poorer DFS at 5 years than ypN0 (73.5% vs 88.4%), and moreover, the 5-year DFS of those with micrometastases was comparable to that of pN1 (74.7% vs 69.5%). Analysis of the NCDB data from this study revealed ITCs with a 1.9-fold and micrometastases with a 2.2-fold increased risk of death compared with ypN0. In the cN1 cohort, the relative increase in mortality associated with residual ITCs was 81%, and 97% with micrometastases.[30]

A prospective registry out of Memorial Sloan Kettering Cancer Center (MSKCC), examining SLNB after NAC, found that low-volume residual axillary disease on SLNB in cN + patients after NAC was associated with high likelihood of non-SLN positivity on completion ALND. A total of 711 cancers were evaluated and 171 patients underwent completion ALND after positive SLNB (either on frozen section or on permanent pathologic condition). In this population, the presence of ITCs and micrometastases on SLNB was associated with additional non-SLN axillary disease in 17% and 64%, respectively,[31] supporting the continued recommendation for completion ALND with low-volume residual axillary disease after NAC.

The *OPBC-04/EUBREAST-06/OMA Study* recently presented at SABCS in December 2022 has begun to examine the long-term outcomes of cN + after NAC that underwent limited axillary surgery. In this international multicenter study, the investigators collected data on axillary recurrence, LRR, and any invasive recurrence in patients that underwent either SLNB or TAD only after NAC and were ypN0. For the entire cohort, axillary recurrence was only 1.1%, LRR 3.1%, and any invasive recurrence 10% at 5 years.[32] Furthermore, they found no difference in axillary recurrence rates at 2 years between the TAD and SLNB groups (0% vs 0.9%, respectively, $P = .19$).[32] A retrospective study out of MSKCC also found that nodal recurrence was low in patients cN1 rendered cN0 after NAC undergoing SLNB alone. These patients had removal of at least 3 SLN using dual tracer, without targeted resection of the biopsied node, with a median follow-up of 40 months. Of 234 patients with at least 3 ypN0 SLN, only 1 (0.4%) had nodal recurrence (synchronous with local recurrence). Notably, this was in a patient that refused adjuvant radiation therapy.[33] This further suggesting the safety of limited axillary surgery after NAC with pCR.

Axillary Radiation

Classically many cN + patients will receive adjuvant nodal irradiation (RNI) regardless of their response to chemotherapy. Currently, there are 2 large, ongoing studies that may support the future use of adjuvant RNI for possible axillary de-escalation over ALND in patients with residual nodal disease after NAC. NSABP B-51/RTOG 1304 is a randomized, phase 3 multicenter trial enrolling cT1-3, N1 patients that convert to pathologically node negative (ypN0 or ypN0(i+)) status determined by SLNB, TAD, or ALND after NAC. The study randomizes patients to either RNI or no RNI (breast conservation therapy [BCT] patients will still undergo whole breast irradiation). The primary endpoint is to determine if adjuvant radiation with RNI improves invasive recurrence-free interval, OS, and LRR with assessments at 3, 6, 12, and 24 months.[34] The trial is now closed to enrollment and is currently following enrolled patients. Alliance A011202 is a complementary randomized, phase 3 multicenter noninferiority trial enrolling cT1-3, N1, M0 patients that receive NAC and have positive SLNB (ypN1mi and ypN1) identified at surgery. Enrolled patients with positive SLNB will be randomized to no further axillary surgery versus completion ALND. Both study groups will receive RNI. Primary endpoints of the trial include recurrence-free interval, LRR, and OS at 5 year follow-up.[35] This study has also reached its enrollment target and is collecting outcomes data. Pending the results of this trial, it may justify the use of RNI in lieu of ALND for patients with residual axillary disease after NAC. These trials have the potential to impact locoregional therapy decisions after NAC in critical ways. However, ALND should still be performed when residual nodal disease is identified, no matter how small volume, until the trial results are published.

SUMMARY

In conclusion, axillary de-escalation following NAC in cN + patients is still an evolving subject matter as we determine how best to safely minimize axillary treatment. A voluntary survey distributed to members of the American Society of Breast Surgeons (response rate 21% of 3090, n = 642) in 2017 found that use of SLNB after NAC in cN + patients increased after publication of *SENTINA*, *ACOSOG Z1071*, and *SN FNAC*. However, those not changing their practice to incorporate SLNB for this cohort cited concerns regarding the lack of outcome data and FNR as the biggest reasons.[36]

Overall, the National Comprehensive Cancer Network (NCCN) lists level 2B evidence for the omission of ALND in highly selected patients that convert to cN0 after NAC and undergo TAD with no residual disease. Furthermore, current NCCN guidelines recommend clip placement in biopsied positive node before NAC in order to confirm the removal of that node at the time of surgery.[37] However, the NCCN panel does note the FNR of SLNB can be reduced with the removal of more than 3 SLN, use of dual tracer for SLN mapping, and resection of the clipped node.[37] Although many of the trials discussed focus on the accuracy of determining axillary response, there is very scarce data on oncologic outcomes.

This should be discussed with patients before considering minimizing axillary surgery so they understand where there is data to support the practice, and where there are gaps. Ongoing trials that will be reported in the future may help better clarify where de-escalation is appropriate and the impact.

CLINICS CARE POINTS

- SLNB is feasible in cN + after NAC, if done with techniques shown to reduce the FNR such as the use of dual tracer technique, removal of 2 or more nodes, and the use of IHC.
- Performing TAD in cN + patients after NAC has consistently demonstrated an FNR less than that of SLNB alone.
- Patient selection is important when considering axillary de-escalation. Patients presenting with extensive disease burden (cN2-N3) should be excluded from this approach since reported trials were limited to patients presenting with cN1 disease. Long-term outcomes of minimal axillary surgery are limited, but even low volume residual disease portends a poorer prognosis than ypN0.
- Studies are still ongoing but in the future axillary radiation (XRT) may be a reasonable alternative to ALND in patients with residual nodal disease.

FUNDING SOURCE

Cancer Center Support Grant (NCI Grant P30 CA016672).

DISCLOSURE

The authors have nothing to disclose.

REFERENCES

1. Johnson AR, Kimball S, Epstein S, et al. Lymphedema Incidence After Axillary Lymph Node Dissection: Quantifying the Impact of Radiation and the Lymphatic Microsurgical Preventive Healing Approach. Ann Plast Surg 2019;82(4S Suppl 3): S234-41.
2. Nguyen TT, Hoskin TL, Habermann EB, et al. Breast Cancer-Related Lymphedema Risk is Related to Multidisciplinary Treatment and Not Surgery Alone: Results from a Large Cohort Study. Ann Surg Oncol 2017;24(10):2972-80.
3. Gillespie TC, Sayegh HE, Brunelle CL, et al. Breast cancer-related lymphedema: risk factors, precautionary measures, and treatments. Gland Surg 2018;7(4): 379-403.
4. Tummel E, Ochoa D, Korourian S, et al. Does Axillary Reverse Mapping Prevent Lymphedema after Lymphadenectomy? Ann Surg 2017;265(5):987-92.
5. Schmid P, Cortes J, Pusztai L, et al. Pembrolizumab for Early Triple-Negative Breast Cancer. N Engl J Med 2020;382(9):810-21.
6. Gianni L, Pienkowski T, Im YH, et al. Efficacy and safety of neoadjuvant pertuzumab and trastuzumab in women with locally advanced, inflammatory, or early HER2-positive breast cancer (NeoSphere): a randomised multicentre, open-label, phase 2 trial. Lancet Oncol 2012;13(1):25-32.
7. Schneeweiss A, Chia S, Hickish T, et al. Pertuzumab plus trastuzumab in combination with standard neoadjuvant anthracycline-containing and anthracycline-free chemotherapy regimens in patients with HER2-positive early breast cancer: a randomized phase II cardiac safety study (TRYPHAENA). Ann Oncol 2013; 24(9):2278-84.
8. Kuerer HM, Sahin AA, Hunt KK, et al. Incidence and Impact of Documented Eradication of Breast Cancer Axillary Lymph Node Metastases Before Surgery

in Patients Treated With Neoadjuvant Chemotherapy. Ann Surg 1999; 230(1):72.

9. Buzdar AU, Ibrahim NK, Francis D, et al. Significantly Higher Pathologic Complete Remission Rate After Neoadjuvant Therapy With Trastuzumab, Paclitaxel, and Epirubicin Chemotherapy: Results of a Randomized Trial in Human Epidermal Growth Factor Receptor 2–Positive Operable Breast Cancer. J Clin Oncol 2005;23(16):3676–85.

10. Dominici LS, Negron Gonzalez VM, Buzdar AU, et al. Cytologically proven axillary lymph node metastases are eradicated in patients receiving preoperative chemotherapy with concurrent trastuzumab for HER2-positive breast cancer. Cancer 2010;116(12):2884–9.

11. Chagpar AB, Martin RC, Scoggins CR, et al. Factors predicting failure to identify a sentinel lymph node in breast cancer. Surgery 2005;138(1):56–63.

12. Straver ME, Meijnen P, van Tienhoven G, et al. Sentinel Node Identification Rate and Nodal Involvement in the EORTC 10981-22023 AMAROS Trial. Ann Surg Oncol 2010;17(7):1854–61.

13. Boughey JC, Suman VJ, Mittendorf EA, et al. Factors Affecting Sentinel Lymph Node Identification Rate After Neoadjuvant Chemotherapy for Breast Cancer Patients Enrolled in ACOSOG Z1071 (Alliance). Ann Surg 2015;261(3):547–52.

14. Hunt KK, Yi M, Mittendorf EA, et al. Sentinel lymph node surgery after neoadjuvant chemotherapy is accurate and reduces the need for axillary dissection in breast cancer patients. Ann Surg 2009;250(4):558–64.

15. Classe JM, Bordes V, Campion L, et al. Sentinel lymph node biopsy after neoadjuvant chemotherapy for advanced breast cancer: Results of ganglion sentinelle et chimiothérapie neoadjuvante, a French prospective multicentric study. J Clin Oncol 2009;27(5):726–32.

16. Kuehn T, Bauerfeind I, Fehm T, et al. Sentinel-lymph-node biopsy in patients with breast cancer before and after neoadjuvant chemotherapy (SENTINA): A prospective, multicentre cohort study. Lancet Oncol 2013;14(7):609–18.

17. Boughey JC, Suman VJ, Mittendorf EA, et al. Sentinel lymph node surgery after neoadjuvant chemotherapy in patients with node-positive breast cancer: The ACOSOG Z1071 (alliance) clinical trial. JAMA 2013;310(14):1455–61.

18. Boileau JF, Poirier B, Basik M, et al. Sentinel node biopsy after neoadjuvant chemotherapy in biopsy-proven node-positive breast cancer: The SN FNAC study. J Clin Oncol 2015;33(3):258–63.

19. Boughey J, et al. Methods impacting the false negative rate of sentinel lymph node surgery in patients presenting with node positive breast cancer (T0-T4,N1-2) who receive neoadjuvant chemotherapy – Results from a prospective trial – ACOSOG Z1071 (Alliance). In: San Antonio Breast Cancer Symposium 2014. ; 2014 Available at: http://eposter.abstractsonline.com/sabcs. Accessed January 30, 2015.

20. Boughey JC, Ballman Kv, Le-Petross HT, et al. Identification and Resection of Clipped Node Decreases the False-negative Rate of Sentinel Lymph Node Surgery in Patients Presenting With Node-positive Breast Cancer (T0–T4, N1–N2) Who Receive Neoadjuvant Chemotherapy. Ann Surg 2016;263(4):802–7.

21. Caudle AS, Yang WT, Mittendorf EA, et al. Selective Surgical Localization of Axillary Lymph Nodes Containing Metastases in Patients With Breast Cancer: A Prospective Feasibility Trial. JAMA Surg 2015;150(2):137.

22. Caudle AS, Yang WT, Krishnamurthy S, et al. Improved axillary evaluation following neoadjuvant therapy for patientswith node-positive breast cancer using

selective evaluation of clipped nodes: Implementation of targeted axillary dissection. J Clin Oncol 2016;34(10):1072–8.

23. Kuemmel S, Heil J, Rueland A, et al. A Prospective, Multicenter Registry Study to Evaluate the Clinical Feasibility of Targeted Axillary Dissection (TAD) in Node-positive Breast Cancer Patients. Ann Surg 2022;276(5):e553–62.

24. Simons JM, van Nijnatten TJA, van der Pol CC, et al. Diagnostic Accuracy of Radioactive Iodine Seed Placement in the Axilla with Sentinel Lymph Node Biopsy after Neoadjuvant Chemotherapy in Node-Positive Breast Cancer. JAMA Surg 2022;157(11):991–9.

25. Donker M, Straver ME, Wesseling J, et al. Marking axillary lymph nodes with radioactive iodine seeds for axillary staging after neoadjuvant systemic treatment in breast cancer patients the mari procedure. Ann Surg 2015;261(2):378–82. https://doi.org/10.1097/SLA.0000000000000558.

26. EUBREAST Network: AXillary Surgery After Neoadjuvant Treatment (AXSANA). EUBREAST Network. Accessed January 1, 2023. Available at: https://www.eubreast.com/?Trials/AXSANA.

27. Loaec C, Frenel J, Renaudeau C, et al. Safely Avoiding Axillary Lymphadenectomy after Neoadjuvant Chemotherapy for Patients with Proven Axillary Lymph Node Involvement Early Breast Cancer? The French Multicenter Prospective Ongoing GANEA 3 Study. Clin Surg 2020;5. Available at: http://clinicsinsurgery.com/.

28. Galimberti V, Cole BF, Zurrida S, et al. Axillary dissection versus no axillary dissection in patients with sentinel-node micrometastases (IBCSG 23–01): a phase 3 randomised controlled trial. Lancet Oncol 2013;14(4):297–305.

29. Giuliano AE, Ballman Kv, McCall L, et al. Effect of axillary dissection vs no axillary dissection on 10-year overall survival among women with invasive breast cancer and sentinel node metastasis: The ACOSOG Z0011 (Alliance) randomized clinical trial. JAMA, J Am Med Assoc 2017;318(10):918–26.

30. Wong SM, Almana N, Choi J, et al. Prognostic Significance of Residual Axillary Nodal Micrometastases and Isolated Tumor Cells After Neoadjuvant Chemotherapy for Breast Cancer. Ann Surg Oncol 2019;26(11):3502–9.

31. Moo TA, Edelweiss M, Hajiyeva S, et al. Is Low-Volume Disease in the Sentinel Node After Neoadjuvant Chemotherapy an Indication for Axillary Dissection? Ann Surg Oncol 2018;25(6):1488–94.

32. Montagna G, Mrdutt M, Botty A, et al. Oncological Outcomes Following Omission of Axillary Lymph Node Dissection in Node Positive Patients Downstaging To Node Negative with Neoadjuvant Chemotherapy: the OPBC-04/EUBREAST-06/OMA study. Canc Res 2023;83(Suppl 5):GS4–02.

33. Barrio Av, Montagna G, Mamtani A, et al. Nodal Recurrence in Patients with Node-Positive Breast Cancer Treated with Sentinel Node Biopsy Alone after Neoadjuvant Chemotherapy - A Rare Event. JAMA Oncol 2021;7(12):1851–5.

34. Mamounas EP, Bandos H, White JR, et al. NRG Oncology/NSABP B-51/RTOG 1304: Phase III trial to determine if chest wall and regional nodal radiotherapy (CWRNRT) post mastectomy (Mx) or the addition of RNRT to whole breast RT post breast-conserving surgery (BCS) reduces invasive breast cancer recurrence-free interval (IBCR-FI) in patients (pts) with pathologically positive axillary (PPAx) nodes who are ypN0 after neoadjuvant chemotherapy (NC). J Clin Oncol 2019;37(15_suppl):TPS600.

35. Boughey J, Haffty B, Buchholz T, et al. Alliance A011202: A Randomized Phase III Trial Comparing Axillary Lymph Node Dissection to Axillary Radiation in Breast Cancer Patients (cT1-3 N1) Who Have Positive Sentinel Lymph Node Disease

After Receiving Neoadjuvant Chemotherapy. Alliance: For Clinical Trials in Oncology 2019. Available at: https://www.allianceforclinicaltrialsinoncology.org/main/cmsfile?cmsPath=/Public/Annual%20Meeting/files/A011202-Boughey-May2019.pdf. Accessed January 1, 2023.

36. Caudle AS, Bedrosian I, Milton DR, et al. Use of Sentinel Lymph Node Dissection After Neoadjuvant Chemotherapy in Patients with Node-Positive Breast Cancer at Diagnosis: Practice Patterns of American Society of Breast Surgeons Members. Ann Surg Oncol 2017;24(10):2925–34.

37. Rashmi Kumar N, Berardi R, Abraham J, et al. NCCN Guidelines Version 4.2022 Breast Cancer; 2022. https://www.nccn.

Managing the Morbidity
Individualizing Risk Assessment, Diagnosis, and Treatment Options for Upper Extremity Lymphedema

Giacomo Montagna, MD, MPH, Andrea V. Barrio, MD*

KEYWORDS

- Breast cancer-related lymphedema • Risk factors • Racial disparities
- Neoadjuvant chemotherapy • Screening • Relative volume change
- Early intervention • Surgical treatment

KEY POINTS

- BCRL remains a significant problem after axillary surgery for breast cancer.
- The pathogenesis of lymphedema is complex and multi-factorial.
- Race and ethnicity are emerging susceptibility factors for BCRL.
- New surgical techniques to reduce the risk of BCRL are currently being evaluated in randomized clinical trials.

INTRODUCTION

As the prognosis of early breast cancer (BC) continues to improve, patients and physicians are increasingly focused on post-treatment quality of life (QOL). Despite great efforts to de-escalate axillary surgery over the last 30 years,[1–5] breast cancer-related lymphedema (BCRL) remains a frequent and feared chronic sequelae of locoregional treatment, affecting 21-30% of patients undergoing axillary lymph node dissection (ALND)[6,7] and 5-8% of patients undergoing sentinel lymph node biopsy (SLNB).[7–9] BCRL is defined as chronic swelling of the upper extremity caused by the accumulation of protein-rich fluid in the interstitial tissues secondary to the inability of the lymphatic system to adequately transport lymph fluid.[10,11] This entity is characterized by symptoms, including swelling, heaviness, tightness, and/or impaired limb mobility, which may result in pain, reduced function, reduced social well-being, and employment-related challenges in BC survivors.[12] Patients treated for BC are at lifelong risk of

Breast Service, Department of Surgery, Memorial Sloan Kettering Cancer Center, 300 East 66th Street, New York, NY 10065, USA
* Corresponding author.
E-mail address: barrioa@mskcc.org

Surg Oncol Clin N Am 32 (2023) 705–724
https://doi.org/10.1016/j.soc.2023.05.004
1055-3207/23/© 2023 Elsevier Inc. All rights reserved.

developing BCRL, which is an incurable condition that necessitates stressful, time-consuming, and expensive treatment.[13] Although the pathophysiology of BCRL is not fully elucidated, studies have shown that BCRL development is multifactorial and that its risk is modified by locoregional and systemic therapy modalities, and personal factors such as race/ethnicity and body mass index (BMI).[14,15] Understanding the biology behind individual susceptibility to BCRL as well as the impact of each treatment modality is crucial to guide clinical decision making and to providing patients individualized treatment recommendations. Herein, we review risk factors for the development of BCRL focusing on emerging data demonstrating racial/ethnic differences in BCRL risk as well as diagnostic tools, prevention strategies, and treatment modalities.

BREAST CANCER-RELATED LYMPHEDEMA STAGES

The International Society of Lymphedema's (ISL) staging system for BCRL includes 3 distinct stages which are outlined in **Table 1**.[16]

RISK FACTORS FOR BREAST CANCER-RELATED LYMPHEDEMA
Commonly Cited Risk Factors

Extent of axillary surgery
The extent of axillary surgery is the most well established risk factor for BCRL, with a fourfold higher incidence of BCRL after ALND as compared to SLNB alone.[2,17–19] Removal of more lymph nodes and the total number of positive lymph nodes are consistently cited as BCRL risk factors, but are likely corollaries for the extent of dissection or need for multimodality therapy, respectively.[14]

Regional nodal irradiation
Compared to whole breast and chest wall radiation therapy (RT) alone, regional nodal irradiation (RNI), which has gained popularity in recent years, is associated with a higher risk of BCRL. In the MA.20 trial, which randomized node-positive and high-risk node-negative women to whole-breast RT + RNI versus whole-breast RT alone, the risk of lymphedema was increased from 4.5% to 8.4% in patients receiving RNI ($p = 0.001$).[20] In a meta-analysis of 21 trials, the addition of RNI after ALND nearly doubled the BCRL risk (18.2% [ALND + breast/chest wall RT + RNI] versus 9.4% [ALND + breast/chest wall RT alone]).[19] More recent observational data suggest that the contribution of RNI to BCRL development remains minimal compared to the extent of axillary surgery. Naoum and colleagues prospectively observed 1815

Table 1	
The International Society of Lymphedema's staging system for breast cancer-related lymphedema	
Stage 1	Characterized by early, visible swelling, but subsides with the elevation of the extremity. Pitting may also be seen.
Stage 2	Characterized by consistent volume change with pitting. However, in this stage, the elevation of the extremity is rarely able to decrease the swelling. At this stage, tissue fibrosis begins.
Stage 3	Characterized by skin thickening, increase in skinfolds, hyperpigmentation, fat deposits, and warty overgrowths. At this stage, the tissue is more fibrotic than in stage 2, and there is no pitting.

Data from The Diagnosis and Treatment of Peripheral Lymphedema: 2016 Consensus Document of the International Society of Lymphology. Lymphology. 2016;49(4):170-184.

patients and classified them into 4 groups, according to the extent of axillary surgery and receipt of RNI: SLNB alone; SLNB + RNI; ALND alone; and ALND + RNI. The cumulative incidences of BCRL at 5 years were 8.0%, 10.7%, 24.9%, and 30.1%, respectively. After adjustment for age, body mass index (BMI), surgery, and reconstruction type, there was no statistical difference in BCRL risk between the ALND + RNI and ALND-alone groups (hazard ratio 1.20, p = 0.49) and between the SLNB + RNI and SLNB-alone groups (hazard ratio 1.33, p = 0.44).[7] While the aforementioned studies show conflicting results, level I evidence from the randomized MA.20 trial[20] supports a strong association between RNI and BCRL risk.

Body mass index
While higher BMI ($\geq$30 kg/m2) at BC diagnosis has been reported to be independently associated with BCRL development in several studies, the magnitude of risk varies. In a cohort of nearly 800 patients prospectively screened for BCRL, patients with a preoperative BMI$\geq$30 had a twofold to threefold increased risk of BCRL development compared to leaner patients.[21] In 2 other retrospective series evaluating BCRL risk in BC survivors, increasing BMI had a modest independent effect on BCRL risk (odds ratio [OR] 1.05-1.065),[22,23] suggesting a limited contribution of BMI to BCRL development.

In addition, among patients who already have BCRL, weight gain or weight loss does not seem to decrease the severity of BCRL.[15,24] In the WISER study, 351 overweight BC survivors with BCRL were randomized to 1 of 4 groups: control group; exercise group; weight loss group; and combined exercise and weight loss group. The authors found that engagement in 12 months of an exercise or weight loss program did not have an effect on BCRL outcomes (clinical assessment, symptoms, BCRL exacerbations, cellulitis, or limb volume).[24]

Taxane-based chemotherapy
Taxane-based chemotherapy is the most commonly used chemotherapy regimen in early BC, and it is associated with fluid retention during treatment.[25] However, its effect on BCRL is controversial. In a prospective cohort study of BC patients, Kilbreath and colleagues[26] found that arm swelling at 6 and 12 months was associated with receipt of adjuvant taxane therapy. Similarly, Zhu and colleagues[27] found that docetaxel-based chemotherapy was associated with BCRL development compared to non-docetaxel-based chemotherapy (32% versus 20%, p = 0.011). Conversely, Swaroop and colleagues[28] failed to identify an association between taxane-based chemotherapy and BCRL in their prospective cohort of over 1100 BC patients. Thus, while it is clear that taxanes, specifically docetaxel, cause fluid retention and edema, there is not a clear consensus that taxane-based chemotherapy is a risk factor for BCRL.

Subclinical lymphedema
Subclinical lymphedema (SCL), defined as an increase in arm volume of <10% after surgery, has been shown to be associated with subsequent BCRL development. Bucci and colleagues analyzed a cohort of 1790 women who underwent either ALND or SLNB and found that patients who experienced SCL were more likely to progress to BCRL than those without SCL. In that study, nearly 40% of patients treated with ALND experienced SCL, and 39% of these patients progressed to BCRL. Of those who underwent SLNB, approximately 25% experienced SCL, and 12% of these patients progressed to BCRL.[29,30] These findings are of particular importance in light of emerging evidence demonstrating the benefit of BCRL screening programs and early intervention in reducing the risk of developing chronic BCRL. In a

recent meta-analysis of 23 studies, participation in a prospective BCRL screening program significantly reduced the risk of developing chronic BCRL (hazard ratio 0.31, 95% confidence interval [CI] 0.10-0.95) compared to those who received usual care,[11] highlighting the importance of screening for early detection.

Emerging Risk Factors

Race/ethnicity

Most studies evaluating BCRL have not reported the racial or ethnic breakdown of their study populations; therefore, until recently, there have been limited clinical data on the impact of race/ethnicity on BCRL risk. Montagna and colleagues prospectively evaluated incidence and risk factors for BCRL in a diverse cohort of 276 women treated with ALND at Memorial Sloan Kettering Cancer Center (MSKCC) (New York, NY, USA). The 2-year cumulative incidence of BCRL was 23.8%, with significant differences based on self-identified race and ethnicity (37.2% [Black], 27.7% [Hispanic], 22.5% [Asian], and 19.8% [White], p = 0.004) (**Fig. 1**). After adjustment for multiple risk factors, including BMI, Black race and Hispanic ethnicity (compared to White race) were the strongest predictors of BCRL development (OR 3.88, 95% CI 2.14–7.08; and OR 3.01, 95% CI 1.10–7.62, respectively; p < 0.001 for each).[15] Notably, only 16 women in the study identified as Hispanic, and therefore the findings in this cohort require confirmation in a larger dataset.

Similar results were found in the Carolina Breast Cancer Study Phase 3 study (a population-based cohort of women with invasive BC), which evaluated self-reported BCRL in a cohort of 2645 women treated between 2008 and 2013, focusing on the effect of age and race on BCRL development. At a median follow-up of 7 years, 26% of Black women developed BCRL as compared to 17% of non-Black women,[31] supporting the findings in the MSKCC study.

The cellular mechanisms that drive the increased BCRL risk in Black women are unknown, but are likely multifactorial, and may be related to a baseline increased propensity for inflammation and fibrosis, which are evident in a variety of clinical settings, such as a higher incidence of inflammatory skin disease and systemic inflammatory markers,[32] and a higher incidence of fibrotic disorders, such as hypertrophic scar formation, kidney fibrosis, scleroderma, and pulmonary fibrosis.[33] Further studies evaluating the mechanisms driving BCRL risk in Black women may help elucidate the mechanism for all women.

Inflammation

Avraham and colleagues[34] have demonstrated that inflammation is critical for adipose deposition in mouse models, which contributes to lymphedema progression; however, the inflammatory mediators that modulate lymphedema risk are not well defined. Crown-like structures of the breast (CLS-B), characterized by macrophages (typically identified using CD68 staining, a pan-macrophage marker) surrounding a dying adipocyte, are a sign of adipose tissue inflammation and may be a marker of systemic inflammation.[35] In preliminary studies, Barrio and colleagues have found that baseline tissue inflammation, determined by the presence of CLS-B, at the time of ALND correlates with BCRL development and Black race. In a prospective cohort of 281 BC patients treated with ALND at MSKCC, CLS-B was more commonly identified in Black women compared to White women (68% versus 46%, p = 0.016). In addition, BCRL developed in 28.1% of women with CLS-B and 12.8% of women without CLS-B (p = 0.012). However, after adjustment for other risk factors, Black race, but not CLS-B, was independently associated with BCRL development, suggesting that CLS-B is likely not the only inflammatory mechanism that modulates racial differences in BCRL risk.[36]

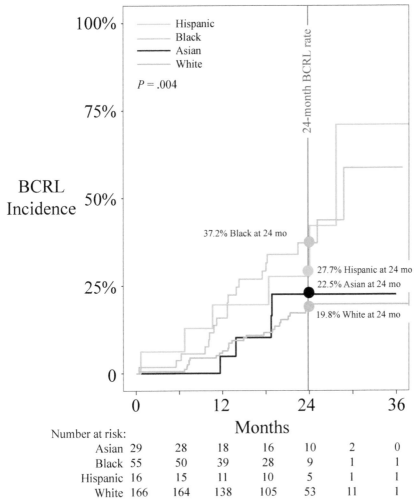

Fig. 1. Competing risk analysis of BCRL in a prospective cohort of patients treated with ALND, by race/ethnicity. The red vertical line indicates the 24-month BCRL rate. ALND, axillary lymph node dissection; BCRL, breast cancer-related lymphedema. (*Adapted from* Montagna G, Zhang J, Sevilimedu V, et al. Risk Factors and Racial and Ethnic Disparities in Patients With Breast Cancer-Related Lymphedema. JAMA Oncol. 2022;8(8):1195-1200.)

Neoadjuvant chemotherapy

The effect of neoadjuvant chemotherapy (NAC) on BCRL risk has not been well studied. Given the increasing utilization of NAC in early-stage BC, evaluating the long-term morbidity of this treatment is timely. In the MSKCC prospective cohort study, Montagna and colleagues also demonstrated that receipt of NAC (as compared to upfront surgery) was independently associated with BCRL risk in patients treated with ALND. Among 276 patients, the 2-year BCRL rate was higher among patients treated with NAC compared to upfront surgery (29.3% versus 11.1%, p = 0.01) (**Fig. 2**) and the association persisted after adjustment for other risk factors (OR 2.10, 95% CI 1.16–3.95, p = 0.01).[15]

While the association between NAC and increased BCRL risk has been previously reported,[37–41] only 1 prior study directly compared patients treated with NAC versus

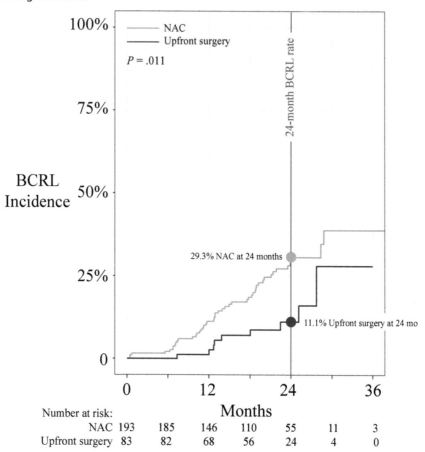

Fig. 2. Competing risk analysis of BCRL in a prospective cohort of patients treated with ALND, by treatment group. The red vertical dashed indicates the 24-month BCRL rate. BCRL, breast cancer-related lymphedema. (*Adapted from* Montagna G, Zhang J, Sevilimedu V, et al. Risk Factors and Racial and Ethnic Disparities in Patients With Breast Cancer-Related Lymphedema. JAMA Oncol. 2022;8(8):1195-1200.)

upfront surgery, and demonstrated a BCRL rate of 41.6% among patients treated with NAC versus 21.7% with upfront surgery at a median follow-up of 5.1 years.[37] In a sub-study of the multicenter American College of Surgeons Oncology Group (ACOSOG) Z1071 prospective single-arm trial in which patients received NAC followed by ALND, Armer and colleagues[39] reported that of 486 participants, 60.3% had a ≥10% increase in limb volume as measured with circumferential arm measurements, at a median follow-up of 3 years. Notably, the ACOSOG Z1071 sub-study failed to obtain baseline arm measurements, potentially overestimating BCRL rates; however, these studies collectively demonstrate a higher BCRL rate among patients receiving NAC followed by subsequent ALND.

These findings are clinically relevant, as the likelihood of nodal pathological complete response (pCR) and ALND avoidance with NAC in clinically node-positive patients varies by receptor subtype.[42,43] Hormone receptor-positive (HR+)/HER2 negative (HER2-) tumors have the lowest reported rates of nodal pCR (approximately 20%),[42] exposing all patients with residual disease, for whom ALND is indicated, to an increased risk of BCRL.[15] In addition, given the lack of benefit of chemotherapy observed among women with 1-3 positive nodes and a low Oncotype DX Breast Recurrence Score (Exact Sciences, Redwood City, CA), as demonstrated in the Southwest Oncology Group (SWOG) S1007/RxPONDER trial, many postmenopausal node-positive HR+/HER2- BC patients may not need chemotherapy (or NAC).[44] Therefore, careful patient selection for NAC and alternatives to avoid ALND in node-positive patients unlikely to downstage are needed to reduce BCRL risk.

Locally advanced breast cancer

Not surprisingly, high-risk patients, such as those with locally advanced tumors or inflammatory breast cancer (IBC), for which more aggressive locoregional therapy is necessary, are at higher risk of developing BCRL. Farley and colleagues[45] recently reported on a cohort of 83 patients diagnosed with IBC between 2016 and 2019 who were treated with trimodality therapy (NAC followed by modified radical mastectomy and adjuvant chest wall and RNI) at The University of Texas MD Anderson Cancer Center. In their study, at a median follow-up of 33 months, the incidence of BCRL was 50.6%, far higher than observed in patients with early-stage BC.

While improvements in systemic therapy regimens have led to an increased likelihood of nodal pCR, particularly in patients with HER2+ and triple negative tumors,[43,46–52] it is unknown whether surgical de-escalation in the axilla can be extended to patients with LABC. Two ongoing trials are evaluating the detection rate and accuracy of SLNB and targeted axillary dissection (TAD) in patients with advanced regional disease and IBC.[53,54] Until these results are available, ALND remains the standard of care in this patient population, with consideration for prospective lymphedema screening to identify subclinical and clinical lymphedema, and provide early intervention.

Timing of Breast Cancer-Related Lymphedema

If BCRL occurred as a result of lymphatic injury alone, the onset would be immediate. Due to other factors that contribute to BCRL risk, including patient, clinical, and treatment factors as outlined above, onset of BCRL is typically delayed. McDuff and colleagues evaluated the timing of BCRL onset in a cohort of 2171 prospectively screened women. BCRL onset peaked between 12 and 30 months after surgery, but the timing of onset varied with locoregional treatment. BCRL risk was highest at 6-12 months in the ALND group, at 18-24 months in the ALND + RNI group, and at 36-48 months in the SLNB + RNI group.[55] These results highlight the importance of longitudinal BCRL screening programs with ongoing follow-up for a minimum of 3 years.

BREAST CANCER-RELATED LYMPHEDEMA DIAGNOSIS

Over the last decade, several new diagnostic tools for the diagnosis of BCRL have been introduced. Current national and international societies endorse prospective screening beginning at the time of BC diagnosis, with baseline measurements performed prior to surgery[56–61]; however, consensus on the diagnostic criteria and screening method is currently lacking.[62]

Diagnostic Criteria

Absolute volume difference versus relative volume change

There are 2 different diagnostic criteria for classifying limb volume difference: absolute volume difference and relative volume change (RVC) (which calculates the percent volume difference between arms). BCRL can be defined as an absolute increase in arm volume of 200 mL or 2 cm, or an increase in arm volume of 10% after adjusting for baseline measurements.[62] These 2 approaches were compared in a study utilizing preoperative baseline perometry measurements of 677 patients and longitudinal measurements taken following treatment. The authors found that an absolute change in arm volume of 200 mL corresponded to a range of RVC, which was dependent upon initial body size. In patients with a small baseline arm volume (eg, 2000 mL), an arm volume increase of 200 mL corresponded to a larger increase in RVC (10%), compared to patients with a larger baseline arm volume (5000 mL), where an arm volume increase of 200 mL corresponded to a much smaller increase in RVC (4%).[63] Therefore, RVC rather than absolute differences should be used to diagnose BCRL, as the former method is not affected by body size,[62] resulting in more accurate diagnosis. Although variation exists, BCRL is most commonly defined as an RVC$\geq$10% more than 3 months after surgery.

The importance of baseline measurements
Objective limb measurements should be performed at baseline and at regular follow-up intervals for best diagnostic accuracy.[56,59,60] Lack of baseline measurements may result in incorrect diagnoses of BCRL due to a natural asymmetry between arms that exists in a substantial proportion of patients.[14] In a prospective cohort of 1028 BC patients, Sun and colleagues[64] demonstrated that preoperatively, 28% and 3% of patients had an asymmetry between arms of $\geq$5% and $\geq$10%, respectively. Without taking these variations into consideration, misdiagnosis occurred in 40-50% of patients.

Subjective lymphedema
Symptoms are an integral part of screening, and are used in conjunction with objective measurements and clinical examination to diagnose BCRL.[62] However, the correlation between patient-perceived and objective lymphedema is poor. McLaughlin and colleagues[65] evaluated 936 consecutive patients who underwent SLNB or SLNB followed by ALND at MSKCC and found that only 41% of patients reporting arm swelling had measured BCRL. Recent studies have also demonstrated that worse QOL after axillary surgery may occur even in the absence of measured lymphedema. Zhang and colleagues[66] evaluated the effect of ALND on QOL over time in a prospective cohort of 242 women utilizing the ULL-27 validated lymphedema survey, and found that a decrease in QOL was independent of arm volume. While studies evaluating the impact of subjective symptoms on subsequent BCRL development are forthcoming, these results highlight the importance of incorporating subjective symptoms into screening programs, and of integrating referral of patients to lymphedema therapy based on symptoms alone to improve long-term QOL.

Measurement Tools

Objective diagnostic methods for breast cancer-related lymphedema
There is no standardized diagnostic method for BCRL screening, but there are several reliable and valid measurement tools to diagnose BCRL, including volume displacement, circumferential arm measurements using tape measure, bioimpedance, and perometer. A brief review of the most commonly used methods, including their pros and cons, is provided in **Table 2**. The method utilized for screening should be one that is available/accessible to the practitioner, with use of a single method per patient, as the screening tools are not interchangeable.

Volumetric Arm Measurements Versus Bioimpedance

While volume displacement, circumferential arm measurements, and perometer all provide a volumetric measurement for the extremity, bioimpedance (BIS) measures

Table 2
Commonly used diagnostic methods for breast cancer-related lymphedema

Diagnostic Technique	Description	Pros	Cons
Volume displacement	Insertion of the arm into a water-filled volumeter causes a water volume equal to the inserted arm to be displaced and captured as overflow.[101]	• Once considered the "gold standard" • Accurate • Inexpensive	• Time consuming • Unhygienic
Circumferential arm measurement/Tape measure	Circumferential measures are taken every 4 cm or 10 cm along the length of the arm using a tape measure (TM), and are converted to arm volume using the truncated cone formula and a commercially available software program.[102–104]	• Easily accessible • Inexpensive • Reliable with training	• Time consuming • Inter/intra-rater variability
Bioimpedance (BIS)	BIS assesses tissue resistance to an electrical current and converts it into a score reflecting interstitial fluid content.[105]	• Quick • Inexpensive • Can detect SCL	• Wide range of sensitivity • Questionable accuracy • High false-positive rate
Perometer	The Perometer (Pero-System Messgeraete GmbH, Wuppertal, Germany) uses infrared sensors to measure limb circumference, contour, cross-sectional area, and volume.[106]	• Quick • Highly reproducible • Accurate • Can detect SCL	• Expensive • Large footprint for perometer • Not easy to acquire

resistance to flow of an electrical current, and instead provides an impedance ratio. A touted advantage of BIS is its ability to detect SCL[67]; however, the lack of correlation between the impedance ratio and an objective volume measurement, as well as the multiple varying definitions for BCRL utilizing BIS in the literature, raises some questions regarding the accuracy of this technique as a stand-alone method for BCRL diagnosis.

BIS has recently gained popularity given findings from the PREVENT trial, which randomized 963 newly diagnosed BC patients treated with SLNB or ALND to prospective surveillance utilizing BIS or tape measure. At a median follow-up of 32.9 months, the authors reported that patients screened with BIS (compared to tape measure) were less likely to develop chronic BCRL (7.9% versus 19.2%, p = 0.016). However, these findings are difficult to interpret, given that groups were not well balanced (more ALND patients in the tape measure arm), and that patients treated with BIS were also less likely to have SCL or receive intervention with a compression garment, raising questions about the methodology of the study.[68,69]

Gillespie and colleagues[70] compared perometry and BIS for the early identification of BCRL in a cohort of 138 prospectively screened patients, and showed poor correlation between abnormal measurements (r = 0.195). A recent prospective study by Diskin and colleagues[71] in patients treated with ALND showed that BIS was abnormal in 94% of patients diagnosed with BCRL by perometry; however, a large proportion of patients with an abnormal BIS (and normal arm volume) (n = 126/175) never went on to develop clinical BCRL at a median follow-up of 1.8 years from abnormal BIS, with a false-positive rate of 59%. Given the concern regarding the potential overdiagnosis of BCRL in patients screened with BIS measurements alone (in the absence of increased arm volume), the authors encourage its use together with a volumetric measurement for lymphedema screening.

DECREASING THE RISK OF BREAST CANCER-RELATED LYMPHEDEMA

Over the last year, several studies have investigated prophylactic strategies to reduce BCRL risk among high-risk patients. These interventions can be divided into patient-initiated or provider-initiated measures.

Patient-Initiated Interventions

Weight loss
Although a high preoperative BMI was previously discussed as a risk factor for BCRL, the impact of overall postoperative weight loss or gain has long been debated in the literature, with some studies demonstrating an increase in BCRL with weight gain, and others refuting this observation.[9,21,72,73] Roberts and colleagues[74] evaluated the effect of weight loss versus net weight gain in a prospective cohort of 1161 patients treated between 2005 and 2020, and demonstrated that net weight loss versus weight gain from baseline to last follow-up was not protective against developing BCRL (hazard ratio 1.38, 95% CI 0.89–2.13, p = 0.152). Therefore, while patients should be counseled that weight loss may not decrease risk of BCRL development, it is still encouraged for patients who are overweight at BC diagnosis, due to the overall health benefits and possible association with reduction in BC recurrence.[75,76]

Prophylactic garment use
Studies have demonstrated that prophylactic manual lymphatic drainage does not prevent BCRL in patients at high risk,[77] but the use of prophylactic compression garments to prevent BCRL has been controversial. Paramanandam and colleagues conducted a randomized trial to determine whether prophylactic use of compression

sleeves prevents arm swelling in women treated with ALND. A total of 307 women were randomized to either receive usual postoperative care or usual care plus 2 compression sleeves to wear until 3 months following the completion of adjuvant therapy. Arm measurements were performed with BIS and tape measurement at baseline, postoperatively, and longitudinally at 6-month intervals for 1 year. The hazard ratio for arm swelling in the compression group compared to the control group was 0.61 (95% CI 0.43–0.85, p = 0.004) as measured by bioimpedance spectroscopy and 0.56 (95% CI 0.33–0.96, p = 0.034) as measured by relative arm volume increase (tape measure). After 1 year, the compression group had a lower cumulative incidence of arm swelling as measured by bioimpedance spectroscopy (42% versus 52%) and relative arm volume increase/tape measure (14% versus 25%).[78] Limitations of the study include short follow-up and lack of data on compliance with the sleeve. While these data provide needed information on the benefit of compression sleeves in high-risk patients, compliance with the sleeve may make uptake of this intervention challenging.

Exercise programs
In 2009 Schmitz and colleagues published the results of the Physical Activity and Lymphedema Trial (PAL), a 12-month, randomized controlled trial (RCT) of twice-per-week weight lifting or standard care in survivors of BC both at risk for and with BCRL. They found that a slowly progressive facility-based weightlifting program decreased BCRL by 35% in patients at risk for lymphedema. Patients with BCRL participating in the weightlifting program had fewer BCRL flare-ups and reduced symptoms compared with those in the control group, but there was no difference in arm swelling between the 2 groups.[79,80] They concluded that an individually prescribed, initially supervised, and slowly progressed aerobic and resistance exercise program does not incite or worsen BRCL.[80] In the recent PROSPER trial from the United Kingdom, the investigators evaluated whether an extensive exercise program improved upper limb disability, as measured by the DASH [*Disability of Arm, Hand, and Shoulder*] questionnaire, compared to standard of care in women at high risk of developing arm disability. The authors found that the PROSPER exercise program was clinically effective with improved limb function after exercise compared to usual care,[81] supporting the benefit of exercise programs among BC survivors in reducing shoulder dysfunction.

Provider-Initiated Intervention (Surgery to Reduce the Risk of Breast Cancer-Related Lymphedema)

Axillary reverse mapping
The axillary reverse mapping (ARM) technique stems from the theory of 2 distinct lymphatic pathways draining the ipsilateral breast and arm.[82,83] With the injection of tracer into the volar aspect of the upper arm, draining lymph nodes can be identified and preserved during SLNB or ALND, potentially decreasing the risk of BCRL. Since crossover lymph nodes (lymph nodes draining both breast and upper extremity) occur in up to 10% of patients, the oncological safety of ARM has been questioned by many. In a meta-analysis of 24 prospective studies evaluating ARM after SLNB (n = 11) and ALND (n = 18), the pooled crossover rate was 8.3% and the pooled rate of metastatic arm nodes was 16.9%.[84] In terms of efficacy of the technique in reducing BCRL risk, a systematic review of 8 studies, each with at least 50 patients having ARM plus SLNB or ARM plus ALND, found that BCRL rates varied widely, occurring in 0-6% of ARM plus SLNB and 5.9-24% of ARM plus ALND patients,[85] which is not substantially different than the BCRL rates reported in the literature for SLNB and ALND performed without ARM. In a more recent meta-analysis of 5 RCTs of 1696 patients, 802 receiving

ALND + ARM and 894 receiving standard ALND, the pooled BCRL incidence was 4.8% in the ALND + ARM group and 18.8% (164/873) in the ALND group (p < 0.0001). The Alliance A221702 is a large ongoing randomized trial evaluating SLNB or ALND with and without ARM which will provide needed prospective level I evidence regarding the efficacy of this technique for the prevention of BCRL.[86]

Immediate lymphatic reconstruction

Immediate lymphatic reconstruction (ILR) for lymphedema prevention consists of both ARM to identify arm lymphatics, combined with ILR to re-anastomose the arm lymphatics to axillary vein branches. This can restore the continuity of lymphatic flow by diverting it to the venous system and, theoretically, reducing the incidence of BCRL. ILR in the axillary region was first described by Boccardo and colleagues[87] when they described the Lymphatic Microsurgical Preventative Healing Approach (LYMPHA). In their initial study, they randomized 46 consecutive patients treated with ALND to ILR or standard of care. At a median follow-up of 4 years they reported an overall BCRL rate of 4.05% following ILR, compared to 30.4% in the non-ILR group.[88] Other non-randomized studies have also shown decreased rates of BCRL when ILR was used in the prophylactic setting.[89–91] RCTs evaluating the efficacy of this approach are ongoing and will provide robust data to support or refute the routine use of ILR in high-risk patients.[92]

TREATMENT

Treatment of BCRL aims at mitigating symptoms and improving QOL of BC survivors. Treatment options can be divided into conservative and surgical.

Conservative Option

Conservative management consists of a reduction phase and a maintenance phase. The reduction phase aims to decrease limb volume and symptoms through complete decongestive therapy (CDT), which is a combination of manual lymphatic drainage (MLD), multiple layer compression bandaging, exercise, skin care, and patient education. Once maximal volume and symptom reduction is achieved, the maintenance phase begins. This includes a transition from multiple-layer bandaging to compression garments, self-MLD, exercise, and skin care.[14] Compression alone may be used to prevent swelling progression in patients with subclinical BCRL, and it may reduce limb volume with or without MLD in those with BCRL.[93]

Surgical Options

Surgical interventions can be classified as follows:

- Reductive (resection of fibrotic lymphatic tissue)
- Reconstructive (reanastomosis of lymphatic vessels to veins, vascularized lymph node transfer which can be done in combination with breast reconstruction)[14,94]

Suction-assisted protein lipectomy is effective at removing nearly 100% of excess limb volume in advanced stages of BCRL. However, it subsequently mandates strict adherence to lifelong compression therapy to maintain volume reductions because it does not improve lymphatic function.[95]

Reconstructive techniques aim to restore lymphatic flow and are predicated on some level of existing residual lymphatic function. As a result, they are more effective in earlier stage I or II BCRL. Emerging data are heterogeneous with respect to indications, benefit, follow-up, and outcomes, making standard implementation difficult.[14]

Vascularized lymph node transfer
Vascularized lymph node transfer (VLNT) is based on transferring lymph nodes from one location (i.e., groin or omentum) into the affected extremity to replace the lymph nodes removed during an ALND. Lymph nodes are harvested from a donor site with their supporting artery and vein, and are transferred to the recipient site.[96] Data on the efficacy of this technique are promising but limited. Patel and colleagues evaluated arm swelling and QOL using a lymphedema-specific quality-of-life questionnaire (LYM-QOL) among 25 patients treated with VLNT and found improvement in both limb volume and quality-of-life scores. Recently, a group at MSKCC reported on the efficacy and safety of VLNT on 89 patients. At a median follow-up of 24 months, they found improvement in all outcome measures (Lymphedema Life Impact Scale, limb volume, BIS score, cellulitis, and need for arm compression).[97–99] Long-term follow-up of large prospective studies evaluating BCRL outcomes, donor site complications, and QOL after VLNT will provide further data on the efficacy of this approach.[100]

SUMMARY

The development of BCRL is multifactorial. New studies have highlighted that race and ethnicity impact the risk of BCRL development. Future studies should focus on understanding the biological reasons behind the increased susceptibility of certain racial minorities to BCRL. Surveillance, early detection, exercise programs, and (possibly) arm compression can reduce the risk of BCRL and should be implemented in clinical practice. Surgical techniques to preserve and restore lymphatic drainage in the prevention setting are currently being evaluated in randomized clinical trials and may become transformative in reducing BCRL risk for high-risk patients.

CLINICS CARE POINTS

Based on the available data, the authors recommend:
- BCRL screening for patients considered to be at high risk for BCRL development
- All patients should have baseline (preoperative) arm measurements
- Use of 1 single screening method (whichever method is accessible in your present environment)
- If BIS is used as a screening modality, recommend the use of a second method to assess arm volume to avoid potential overdiagnosis
- As screening methods are not interchangeable, do not switch screening method for an individual patient over time, if possible
- Work closely with a lymphedema therapist to allow for easy access to care

DISCLOSURE

All authors have no disclosures to report.

REFERENCES

1. Veronesi U, Paganelli G, Viale G, et al. A randomized comparison of sentinel-node biopsy with routine axillary dissection in breast cancer. N Engl J Med 2003;349(6):546–53.
2. Krag DN, Anderson SJ, Julian TB, et al. Sentinel-lymph-node resection compared with conventional axillary-lymph-node dissection in clinically node-negative patients with breast cancer: overall survival findings from the NSABP B-32 randomised phase 3 trial. Lancet Oncol 2010;11(10):927–33.

3. Giuliano AE, Ballman KV, McCall L, et al. Effect of axillary dissection vs no axillary dissection on 10-year overall survival among women with invasive breast cancer and sentinel node metastasis: the ACOSOG Z0011 (Alliance) randomized clinical trial. JAMA 2017;318(10):918–26.

4. Bartels SAL, Donker M, Poncet C, et al. Radiotherapy or surgery of the axilla after a positive sentinel node in breast cancer: 10-year results of the randomized controlled EORTC 10981-22023 AMAROS trial. J Clin Oncol 2022;41(12):2159–65.

5. Galimberti V, Cole BF, Viale G, et al. Axillary dissection versus no axillary dissection in patients with breast cancer and sentinel-node micrometastases (IBCSG 23-01): 10-year follow-up of a randomised, controlled phase 3 trial. Lancet Oncol 2018;19(10):1385–93.

6. DiSipio T, Rye S, Newman B, et al. Incidence of unilateral arm lymphoedema after breast cancer: a systematic review and meta-analysis. Lancet Oncol 2013;14(6):500–15.

7. Naoum GE, Roberts S, Brunelle CL, et al. Quantifying the impact of axillary surgery and nodal irradiation on breast cancer-related lymphedema and local tumor control: long-term results from a prospective screening trial. J Clin Oncol 2020;38(29):3430–8.

8. Lucci A, McCall LM, Beitsch PD, et al. Surgical complications associated with sentinel lymph node dissection (SLND) plus axillary lymph node dissection compared with SLND alone in the American College of Surgeons Oncology Group Trial Z0011. J Clin Oncol 2007;25(24):3657–63.

9. McLaughlin SA, Wright MJ, Morris KT, et al. Prevalence of lymphedema in women with breast cancer 5 years after sentinel lymph node biopsy or axillary dissection: objective measurements. J Clin Oncol 2008;26(32):5213–9.

10. Rockson SG. Lymphedema after breast cancer treatment. N Engl J Med 2018;379(20):1937–44.

11. Rafn BS, Christensen J, Larsen A, et al. Prospective surveillance for breast cancer-related arm lymphedema: a systematic review and meta-analysis. J Clin Oncol 2022;40(9):1009–26.

12. Pusic AL, Cemal Y, Albornoz C, et al. Quality of life among breast cancer patients with lymphedema: a systematic review of patient-reported outcome instruments and outcomes. J Cancer Surviv 2013;7(1):83–92.

13. Fu MR. Breast cancer-related lymphedema: Symptoms, diagnosis, risk reduction, and management. World J Clin Oncol 2014;5(3):241–7.

14. Gunn J, Lemini R, Partain K, et al. Trends in utilization of sentinel node biopsy and adjuvant radiation in women $\geq$ 70. Breast J 2020;26(7):1321–9.

15. Montagna G, Zhang J, Sevilimedu V, et al. Risk factors and racial and ethnic disparities in patients with breast cancer-related lymphedema. JAMA Oncol 2022;8(8):1195–200.

16. Executive C. The Diagnosis and treatment of peripheral lymphedema: 2016 consensus document of the international society of lymphology. Lymphology 2016;49(4):170–84.

17. Boughey JC, Suman VJ, Mittendorf EA, et al. Sentinel lymph node surgery after neoadjuvant chemotherapy in patients with node-positive breast cancer: the ACOSOG Z1071 (Alliance) clinical trial. JAMA 2013;310(14):1455–61.

18. Galimberti V, Cole BF, Zurrida S, et al. Axillary dissection versus no axillary dissection in patients with sentinel-node micrometastases (IBCSG 23-01): a phase 3 randomised controlled trial. Lancet Oncol 2013;14(4):297–305.

19. Shaitelman SF, Chiang YJ, Griffin KD, et al. Radiation therapy targets and the risk of breast cancer-related lymphedema: a systematic review and network meta-analysis. Breast Cancer Res Treat 2017;162(2):201–15.

20. Whelan TJ, Olivotto IA, Levine MN. Regional nodal irradiation in early-stage breast cancer. N Engl J Med 2015;373(19):1878–9.

21. Jammallo LS, Miller CL, Singer M, et al. Impact of body mass index and weight fluctuation on lymphedema risk in patients treated for breast cancer. Breast Cancer Res Treat 2013;142(1):59–67.

22. Martinez-Jaimez P, Armora Verdu M, Forero CG, et al. Breast cancer-related lymphoedema: Risk factors and prediction model. J Adv Nurs 2022;78(3): 765–75.

23. Liu YF, Liu JE, Zhu Y, et al. Development and validation of a nomogram to predict the risk of breast cancer-related lymphedema among Chinese breast cancer survivors. Support Care Cancer 2021;29(9):5435–45.

24. Schmitz KH, Troxel AB, Dean LT, et al. Effect of home-based exercise and weight loss programs on breast cancer-related lymphedema outcomes among overweight breast cancer survivors: the WISER survivor randomized clinical trial. JAMA Oncol 2019;5(11):1605–13.

25. Hugenholtz-Wamsteker W, Robbeson C, Nijs J, et al. The effect of docetaxel on developing oedema in patients with breast cancer: a systematic review. Eur J Cancer Care 2016;25(2):269–79.

26. Kilbreath SL, Refshauge KM, Beith JM, et al. Risk factors for lymphoedema in women with breast cancer: a large prospective cohort. Breast 2016;28:29–36.

27. Zhu W, Li D, Li X, et al. Association between adjuvant docetaxel-based chemotherapy and breast cancer-related lymphedema. Anti Cancer Drugs 2017;28(3): 350–5.

28. Swaroop MN, Ferguson CM, Horick NK, et al. Impact of adjuvant taxane-based chemotherapy on development of breast cancer-related lymphedema: results from a large prospective cohort. Breast Cancer Res Treat 2015;151(2):393–403.

29. Bucci LK, Brunelle CL, Bernstein MC, et al. Subclinical lymphedema after treatment for breast cancer: risk of progression and considerations for early intervention. Ann Surg Oncol 2021;28(13):8624–33.

30. Bucci LK, Taghian AG. ASO author reflections: the promising potential of early intervention for subclinical lymphedema in women who underwent nodal surgery for breast cancer. Ann Surg Oncol 2021;28(13):8634–5.

31. Ren Y, Kebede MA, Ogunleye AA, et al. Burden of lymphedema in long-term breast cancer survivors by race and age. Cancer 2022;128(23):4119–28.

32. Dayan JH, Ly CL, Kataru RP, et al. Lymphedema: pathogenesis and novel therapies. Annu Rev Med 2018;69:263–76.

33. Hellwege JN, Torstenson ES, Russell SB, et al. Evidence of selection as a cause for racial disparities in fibroproliferative disease. PLoS One 2017;12(8): e0182791.

34. Avraham T, Zampell JC, Yan A, et al. Th2 differentiation is necessary for soft tissue fibrosis and lymphatic dysfunction resulting from lymphedema. FASEB J 2013;27(3):1114–26.

35. Iyengar NM, Zhou XK, Gucalp A, et al. Systemic correlates of white adipose tissue inflammation in early-stage breast cancer. Clin Cancer Res 2016;22(9): 2283–9.

36. Barrio AV, Montagna G, Sevilimedu V, et al. Does breast inflammation contribute to lymphedema risk in patients treated with haxillary lymph node dissection? San Antonio, TX: San Antonio Breast Cancer Symposium; 2022.

37. Jung SY, Shin KH, Kim M, et al. Treatment factors affecting breast cancer-related lymphedema after systemic chemotherapy and radiotherapy in stage II/III breast cancer patients. Breast Cancer Res Treat 2014;148(1):91–8.
38. Kim M, Park IH, Lee KS, et al. Breast cancer-related lymphedema after neoadjuvant chemotherapy. Cancer Res Treat 2015;47(3):416–23.
39. Armer JM, Ballman KV, McCall L, et al. Lymphedema symptoms and limb measurement changes in breast cancer survivors treated with neoadjuvant chemotherapy and axillary dissection: results of American College of Surgeons Oncology Group (ACOSOG) Z1071 (Alliance) substudy. Support Care Cancer 2019;27(2):495–503.
40. Warren LE, Miller CL, Horick N, et al. The impact of radiation therapy on the risk of lymphedema after treatment for breast cancer: a prospective cohort study. Int J Radiat Oncol Biol Phys 2014;88(3):565–71.
41. Bevilacqua JL, Kattan MW, Changhong Y, et al. Nomograms for predicting the risk of arm lymphedema after axillary dissection in breast cancer. Ann Surg Oncol 2012;19(8):2580–9.
42. Boughey JC, Ballman KV, McCall LM, et al. Tumor biology and response to chemotherapy impact breast cancer-specific survival in node-positive breast cancer patients treated with neoadjuvant chemotherapy: long-term follow-up from ACOSOG Z1071 (Alliance). Ann Surg 2017;266(4):667–76.
43. Montagna G, Mamtani A, Knezevic A, et al. Selecting node-positive patients for axillary downstaging with neoadjuvant chemotherapy. Ann Surg Oncol 2020; 27(11):4515–22.
44. Kalinsky K, Barlow WE, Gralow JR, et al. 21-gene assay to inform chemotherapy benefit in node-positive breast cancer. N Engl J Med 2021;385(25):2336–47.
45. Farley CR, Irwin S, Adesoye T, et al. Lymphedema in inflammatory breast cancer patients following trimodal treatment. Ann Surg Oncol 2022;29(10):6370–8.
46. Kuerer HM, Newman LA, Smith TL, et al. Clinical course of breast cancer patients with complete pathologic primary tumor and axillary lymph node response to doxorubicin-based neoadjuvant chemotherapy. J Clin Oncol 1999;17(2):460–9.
47. Boughey JC, McCall LM, Ballman KV, et al. Tumor biology correlates with rates of breast-conserving surgery and pathologic complete response after neoadjuvant chemotherapy for breast cancer: findings from the ACOSOG Z1071 (Alliance) Prospective Multicenter Clinical Trial. Ann Surg 2014;260(4):608–14 [discussion: 614-606].
48. Gianni L, Pienkowski T, Im YH, et al. Efficacy and safety of neoadjuvant pertuzumab and trastuzumab in women with locally advanced, inflammatory, or early HER2-positive breast cancer (NeoSphere): a randomised multicentre, open-label, phase 2 trial. Lancet Oncol 2012;13(1):25–32.
49. van Ramshorst MS, van der Voort A, van Werkhoven ED, et al. Neoadjuvant chemotherapy with or without anthracyclines in the presence of dual HER2 blockade for HER2-positive breast cancer (TRAIN-2): a multicentre, open-label, randomised, phase 3 trial. Lancet Oncol 2018;19(12):1630–40.
50. Schneeweiss A, Chia S, Hickish T, et al. Pertuzumab plus trastuzumab in combination with standard neoadjuvant anthracycline-containing and anthracycline-free chemotherapy regimens in patients with HER2-positive early breast cancer: a randomized phase II cardiac safety study (TRYPHAENA). Ann Oncol 2013; 24(9):2278–84.
51. Loibl S, O'Shaughnessy J, Untch M, et al. Addition of the PARP inhibitor veliparib plus carboplatin or carboplatin alone to standard neoadjuvant

chemotherapy in triple-negative breast cancer (BrighTNess): a randomised, phase 3 trial. Lancet Oncol 2018;19(4):497–509.

52. Schmid P, Cortes J, Pusztai L, et al. Pembrolizumab for Early Triple-Negative Breast Cancer. N Engl J Med 2020;382(9):810–21.

53. Available at: https://clinicaltrials.gov/ct2/show/NCT03255577. Sentinel Lymph Node Biopsy After Neoadjuvant Chemotherapy For Locally Advanced Breast Cancer. Accessed December 15, 2022.

54. Available at: https://clinicaltrials.gov/ct2/show/NCT05462457. TAD in Primary Breast Cancer With Initially $\geq$ 3 Suspicious Lymph Nodes (SenTa 2). Accessed December 12, 2022.

55. McDuff SGR, Mina AI, Brunelle CL, et al. Timing of lymphedema after treatment for breast cancer: when are patients most at risk? Int J Radiat Oncol Biol Phys 2019;103(1):62–70.

56. Brunelle C, Skolny M, Ferguson C, et al. Establishing and sustaining a prospective screening program for breast cancer-related lymphedema at the massachusetts general hospital: lessons learned. J Personalized Med 2015;5(2):153–64.

57. Stout Gergich NL, Pfalzer LA, McGarvey C, et al. Preoperative assessment enables the early diagnosis and successful treatment of lymphedema. Cancer 2008;112(12):2809–19.

58. McLaughlin SA, Staley AC, Vicini F, et al. Considerations for clinicians in the diagnosis, prevention, and treatment of breast cancer-related lymphedema: recommendations from a multidisciplinary expert ASBrS Panel : part 1: definitions, assessments, education, and future directions. Ann Surg Oncol 2017; 24(10):2818–26.

59. National Lymphedema Network. Position paper: The diagnosis and treatment of lymphedema. https://lymphnet.org/position-papers. Accessed June 9, 2023.

60. International Society of Lymphology. The diagnosis and treatment of peripheral lymphedema: 2013 Consensus Document of the International Society of Lymphology. Lymphology 2013;46(1):1–11.

61. Available at: https://oncolife.com.ua/doc/nccn/Survivorship.pdf. Freedman-Cass. D, McMillian N, Baker SK, et al: NCCN Clinical Practice Guidelines in Oncology (NCCN Guideline): Version 3.2017 Survivorship. Accessed June 9, 2023.

62. Kassamani YW, Brunelle CL, Gillespie TC, et al. Diagnostic criteria for breast cancer-related lymphedema of the upper extremity: the need for universal agreement. Ann Surg Oncol 2022;29(2):989–1002.

63. Ancukiewicz M, Miller CL, Skolny MN, et al. Comparison of relative versus absolute arm size change as criteria for quantifying breast cancer-related lymphedema: the flaws in current studies and need for universal methodology. Breast Cancer Res Treat 2012;135(1):145–52.

64. Sun F, Skolny MN, Swaroop MN, et al. The need for preoperative baseline arm measurement to accurately quantify breast cancer-related lymphedema. Breast Cancer Res Treat 2016;157(2):229–40.

65. McLaughlin SA, Wright MJ, Morris KT, et al. Prevalence of lymphedema in women with breast cancer 5 years after sentinel lymph node biopsy or axillary dissection: patient perceptions and precautionary behaviors. J Clin Oncol 2008;26(32):5220–6.

66. Zhang JQ, Montagna G, Sevilimedu V, et al. Longitudinal prospective evaluation of quality of life after axillary lymph node dissection. Ann Surg Oncol 2022 (Epub ahead of print).

67. Ridner SH, Dietrich MS, Spotanski K, et al. A prospective study of I-dex values in breast cancer patients pretreatment and through 12 months postoperatively. Lymphatic Res Biol 2018;16(5):435–41.

68. Ridner SH, Dietrich MS, Boyages J, et al. A comparison of bioimpedance spectroscopy or tape measure triggered compression intervention in chronic breast cancer lymphedema prevention. Lymphatic Res Biol 2022;20(6):618–28.

69. Barrio AV, Brunelle C, Morrow M, et al. Letter to Editor re: Ridner et al.: "A randomized trial evaluating bioimpedance spectroscopy versus tape measurement for the prevention of lymphedema following treatment for breast cancer: interim analysis". Ann Surg Oncol 2019;26(Suppl 3):863–4.

70. Gillespie TC, Roberts SA, Brunelle CL, et al. Comparison of perometry-based volumetric arm measurements and bioimpedance spectroscopy for early identification of lymphedema in a prospectively-screened cohort of breast cancer patients. Lymphology 2021;54(1):1–11.

71. Diskin B, Axelrod B, Sevilimedu V, et al. Diagnosing Lymphedema after Axillary Surgery: Which Method is Superior? 2023 Society of Surgical Oncology Annual Meeting 2023; Boston, MA.

72. Petrek JA, Senie RT, Peters M, et al. Lymphedema in a cohort of breast carcinoma survivors 20 years after diagnosis. Cancer 2001;92(6):1368–77.

73. Goldberg JI, Wiechmann LI, Riedel ER, et al. Morbidity of sentinel node biopsy in breast cancer: the relationship between the number of excised lymph nodes and lymphedema. Ann Surg Oncol 2010;17(12):3278–86.

74. Roberts SA, Gillespie TC, Shui AM, et al. Weight loss does not decrease risk of breast cancer-related arm lymphedema. Cancer 2021;127(21):3939–45.

75. Chlebowski RT, Blackburn GL, Thomson CA, et al. Dietary fat reduction and breast cancer outcome: interim efficacy results from the Women's Intervention Nutrition Study. J Natl Cancer Inst 2006;98(24):1767–76.

76. Chlebowski RT, Reeves MM. Weight loss randomized intervention trials in female cancer survivors. J Clin Oncol 2016;34(35):4238–48.

77. Stuiver MM, ten Tusscher MR, Agasi-Idenburg CS, et al. Conservative interventions for preventing clinically detectable upper-limb lymphoedema in patients who are at risk of developing lymphoedema after breast cancer therapy. Cochrane Database Syst Rev 2015;(2):CD009765.

78. Paramanandam VS, Dylke E, Clark GM, et al. Prophylactic use of compression sleeves reduces the incidence of arm swelling in women at high risk of breast cancer-related lymphedema: a randomized controlled trial. J Clin Oncol 2022; 40(18):2004–12.

79. Schmitz KH, Ahmed RL, Troxel A, et al. Weight lifting in women with breast-cancer-related lymphedema. N Engl J Med 2009;361(7):664–73.

80. Schmitz KH, Ahmed RL, Troxel AB, et al. Weight lifting for women at risk for breast cancer-related lymphedema: a randomized trial. JAMA 2010;304(24): 2699–705.

81. Bruce J, Mazuquin B, Canaway A, et al. Exercise versus usual care after nonreconstructive breast cancer surgery (UK PROSPER): multicentre randomised controlled trial and economic evaluation. BMJ 2021;375:e066542.

82. Thompson M, Korourian S, Henry-Tillman R, et al. Axillary reverse mapping (ARM): a new concept to identify and enhance lymphatic preservation. Ann Surg Oncol 2007;14(6):1890–5.

83. Nos C, Kaufmann G, Clough KB, et al. Combined axillary reverse mapping (ARM) technique for breast cancer patients requiring axillary dissection. Ann Surg Oncol 2008;15(9):2550–5.

84. Han C, Yang B, Zuo WS, et al. The feasibility and oncological safety of axillary reverse mapping in patients with breast cancer: a systematic review and meta-analysis of prospective studies. PLoS One 2016;11(2):e0150285.

85. Ahmed M, Rubio IT, Kovacs T, et al. Systematic review of axillary reverse mapping in breast cancer. Br J Surg 2016;103(3):170–8.

86. Available at: https://clinicaltrials.gov/ct2/show/record/NCT03927027. Axillary Reverse Mapping in Preventing Lymphedema in Patients With Breast Cancer Undergoing Axillary Lymph Node Dissection. Accessed January 8, 2023.

87. Boccardo FM, Casabona F, Friedman D, et al. Surgical prevention of arm lymphedema after breast cancer treatment. Ann Surg Oncol 2011;18(9):2500–5.

88. Boccardo F, Casabona F, De Cian F, et al. Lymphatic microsurgical preventing healing approach (LYMPHA) for primary surgical prevention of breast cancer-related lymphedema: over 4 years follow-up. Microsurgery 2014;34(6):421–4.

89. Schwarz GS, Grobmyer SR, Djohan RS, et al. Axillary reverse mapping and lymphaticovenous bypass: Lymphedema prevention through enhanced lymphatic visualization and restoration of flow. J Surg Oncol 2019;120(2):160–7.

90. Feldman S, Bansil H, Ascherman J, et al. Single Institution experience with lymphatic microsurgical preventive healing approach (LYMPHA) for the primary prevention of lymphedema. Ann Surg Oncol 2015;22(10):3296–301.

91. Ozmen T, Lazaro M, Zhou Y, et al. Evaluation of simplified lymphatic microsurgical preventing healing approach (S-LYMPHA) for the prevention of breast cancer-related clinical lymphedema after axillary lymph node dissection. Ann Surg 2019;270(6):1156–60.

92. Available at: https://clinicaltrials.gov/ct2/show/NCT04241341. Does immediate lymphatic reconstruction decrease the risk of lymphedema after axillary lymph node dissection. Accessed January 8, 2023.

93. McNeely ML, Magee DJ, Lees AW, et al. The addition of manual lymph drainage to compression therapy for breast cancer related lymphedema: a randomized controlled trial. Breast Cancer Res Treat 2004;86(2):95–106.

94. Chang EI. Optimizing treatment of breast cancer related lymphedema using combined DIEP flap and lymphedema Surgery. Arch Plast Surg 2022;49(2): 150–7.

95. Granzow JW. Lymphedema surgery: the current state of the art. Clin Exp Metastasis 2018;35(5–6):553–8.

96. Gould DJ, Mehrara BJ, Neligan P, et al. Lymph node transplantation for the treatment of lymphedema. J Surg Oncol 2018;118(5):736–42.

97. Brown S, Mehrara BJ, Coriddi M, et al. A prospective study on the safety and efficacy of vascularized lymph node transplant. Ann Surg 2022;276(4):635–53.

98. Nguyen AT, Chang EI, Suami H, et al. An algorithmic approach to simultaneous vascularized lymph node transfer with microvascular breast reconstruction. Ann Surg Oncol 2015;22(9):2919–24.

99. Saaristo AM, Niemi TS, Viitanen TP, et al. Microvascular breast reconstruction and lymph node transfer for postmastectomy lymphedema patients. Ann Surg 2012;255(3):468–73.

100. Available at: https://clinicaltrials.gov/ct2/show/NCT03248310. A study comparing quality of life in patients with lymphedema who undergo surgical treatment versus non-surgical management. Accessed June 9, 2023.

101. Mayrovitz HN. Noninvasive measurements of breast cancer-related lymphedema. Cureus 2021;13(11):e19813.

102. Armer JM, Stewart BR. A comparison of four diagnostic criteria for lymphedema in a post-breast cancer population. Lymphatic Res Biol 2005;3(4):208–17.

Incorporating Tumor Biology to Select Patients for the Omission of Radiation Therapy

Lior Z. Braunstein, MD

KEYWORDS

- Breast conservation • Breast cancer • Breast radiotherapy
- Omission of radiotherapy • Precision radiotherapy

KEY POINTS

- Adjuvant breast radiotherapy is a critical component of breast conservation therapy (BCT).
- Given the heterogeneity of breast cancer as a class comprising many disparate diseases each with its own natural history and risk profile, some breast conservation patients may enjoy exceedingly favorable outcomes following breast conservation surgery alone (without radiotherapy).
- Contemporary trials seek to identify subgroups of breast conservation patients who may safely forego radiotherapy without an inordinate decrement in disease control.
- Whereas prior-generation trials focused on clinicopathologic features for risk stratification, contemporary studies seek to employ molecular biomarkers to identify those patients who need not undergo radiotherapy.

Adjuvant radiation therapy (RT) following breast-conserving surgery (BCS) has long been known to improve local, regional, and distant disease control among those with invasive breast cancer.[1–3] This observation, now borne out by an extensive body of literature, has cemented adjuvant breast RT as a central element following lumpectomy– the combination being known as breast conservation therapy (BCT). Although radiotherapy is effective and well-tolerated in contemporary studies, it nonetheless may pose an inconvenience to patients and carries a minute, yet measurable, risk of long-term toxicity such as cardio/pulmonary injury or iatrogenic secondary malignancies. Moreover, retrospective reports and large meta-analyses[3] clearly suggest that not all patients stand to benefit equally from RT, with certain clinicopathologic features portending excellent outcomes regardless of the adjuvant treatment approach.[4] Consequently, several groups over the years have sought to identify which low-risk patients might be safely spared the morbidity and expense of RT. In one early such

Department of Radiation Oncology, Memorial Sloan Kettering Cancer Center, 1275 York Avenue, Box 22, New York, NY 10065, USA
E-mail address: BRAUNSTL@mskcc.org

Surg Oncol Clin N Am 32 (2023) 725–732
https://doi.org/10.1016/j.soc.2023.05.006
1055-3207/23/© 2023 Elsevier Inc. All rights reserved.

study, several Harvard centers prospectively accrued a cohort of 87 women with T1N0 invasive breast cancer who were treated with BCS alone from 1986 to 1992.[5,6] Despite favorable feature selection (unicentric disease, margins ≥1 cm, no lymphovascular invasion) the local recurrence rate was an unacceptably-high 23% at a median follow-up of 86 months. This was significantly worse than would be expected for a low-risk population, thus supporting the maintenance of the status quo of adjuvant RT, among even this favorable subgroup. Of note, this study included a non-trivial stratum of patients <50 years of age, and estrogen-receptor (ER) status was unknown in 50% of cases. In another study seeking to question the role of RT following lumpectomy, the National Surgical Adjuvant Breast and Bowel Project (NSABP) B-21 trial sought to evaluate whether the local control benefit afforded by tamoxifen could obviate the need for adjuvant RT.[7] In B-21, 1009 women who had received lumpectomy for tumors ≤ 1 cm underwent three-way randomization: to adjuvant tamoxifen, RT, or the combination. At 8 years, the cumulative incidence of local recurrence (LR) was 16.5% for those who received tamoxifen alone, 9.3% for those receiving RT, and 2.8% for those who received both ($P = .01$). Thus, the investigators concluded that despite otherwise rigorous selection, this population remained at sufficient risk of local failure to maintain the role of adjuvant RT. Of note, as an in the Harvard trial above, despite the implications of tamoxifen in this trial, ER status was unknown among nearly 30% of patients, and ~20% were <50 years of age, suggesting a slightly higher risk population than would be considered feasible for RT omission by current standards. Since older age at breast cancer diagnosis has long heralded more favorable breast cancer outcomes (such as reduced LRR even when adjusted for clinicopathologic features and biologic subtype), a Canadian trial evaluated only women ≥ 50 years of age.[2] From 1992 to 2000, 769 women with T1 or T2 breast cancers were randomized to tamoxifen alone or in combination with RT. The 5-year rate of LR was 7.7% for those who received tamoxifen alone versus 0.6% for those who received both tamoxifen and RT ($P < .001$), again demonstrating the added local benefit of RT, as has been the case in every study to date. Further subgroup analyses of the most favorable patients with T1 ER + tumors revealed that the local recurrence rate at 8-year remained, again, unacceptable at 15.2%. Several smaller historical studies have similarly sought to omit radiotherapy for subsets of patients with breast cancer. A study from Finland enrolled 264 segmentectomy patients with small, unifocal tumors, randomizing them to receive RT or no RT.[8] With a median follow-up of 12 years, LR was seen among 12% of those who received RT versus 27% in those who did not receive RT. A similar German trial utilized a 2 × 2 factorial design to study the influence of both RT and tamoxifen on local control.[9] Though it was not powered to detect an interaction between RT and tamoxifen, 10-year LR was 34% among those receiving lumpectomy alone versus 10% among those who also underwent adjuvant RT. Notably, the addition of tamoxifen improved these rates to 7% LR without RT and 5% LR with RT, but importantly the sample was insufficient to make definitive conclusions about interactions between the 2 treatments or the independent role of tamoxifen.

The Italian study, Milan 3, enrolled 579 quadrantectomy patients with tumors <2.5 cm, randomizing them to receive RT or no RT.[10] On this relatively large study, the 10-year cumulative incidence of LR was 5.8% among those treated with RT versus 23.5% among those who were not ($P < .001$). This difference was particularly notable among patients ≤45 years of age, although there was no apparent difference among those >65 year old ($P = .326$).

It is important to note that the studies described above were unable to rigorously evaluate breast cancer ER-status or to dissect other molecular signatures/transcriptional profiles which are now in common use as more recent innovations. As discussed later in discussion, the contemporary utilization of molecular biomarkers has greatly improved the ability to risk-stratify patients prior to enrollment on such trials, of which there are now several aiming to limit the use of RT in appropriately selected populations.

To that end, Cancer and Leukemia Group B (CALGB) conducted among the only studies to date showing the feasibility of omitting RT following lumpectomy.[4,11] CALGB 9343 accrued 636 women from 1994 to 1999. All subjects were ≥ 70 year old, with T1 ER + breast carcinoma following lumpectomy. Patients were randomized to adjuvant therapy comprising 2 arms: tamoxifen with RT or tamoxifen alone. As seen in prior studies, the 10-year rate of local and regional recurrence (LRR) was significantly different between the 2 groups: 2% among those receiving tamoxifen with RT versus 10% for those receiving tamoxifen alone. Importantly, no significant differences were observed with regard to distant metastases or overall survival between treatment options. While the noted difference in LRR was statistically significant, the small absolute local benefit of RT, along with the absence of a survival benefit, have been interpreted as sufficient evidence to reasonably offer those over 70 years of age the option of omitting RT should they plan to pursue anti-estrogen therapy.

Contemporary advances in imaging, systemic therapy, margin assessment, and molecular analysis have changed the BCT landscape, now reducing LRR rates for early breast cancer to below 5% to 10% in many reports.[12–14] In contrast, the studies cited above that attempted to identify low-risk subgroups were largely conducted with now-outdated approaches, yielding higher-than-expected LRR rates even among the most favorable patients. Standard treatment approaches and risk-stratification techniques have since been refined considerably, with efforts to de-escalate treatment for the lowest-risk patients.[15] Molecular profiling approaches have also since revealed that breast cancer is not a single disease entity, but rather a class of distinct biological subtypes. These subtypes carry prognostic and predictive significance with a discrete natural history characterizing each.[16–19] Given the costs and complexity associated with comprehensive transcriptional profiling, surrogate methods are typically used in clinical practice. These generally rely on widespread and validated immunohistochemical (IHC) and histologic techniques that have also been correlated with the relevant transcriptional profiles, and include staining for the estrogen receptor (ER), progesterone receptor (PR), Her2neu overexpression (HER2) and the Ki-67 proliferation marker, with/without an assessment of tumor grade. Among the intrinsic biologic subtypes initially distinguished via molecular profiling, as discussed later in discussion, the most favorable is luminal A, typically defined by immunohistochemistry showing ER+, PR+, and Her2-, along with a low/intermediate histologic grade and/or low Ki-67 proliferation rate.[12,20,21] Accordingly, luminal A tumors appear to confer the lowest risk of LRR among all breast cancers. This recent biologic insight may be the key factor in identifying patients of sufficiently low risk that RT might be reasonably omitted following BCS.

However, with the widespread clinical adoption of IHC-based subtyping, concerns have been raised regarding the fidelity of this technique in capturing the underlying molecular profile and predicting intrinsic tumor biology. As a result, researchers have sought to develop more comprehensive and standardized assays to reliably and reproducibly characterize biologic subtype.

In a landmark transcriptional profiling study, van 't Veer and colleagues collected primary breast tumors from 117 patients and applied supervised classification of DNA microarrays in an effort to identify a transcriptional signature associated with rapid progression to distant metastases.[22] Initially scanning 25,000 genes, only 5000 were seen at ≥2-fold difference across samples and these represented the genes of interest for signature development. These were then clustered based on their patterns to yield a binary classifier that was able to distinguish *BRCA1* carriers from non-carriers and to identify a class enriched for tumors with early distant relapse. In this first study of its kind, the utility of molecular subtyping was on full display.

Subsequent groups went on to identify more comprehensive genetic signatures that yielded the canonical breast cancer intrinsic subtypes known today: luminal A and B, ERBB2+, and basal.[23] These efforts ultimately yielded a commercialized platform now under rigorous study for the clinical-grade molecular profiling of breast cancers.[24]

The PAM-50 (Prediction Analysis of Microarray – 50) is a molecular diagnostic test, performed on RNA extracted from formalin-fixed paraffin-embedded (FFPE) breast tumor tissue samples. FFPE samples are typically produced in the course of standard clinical care, requiring no additional tissue collection or patient interaction. The assay technology chemically labels each mRNA transcript in the sample with a molecular "barcode," facilitating analysis of the expression profile of 50 predictive genes (ie, an analysis instrument determines the relative activity among 50 genes by quantifying the abundance of each barcoded transcript). A classifier algorithm then assigns the resultant expression profile a score and one of the 4 breast cancer biologic subtypes (luminal A, luminal B, HER2, or basal) in accordance with prior validation cohorts. To date, studies using PAM-50 in breast cancer have demonstrated the robust prognostic ability of this assay in several settings. Namely, the PAM-50 Risk of Recurrence (ROR) score has been shown to accurately identify risk profiles in the context of endocrine therapy or chemotherapy,[25–27] while similarly informing current-generation clinical trials regarding which patients might feasibly forgo these treatments. Moreover, several studies now seek to employ this diagnostic test to risk-stratify breast cancer patients who are candidates for RT.

As noted, a series of trials seeks to identify low-risk patients who may feasibly omit RT from their therapeutic plan. In particular, patients with the luminal A breast cancer subtype have the lowest risk of LR and may be well-suited for treatment de-escalation; however, accurately distinguishing this population from less-favorable subtypes has proven challenging using IHC-based techniques.

The PRECISION trial (ClinicalTrials.gov NCT02653755) rapidly completed accrual of approximately 350 patients who omitted radiotherapy following lumpectomy. Patients were 50 to 75 years of age (inclusive) with T1N0 ER + breast cancers treated with lumpectomy, and all underwent Prosigna PAM-50 profiling with ROR ≤40 placing them in the lowest risk subgroup. An early report of the preliminary findings at the 2022 San Antonio Breast Cancer Symposium revealed that the cohort exhibited a 2-year cumulative rate of locoregional recurrence of 0.3%. Longer term results will be forthcoming and may set the groundwork for the use of this molecular profile in radiotherapeutic decision making.

In parallel, an Australian and New Zealand phase 3 randomized trial is similarly evaluating the use of this 50-gene profile in a randomized fashion, looking to accrue 1167 participants with ROR ≤60 for randomization to radiotherapy versus no radiotherapy. The EXPERT trial (EXamining PERsonalised Radiation Therapy for Low-risk Early Breast Cancer; Clinicaltrials.gov NCT02889874) is open and accruing patients ≥ 50 years of age with T1N0 ER + breast cancers, aiming to complete accrual by the end of 2023.

These, and other trials, seek to employ the luminal A subtype, as determined by the PAM-50 assay, to identify low-risk patients to a degree that has not been previously possible. These studies fundamentally hypothesize that this molecular classification, along with the eligibility criteria described above, will yield a sample of patients in whom RT may be safely omitted from the course of BCT without an inordinate decrement in local control. As discussed, investigators plan to use the Prosigna PAM-50 assay to further sub-stratify a known low-risk population (as currently determined by standard clinical and pathologic parameters). While this assay has been validated for generating a risk category and numerical score to assess a patient's risk of distance recurrence, it has not previously been studied for radiation-based treatment decision making.

The well-established and widely used transcriptional profile for systemic therapy decision-making, OncotypeDX, is also under active investigation for radiotherapy decision-making. This 21-gene assay yields a recurrence score (RS) that has been extensively studied for chemotherapy decision-making in the context of early stage node-negative disease[28–30] and higher-stage node-positive disease.[31,32]

Mirroring the PAM-50 assay above, there are also 2 parallel phase II and III studies evaluating OncotypeDX for radiotherapy decisions. The IDEA study (Individualized Decisions for Endocrine Therapy Alone; ClinicalTrials.gov NCT02400190) is a single-arm phase II trial that opened in 2015 and rapidly completed accrual of over 200 participants who underwent lumpectomy for T1N0 ER + disease with Oncotype DX RS ≤ 18 and thereafter omitted radiotherapy. At the first planned interim analysis reported at the American Society for Radiation Oncology (ASTRO) 2019 meeting, the trial reported 400 person-years of follow-up among 200 eligible patients with no disease recurrences.[33]

Concurrent with the IDEA trial, NRG Oncology has initiated NRG BR-007: the De-Escalation of Breast Radiation Trial (DEBRA; ClinicalTrials.gov NCT04852887). This phase III randomized study seeks to enroll 1670 participants, 50 to 70 years of age, with T1N0 ER+ and/or PR+, HER2-breast cancer following lumpectomy. Patients undergo OncotypeDX testing and those with RS ≤ 18 are eligible for randomization to radiotherapy versus no radiotherapy, with all patients presumably required to receive a standard years-long of course of endocrine therapy.

Instead of focusing on transcriptional profiling, the Canadian LUMINA study (NCT01791829) employed a strict Ki-67 cutoff of ≤13.25% (with centralized standardized evaluation) in an effort to identify the lowest risk subgroup among patients with ER + breast cancer who might feasibly forego radiotherapy. This study enrolled 501 patients ≥55 years of age with grade 1 to 2 T1N0 luminal A breast cancer (defined as ER ≥ 1%, PR > 20%, HER2 negative, and Ki67 ≤ 13.25%). At a median follow-up of 5 years, the 5-year rate of LR was 2.3% without radiotherapy, closely mirroring the baseline rate of contralateral breast cancers of 1.9%. Thus, the LUMINA study, among others, has now identified an exceedingly favorable sub-population of patients with breast cancer with excellent outcomes despite the omission of radiotherapy.

With nascent advances in the management of early stage breast cancer, select patients now enjoy increasingly favorable outcomes that call into question the trimodality aggressive treatment paradigms of the past. Indeed, risk stratification by OncotypeDX, Prosigna, Mammaprint, BSI, or others now position some patients for forego chemotherapy where their forebears would have endured months of systemic therapy with its concomitant toxicities. Similarly, breast conservation and sentinel node biopsy have largely supplanted the modified radical mastectomy, inclusive of axillary nodal dissection, for many such early stage patients who now have excellent cosmetic outcomes and profound improvements in quality of life in comparison to decades past. And this march of progress continues onward, now influencing adjuvant radiotherapy practice. Whereas radiation was established by the landmark studies of decades past as a fundamental component of breast conservation, new approaches to risk prediction now promise to empower patients to tailor therapy according to their personal wishes and circumstances.

DISCLOSURE

The author received research materiel support from Nanostring Technologies and Veracyte Inc. for conduct of the PRECISION trial (LZB), and is the Principal Investigator of NRG BR-008 – the HERO trial (L.Z. Braunstein). No other relevant conflicts of interest to disclose.

REFERENCES

1. Fisher B, Anderson S, Bryant J, et al. Twenty-year follow-up of a randomized trial comparing total mastectomy, lumpectomy, and lumpectomy plus irradiation for the treatment of invasive breast cancer. N Engl J Med 2002;347(16):1233–41.
2. Fyles AW, McCready DR, Manchul LA, et al. Tamoxifen with or without breast irradiation in women 50 years of age or older with early breast cancer. N Engl J Med 2004;351(10):963–70.
3. Early Breast Cancer Trialists' Collaborative G, Darby S, McGale P, et al. Effect of radiotherapy after breast-conserving surgery on 10-year recurrence and 15-year breast cancer death: meta-analysis of individual patient data for 10,801 women in 17 randomised trials. Lancet 2011;378(9804):1707–16.
4. Hughes KS, Schnaper LA, Bellon JR, et al. Lumpectomy plus tamoxifen with or without irradiation in women age 70 years or older with early breast cancer: long-term follow-up of CALGB 9343. J Clin Oncol 2013;31(19):2382–7.
5. Schnitt SJ, Hayman J, Gelman R, et al. A prospective study of conservative surgery alone in the treatment of selected patients with stage I breast cancer. Cancer 1996;77(6):1094–100.
6. Lim M, Bellon JR, Gelman R, et al. A prospective study of conservative surgery without radiation therapy in select patients with Stage I breast cancer. Int J Radiat Oncol Biol Phys 2006;65(4):1149–54.
7. Fisher B, Bryant J, Dignam JJ, et al. Tamoxifen, radiation therapy, or both for prevention of ipsilateral breast tumor recurrence after lumpectomy in women with invasive breast cancers of one centimeter or less. J Clin Oncol 2002;20(20):4141–9.
8. Holli K, Hietanen P, Saaristo R, et al. Radiotherapy after segmental resection of breast cancer with favorable prognostic features: 12-year follow-up results of a randomized trial. J Clin Oncol 2009;27(6):927–32.
9. Winzer KJ, Sauerbrei W, Braun M, et al. Radiation therapy and tamoxifen after breast-conserving surgery: updated results of a 2 x 2 randomised clinical trial in patients with low risk of recurrence. European journal of cancer 2010;46(1):95–101.
10. Veronesi U, Marubini E, Mariani L, et al. Radiotherapy after breast-conserving surgery in small breast carcinoma: long-term results of a randomized trial. Ann Oncol 2001;12(7):997–1003.
11. Hughes KS, Schnaper LA, Berry D, et al. Lumpectomy plus tamoxifen with or without irradiation in women 70 years of age or older with early breast cancer. N Engl J Med 2004;351(10):971–7.
12. Arvold ND, Taghian AG, Niemierko A, et al. Age, breast cancer subtype approximation, and local recurrence after breast-conserving therapy. J Clin Oncol 2011;29(29):3885–91.
13. Miles RC, Gullerud RE, Lohse CM, et al. Local recurrence after breast-conserving surgery: multivariable analysis of risk factors and the impact of young age. Ann Surg Oncol 2012;19(4):1153–9.

14. Canavan J, Truong PT, Smith SL, et al. Local recurrence in women with stage I breast cancer: declining rates over time in a large, population-based cohort. Int J Radiat Oncol Biol Phys 2014;88(1):80–6.

15. Smith SL, Truong PT, Lu L, et al. Identification of patients at very low risk of local recurrence after breast-conserving surgery. Int J Radiat Oncol Biol Phys 2014; 89(3):556–62.

16. Perou CM, Sorlie T, Eisen MB, et al. Molecular portraits of human breast tumours. Nature 2000;406(6797):747–52.

17. Sorlie T, Perou CM, Tibshirani R, et al. Gene expression patterns of breast carcinomas distinguish tumor subclasses with clinical implications. Proceedings of the National Academy of Sciences of the United States of America 2001;98(19): 10869–74.

18. Sorlie T, Tibshirani R, Parker J, et al. Repeated observation of breast tumor subtypes in independent gene expression data sets. Proceedings of the National Academy of Sciences of the United States of America 2003;100(14):8418–23.

19. Fan C, Oh DS, Wessels L, et al. Concordance among gene-expression-based predictors for breast cancer. N Engl J Med 2006;355(6):560–9.

20. Nguyen PL, Taghian AG, Katz MS, et al. Breast cancer subtype approximated by estrogen receptor, progesterone receptor, and HER-2 is associated with local and distant recurrence after breast-conserving therapy. J Clin Oncol 2008; 26(14):2373–8.

21. Voduc KD, Cheang MC, Tyldesley S, et al. Breast cancer subtypes and the risk of local and regional relapse. J Clin Oncol 2010;28(10):1684–91.

22. Van't Veer LJ, Dai H, Van De Vijver MJ, et al. Gene expression profiling predicts clinical outcome of breast cancer. nature 2002;415(6871):530–6.

23. Sørlie T, Tibshirani R, Parker J, et al. Repeated observation of breast tumor subtypes in independent gene expression data sets. Proc Natl Acad Sci USA 2003; 100(14):8418–23.

24. Filipits M, Nielsen TO, Rudas M, et al. The PAM50 Risk-of-Recurrence Score Predicts Risk for Late Distant Recurrence after Endocrine Therapy in Postmenopausal Women with Endocrine-Responsive Early Breast CancerPAM50 ROR Score and Late Distant Recurrence in Breast Cancer. Clin Cancer Res 2014; 20(5):1298–305.

25. Dowsett M, Sestak I, Lopez-Knowles E, et al. Comparison of PAM50 risk of recurrence score with oncotype DX and IHC4 for predicting risk of distant recurrence after endocrine therapy. J Clin Oncol 2013;31(22):2783–90.

26. Gnant M, Filipits M, Greil R, et al. Predicting distant recurrence in receptor-positive breast cancer patients with limited clinicopathological risk: using the PAM50 Risk of Recurrence score in 1478 postmenopausal patients of the ABCSG-8 trial treated with adjuvant endocrine therapy alone. Ann Oncol 2014; 25(2):339–45.

27. Filipits M, Nielsen TO, Rudas M, et al. The PAM50 risk-of-recurrence score predicts risk for late distant recurrence after endocrine therapy in postmenopausal women with endocrine-responsive early breast cancer. Clin Cancer Res 2014; 20(5):1298–305.

28. Sparano JA, Paik S. Development of the 21-gene assay and its application in clinical practice and clinical trials. J Clin Oncol 2008;26(5):721–8.

29. Sparano JA, Gray RJ, Makower DF, et al. Prospective validation of a 21-gene expression assay in breast cancer. N Engl J Med 2015;373(21):2005–14.

30. Sparano JA, Gray RJ, Wood WC, et al. TAILORx: Phase III trial of chemoendocrine therapy versus endocrine therapy alone in hormone receptor-positive,

HER2-negative, node-negative breast cancer and an intermediate prognosis 21-gene recurrence score, *J Clin Oncol*, 2018, 36, no. 18_suppl, LBA1-LBA1.

31. Kalinsky K, Barlow WE, Gralow JR, et al. 21-gene assay to inform chemotherapy benefit in node-positive breast cancer. N Engl J Med 2021;385(25):2336–47.
32. Piccart M, Kalinsky K, Gray R, et al. Gene expression signatures for tailoring adjuvant chemotherapy of luminal breast cancer: stronger evidence, greater trust. Ann Oncol 2021;32(9):1077–82.
33. Jagsi R, Griffith K, Harris E, et al. Planned interim analysis results from a prospective multicenter single-arm cohort study of patients receiving endocrine therapy but not radiotherapy after breast-conserving surgery for early-stage breast cancer with favorable biologic features. Int J Radiat Oncol Biol Phys 2019; 105(1):S7–8.

Selecting Triple Negative Breast Cancer Patients for Immunotherapy

Stephanie Downs-Canner, MD[a],
Elizabeth A. Mittendorf, MD, PhD[b,c,d],*

KEYWORDS

- Triple negative breast cancer • Immunotherapy • Neoadjuvant • Pembrolizumab

KEY POINTS

- The approval of preoperative pembrolizumab combined with chemotherapy for early-stage triple-negative breast cancer represents a major advancement in the treatment of this disease.
- Surgical oncologists must carefully assess a patient's clinical stage and comorbidities to optimize patient selection for preoperative immunotherapy.
- Adverse events specifically related to immunotherapy require dedicated screening and treatment to ensure safe surgical outcomes.

INTRODUCTION

In the past several decades, significant advances have been made in our understanding of breast tumor biology. Translation of these findings into new therapeutic options has resulted in significantly improved outcomes for patients with human epidermal growth factor receptor 2 (HER2) overexpressing and hormone receptor-positive (HR+) breast cancers.[1,2] Improvements for patients with triple-negative breast cancer (TNBC) have been slower to be realized. TNBC is notable for its more aggressive clinical course, and it is 3 times more likely to end in death than other subtypes.[3] TNBC

Funding: E.A. Mittendorf acknowledges support as the Rob and Karen Hale Distinguished Chair in Surgical Oncology. S. Downs-Canner reports funding from the National Institutes of Health, award number 1K08CA259533-01A1.
[a] Breast Service, Department of Surgery, Memorial Sloan Kettering Cancer Center, 300 East 66th Street, New York, NY 10065, USA; [b] Division of Breast Surgery, Department of Surgery, Brigham and Women's Hospital, Boston, MA, USA; [c] Breast Oncology Program, Dana-Farber Brigham Cancer Center, 450 Brookline Avenue, Boston, MA 02215, USA; [d] Harvard Medical School, Boston, MA, USA
* Corresponding author. Dana-Farber Brigham Cancer Center, 450 Brookline Avenue, Boston, MA 02215.
E-mail address: emittendorf@bwh.harvard.edu
Twitter: @SDownsCanner (S.D.-C.); @EMittendorfMD (E.A.M.)

Surg Oncol Clin N Am 32 (2023) 733–745
https://doi.org/10.1016/j.soc.2023.05.005
1055-3207/23/© 2023 Elsevier Inc. All rights reserved.

comprises approximately 20% of all breast cancers, disproportionately impacting young and African American women, as well as those residing in the Southern United States.[4,5]

Until recently, standard systemic therapy for TNBC consisted of doxorubicin and cyclophosphamide followed by paclitaxel (AC-T). This regimen is often given in the neoadjuvant setting with an overall pathologic complete response (pCR) rate of approximately 35% based on the Collaborative Trials in Neoadjuvant Breast Cancer (CTNeoBC) pooled analysis.[6] The addition of carboplatin resulted in improved pCR rates in the CALGB 40603, BrighTNess, and GeparSixto trials.[7–9] For those treated with neoadjuvant chemotherapy who do not experience a pCR, the CREATE-X trial showed that adjuvant capecitabine improved overall survival (OS).[10] For patients with high-risk HER2-breast cancer (including TNBC) and a pathogenic mutation in BRCA1 or BRCA2, the Olympia trial showed a significant improvement in disease-free survival (DFS) with the addition of the adjuvant poly (ADP-ribose) polymerase (PARP) inhibitor olaparib.[11]

Another form of treatment that has recently shown benefit in TNBC is immune checkpoint inhibition (ICI) which functions by "releasing the brakes" on the immune system imposed by the tumor microenvironment. To maintain self-tolerance and prevent autoimmunity, immune cells require a second signal to become activated or suppressed. Checkpoint molecules, which include programmed death-1 receptor (PD-1), cytotoxic T-lymphocyte antigen-4 (CTLA-4), and lymphocyte-activation gene-3, are present on both T cells and other immune cells and serve as second signals to prevent immune activation. Ligands for these checkpoint molecules, such as programmed death-ligand 1 (PD-L1) and programmed death-ligand 2 (PD-L2), can be upregulated by tumors. Blocking the interaction between checkpoint molecules and their ligands, by monoclonal antibodies, results in improved antitumor activity (**Fig. 1**).

Monoclonal antibodies targeting checkpoint molecules and their ligands have been effective in multiple different tumor types.[12,13] Among breast cancer subtypes, TNBC has the highest mutational burden and highest percentage of tumor-infiltrating lymphocytes (TILs), making it the ideal breast cancer subtype to treat with ICI.[14–16] In this review, we detail the current evidence supporting the use of immunotherapy in TNBC and the importance of patient selection for treatment with preoperative immunotherapy.

DISCUSSION
Current Evidence

Metastatic breast cancer
The first clinical trials of anti-PD-L1 and/or anti-PD-1 monoclonal antibodies in TNBC included patients with metastatic and locally advanced cancers. Studies of ICI monotherapy showed modest activity.[17–20] The addition of chemotherapy to ICI initially showed mixed results with an improvement in progression-free survival seen in those treated with atezolizumab in addition to chemotherapy in IMpassion 130, but not IMpassion 131.[21,22] The KEYNOTE-355 trial randomized patients with metastatic or inoperable TNBC to pembrolizumab or placebo plus chemotherapy and showed a progression-free survival benefit in patients with PD-L1-positive tumors,[23] leading to Food and Drug Administration (FDA) approval of pembrolizumab for metastatic, PD-L1-positive TNBC in November 2020.

Early-stage breast cancer
After FDA approval of pembrolizumab in the metastatic setting, the KEYNOTE-522 phase III randomized trial tested the combination of preoperative immunotherapy and chemotherapy compared with chemotherapy alone in patients with early-stage

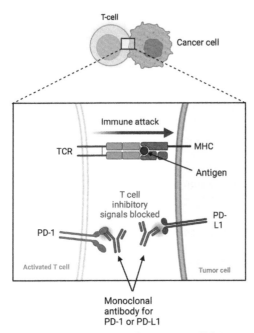

T-cell

Cancer cell

Immune attack

TCR

MHC

Antigen

T cell
inhibitory
signals blocked

PD-1

PD-
L1

Activated T cell

Tumor cell

Monoclonal
antibody for
PD-1 or PD-L1

Fig. 1. Cytotoxic immune cell engagement with a tumor cell (via TCR and MHC-II interaction) will result in tumor cell killing, unless it is inhibited by the interaction between PD-1 and its ligand PDL-1 (on a tumor cell in this example). Monoclonal antibodies to PD-1 or PD-L1 prevent this interaction and allow immune cell engagement with tumor which results in tumor cell death. Checkpoint inhibitors of CTLA-4 and LAG-3 work similarly, by preventing interaction with their respective partners CD-80 and MHC-II. MHC-II, major histocompatibility class II; TCR, T-cell receptor. (Created with BioRender.com.)

TNBC, with coprimary endpoints of pCR and event-free survival (EFS). The study randomized 1174 women with T1cN1-2 or T2-T4N0-2 disease to receive preoperative pembrolizumab plus chemotherapy (paclitaxel and carboplatin followed by adriamycin or epirubicin and cyclophosphamide) or placebo plus chemotherapy. After surgery, all patients completed 1 year of adjuvant pembrolizumab or placebo (**Fig. 2**). At the first preplanned interim analysis, patients in the pembrolizumab arm had a significantly higher pCR rate (64.8%) than those in the placebo arm (51.2%).[24] At the fourth planned interim analysis of KEYNOTE-522, patients treated with pembrolizumab were found to have an improved EFS compared with those treated with placebo (84.5% vs 76.8%).[25] In July 2021, FDA approval was granted for the use of pembrolizumab plus chemotherapy in the preoperative setting, based on positive results of the study's coprimary endpoints. Importantly, and unlike in the metastatic setting, the benefit of pembrolizumab was not dependent on PD-L1 positivity.

Four other major studies evaluated preoperative immunotherapy in TNBC. The phase III IMpassion031 study evaluated the immunotherapeutic agent atezolizumab combined with nab-paclitaxel followed by adriamycin and cyclophosphamide. The trial's coprimary endpoints were pCR rate in the overall population and in the PD-L1+ population. The results were similar to those seen in the KEYNOTE-522 study with an overall improvement in pCR of 17% (58% vs 41%) independent of

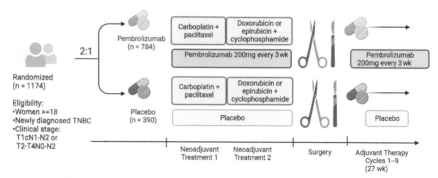

Fig. 2. KEYNOTE-522 Trial design adapted from the study by Schmid and colleagues.[43] (Created with BioRender.com.)

the PD-L1 status. IMpassion031 was a smaller study randomizing 333 patients. It was therefore not powered to detect an EFS benefit; however, at an early analysis after a median of approximately 20 months in follow-up, the authors did report a nonsignificant EFS benefit to receiving atezolizumab (hazard ratio 0.76).[26] A final efficacy analysis after longer follow-up will report EFS as well as other secondary endpoints, including DFS and OS. The GeparNeuvo trial (durvalumab or placebo plus nab-paclitaxel followed by epirubicin and cyclophosphamide) and the Phase III NeoTRIPaPDL1 study (atezolizumab or placebo plus nab-paclitaxel and carboplatin) have demonstrated improved pCR with the addition of immunotherapy to chemotherapy but not nearly the same magnitude as seen in KEYNOTE-522 and IMpassion 031.[27,28] Finally, in the adaptively randomized I-SPY2 trial, the addition of pembrolizumab to standard neoadjuvant chemotherapy resulted in a doubling of pCR rates[29] (**Table 1**).

Complications: Immune-Related Adverse Events

The use of ICI is associated with adverse events related to loss of self-tolerance and resultant autoimmunity. It is critical for the surgeon to be familiar with immune-related adverse events (irAEs) as they may be the first care provider to diagnose these complications. IrAEs in early studies of anti-PD1/anti-PD-L1 and anti-CTLA-4 occurred in up to 70% of patients, with as many as half of affected patients discontinuing treatment at least temporarily.[30] Although most irAEs develop within the first 8 to 12 weeks of treatment initiation, late-onset (after cessation of therapy) and lifelong irAEs are common and underreported.[31]

IrAEs can affect nearly every organ system (**Fig. 3**). In the KEYNOTE-522 trial, 33.5% of patients receiving pembrolizumab experienced an irAE, and 12.9% of these were at least grade 3. The most common irAEs included hypothyroidism (15.1%), hyperthyroidism (5.2%), and adrenal insufficiency (2.6%).[24] Thyroid dysfunction and adrenal insufficiency are generally permanent and require lifelong treatment. These particular irAEs can present at variable timepoints, including between cessation of systemic therapy and surgery. Given the potential to impact anesthetic outcomes, it is recommended to screen for thyroid disfunction and adrenal insufficiency in the perioperative period.[32]

Screening and treatment for immune-related adverse events

The Society for the Immunotherapy of Cancer published guidelines for the evaluation and management of irAEs in breast cancer.[33] For those experiencing an irAE,

Table 1
Phase II/III completed trials for neoadjuvant immunotherapy

	GeparNuevo (Phase II)	IMpassion031 (Phase III)	KEYNOTE-522 (Phase III)	NeoTRIPaPDL1 (Phase III)	I-SPY2 (Phase II)[a]
N	174	333	1174	280	270
Primary endpoint(s)	pCR	pCR	pCR and EFS	pCR and EFS	pCR
Immunotherapy agent	Durvalumab	Atezolizumab	Pembrolizumab	Atezolizumab	Pembrolizumab
Duration immunotherapy	24–26 wk	52 wk	52 wk	24 wk	4 cycles
Chemotherapy backbone	Nab-paclitaxel → EC	Nab-paclitaxel → dd AC	Paclitaxel-carboplatin → AC	Nab-paclitaxel + carbo	Paclitaxel → AC
Change pCR (ITT)	9%	17%	14%	3%	38%
Immunotherapy arm	59%	58%	65%	44%	60%
Placebo arm	44%	41%	51%	41%	22%
EFS difference/hazard ratio		20 mo/0.76 (ns)	15 mo/0.62 ($P < .001$)		

Abbreviations: AC, adriamycin + cyclophosphamide; dd, dose-dense; EC, epirubicin + cyclophosphamide; EFS, event-free survival; ITT, intention to treat; ns, nonsignificant; pCR, pathologic complete response; TNBC, triple-negative breast cancer.
[a] n Includes high-risk hormone receptor+ patients included in trial. pCR data only reported for TNBC patients. Only data from first-arm of study shown.

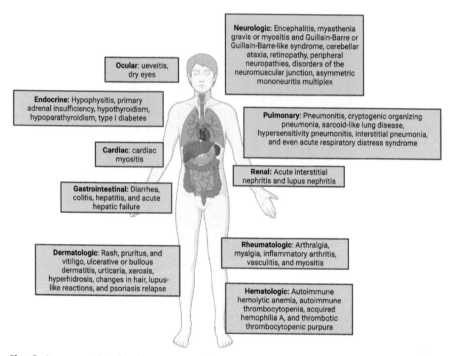

Neurologic: Encephalitis, myasthenia gravis or myositis and Guillain-Barre or Guillain-Barre-like syndrome, cerebellar ataxia, retinopathy, peripheral neuropathies, disorders of the neuromuscular junction, asymmetric mononeuritis multiplex

Ocular: ueveitis, dry eyes

Endocrine: Hypophysitis, primary adrenal insufficiency, hypothyroidism, hypoparathyroidism, type I diabetes

Cardiac: cardiac myositis

Pulmonary: Pneumonitis, cryptogenic organizing pneumonia, sarcoid-like lung disease, hypersensitivity pneumonitis, interstitial pneumonia, and even acute respiratory distress syndrome

Renal: Acute interstitial nephritis and lupus nephritis

Gastrointestinal: Diarrhea, colitis, hepatitis, and acute hepatic failure

Dermatologic: Rash, pruritus, and vitiligo, ulcerative or bullous dermatitis, urticaria, xerosis, hyperhidrosis, changes in hair, lupus-like reactions, and psoriasis relapse

Rheumatologic: Arthralgia, myalgia, inflammatory arthritis, vasculitis, and myositis

Hematologic: Autoimmune hemolytic anemia, autoimmune thrombocytopenia, acquired hemophilia A, and thrombotic thrombocytopenic purpura

Fig. 3. Immune-related adverse events by organ system as described in the literature. (Created with BioRender.com.)

management principles generally consist of consideration of interruption of treatment and the use of steroids or other immunosuppressive medications.[34,35] Severe irAEs (grade 3 or 4) require temporary cessation of immunotherapy and administration of intravenous steoirds, and if not resolved by 4 to 6 weeks, imunotherapy should be discontinued permanently.[36]

The above-referenced guidelines were written before the approval of pembrolizumab for preoperative use in early-stage TNBC. For patients treated in the neoadjuvant setting, it is prudent to screen for specific irAEs to ensure a safe surgery and anesthetic. At a minimum, patients should be screened for thyroid dysfunction and adrenal insufficiency in the perioperative period. After identification of one of these irAEs, an appropriate referral to an endocrinologist, good communication with the anesthesiologist, and careful timing of surgery is necessary to ensure an optimal outcome for the patient.

There are limited data on the appropriate timing of surgery after ICI and the impact of ICI on surgical complications. The published data describe patients with metastatic disease who underwent surgery after treatment with immunotherapy, and there appear to be no specific complications related to the timing of ICI; however, those with more severe irAEs were more likely to experience delays to surgery.[37–42]

Approach to Patient Selection

Knowledge of the enrollment criteria of KEYNOTE-522 is critical in identifying and including eligible patients for preoperative immunotherapy. Surgeons are often the first point of contact for patients, and lack of referral for neoadjuvant chemoimmunotherapy could represent a lost opportunity for this treatment.

Programmed death ligand-1 status
Unlike in the metastatic setting, patients are eligible regardless of PD-L1 status, as improved pCR and EFS were seen in both PD-L1-positive and negative patients, and therefore, PD-L1 staining is not necessary for patient selection.[43]

Optimization of clinical staging evaluation
Patients with clinical T1cN1-2 or T2-4N0-2 TNBC are eligible for treatment with preoperative immunotherapy. Surgeons must thoroughly assess clinical T and N stages to optimize patient selection. Clinical T stage can be determined by physical examination or any breast imaging modality. We favor using the largest measurement to determine eligibility.

Clinical N stage is determined by physical examination and either fine needle aspiration or core needle biopsy of suspicious lymph nodes. Many centers deliberately avoid dedicated axillary imaging in patients with clinical T1 and T2 breast cancers to maximize omission of axillary dissection, according to the ACOSOG Z0011 trial.[44,45] However, for patients with T1c TNBC, N1 disease is an indication for preoperative immunotherapy plus chemotherapy, and a significant portion of T1c patients may have node-positive disease not detected on diagnostic breast imaging or physical examination. In 175 clinical T1cN0 patients treated with surgery first at the Dana-Farber Brigham Cancer Center, 15% had pathologically node-positive disease. A similar group of 18,000 clinical T1cN0 patients identified in the National Cancer Database had pathologic N1 disease in 11% of cases.[46] The routine use of pretreatment axillary ultrasound may identify patients not otherwise eligible for preoperative immunotherapy.

Special populations
There are challenges associated with treating certain patient populations with ICI. Although there are no data specific to ICI use in patients with breast cancer and concomitant human immunodeficiency virus (HIV) infection, prospective studies have demonstrated safety and efficacy of ICI in HIV-positive patients with other solid tumors.[47,48] For patients with an autoimmune disease, flares of autoimmune symptoms can occur and are generally considered manageable without a break in immunotherapy.[49] For patients with solid organ transplantation who develop breast cancer, the use of ICI poses a risk of graft rejection and is generally avoided outside of a clinical trial.[50] Data in pregnant women are lacking; however, preclinical data and case reports suggest that immunotherapy is not safe for use in pregnant women.[51] For older patients, assessment of functional status before the administration of ICI is key. Although trial data suggest that toxicity profiles are similar for older and younger patients, these results must be interpreted with caution, as real-world patients are likely to be less fit than those treated on clinical trials.[52]

Controversies and Future Directions

Optimal chemotherapy backbone
The chemotherapy backbone used in the KEYNOTE-522 trial is relatively toxic. The consequences of combining this backbone with immunotherapy and its associated irAEs must be balanced with the impact on the quality of life of patients. Patient-reported outcome data on quality of life demonstrated no significant difference in patients treated with pembrolizumab or placebo in the KEYNOTE-522 trial; however, real-world data are needed to more accurately capture the impact of immunotherapy on patients likely less fit than a clinical trial population.[53]

The GeparNuevo, I-SPY2, and IMpassion-031 trials discussed above have demonstrated increased pCR rates using a chemotherapy backbone of nab-paclitaxel followed by epirubicin/adriamycin and cyclophosphamide.[26,27,29] An anthracycline-free regimen tested in the Phase II NeoPACT trial was also promising with a pCR rate of 60% when pembrolizumab was combined with carboplatin and docetaxel in the preoperative setting.[54] Minimization of morbidity while optimizing cancer outcomes will continue to be improved upon with the results of these and future studies.

Optimal duration of immunotherapy
After completing 8 cycles of preoperative therapy, patients in the KEYNOTE-522 study were randomized to receive a full year of either placebo or pembrolizumab regardless of response to treatment. Almost half of the patients will achieve pCR after preoperative treatment, and the benefit of completing a full year of adjuvant immunotherapy is not known. The Alliance for Clinical Trials in Oncology OptimICE-PCR study randomizes patients treated with neoadjuvant chemotherapy plus pembrolizumab who experience pCR to complete 1 year of adjuvant pembrolizumab or observation. The study has a primary endpoint of noninferiority of observation compared with adjuvant pembrolizumab.

Patient selection
Nearly half of the patients with TNBC treated with standard chemotherapy alone will experience pCR, and the addition of anti-PD-1 immunotherapy will not result in pCR in 30% to 35% of patients. There are no known biomarkers that predict the response to chemo-immunotherapy in TNBC. It is well established that TILs predict the response to chemotherapy in TNBC.[16] However, in the GeparNuevo study, stromal TILs, tumor mutational burden, and immune gene expression signatures predicted response to any preoperative therapy but did not differentiate between those treated with chemotherapy and those with chemotherapy plus immunotherapy.[55] TILs are a heterogeneous group of immune cells, and the specific composition of TIL infiltrate and its spatial distribution may be more promising biomarkers. In other cancers, the presence of tertiary lymphoid structures is one of the best predictive biomarkers of response to immunotherapy, although this remains to be seen in TNBC.[56,57] Unlike in the metastatic setting, in the phase III studies KEYNOTE-522 and IMpassion-031, PD-L1 expression was not associated with response to immunotherapy.

Circulating tumor DNA or circulating tumor cells (CTCs) may be another promising biomarker to determine response to treatment or predict the benefit of adjuvant pembrolizumab after its use in the neoadjuvant setting. PD-L1 can be detected on CTCs in patients without a metastatic disease.[58] Residual PD-L1-positive CTCs in patients treated with neoadjuvant chemo-immunotherapy could be used to predict the need for adjuvant immunotherapy.[59] In early-stage TNBC, the I-SPY2 trial evaluated ctDNA using the Signatera platform and found that all patients treated with neoadjuvant immunotherapy who experienced pCR cleared ctDNA; in those who did not experience pCR, outcomes were better among those who cleared ctDNA.[60] At least four additional ongoing studies in early-stage TNBC are evaluating the use of ctDNA for the detection of residual disease or relapse, or to guide adjuvant therapy.

Other promising potential biomarkers include mRNA-based signatures and microbiome-informed selection of patients.[33] As patient selection becomes more precise, efficacy will be maximized, and morbidity will be minimized.

Future directions
Ongoing research seeks to identify combinatorial treatments to improve response to immunotherapy and novel immunotherapeutic targets in TNBC and other subtypes of breast cancer. Local ablative therapy, such as radiation or cryoablation may induce a systemic immune response that could synergize with ICI. In the preoperative setting,

multiple studies seek to combine preoperative radiation with immunotherapy.[61] Other studies, predominantly in the metastatic setting, combine ICI with PARP inhibitors for those with and without BRCA 1 or 2 germline mutations[62,63] or with anti-vascular endothelial growth factor (VEGF) monoclonal antibodies.[64] To overcome loss of immunogenicity, bispecific T-cell engagers are in development. Adenosine receptor inhibitors are thought to overcome metabolic reprogramming, resulting in a less-favorable immune microenvironment, and are being combined with immunotherapy in clinical trials.[33] Intralesional oncolytic immunotherapy combined with immunotherapy is currently in trials for metastatic TNBC (NCT03362060). Finally, other immune checkpoint targets such as CTLA-4, Lag-3, TIGIT, and the immune-activating OX40 are under investigation.[33] These and other studies may also improve response to immunotherapy in less immunogenic subtypes of breast cancer, such as HR+ cancers.

SUMMARY

The KEYNOTE-522 study evaluated the addition of the anti-PD-1 monoclonal antibody pembrolizumab to chemotherapy for early-stage TNBC. Patients treated with preoperative pembrolizumab experienced a significant improvement in pCR and an EFS benefit of 7 months, independent of PD-L1 status, leading to FDA approval in July 2021. Eligibility is mainly based on clinical stage, and surgeons and medical oncologists should carefully evaluate T and N stages for optimal inclusion of T1cN1-2 and T2-4N0 patients. IrAEs present a challenge in the management of these patients, and physicians need to be aware of the presentation and timeline of these sometimes-severe complications, which can be permanent. Patient selection and outcomes will continue to improve as we better understand the ideal chemotherapy backbone, the duration and necessity of adjuvant pembrolizumab, and biomarkers to better inform patient selection.

CLINICS CARE POINTS

- Patients with clinical stage T1cN1-N2 and T2-T4N0-N2 TNBC are eligible to be treated with preoperative immunotherapy combined with chemotherapy.
- Dedicated axillary ultrasound in patients with T1c disease may identify additional patients eligible for preoperative immunotherapy through identification of involved nodes.
- Immune-related adverse events can occur at any time, including the period between completion of preoperative therapy and surgery, and therefore, screening for thyroid dysfunction and adrenal insufficiency in the perioperative period is prudent.

DISCLOSURE

E.A. Mittendorf reports compensated service on scientific advisory boards for AstraZeneca, Exact sciences (formerly Genomic Health), Merck, Roche/Genentech; uncompensated service on steering committees for Bristol Myers Squibb, Lilly, and Roche, Switzerland/Genentech and institutional research support from Roche/Genentech (via SU2C grant) and Gilead, United States. She receives research funding from Susan Komen for the cure for which she serves as a scientific advisor. She also reports uncompensated participation as a member of the American Society of Clinical Oncology Board of Directors. S. Downs-Canner reports no conflicts of interest.

REFERENCES

1. Pernas S, Tolaney SM. HER2-positive breast cancer: new therapeutic frontiers and overcoming resistance. Ther Adv Med Oncol 2019;11. 1758835919833519.
2. Nasrazadani A, Thomas RA, Oesterreich S, et al. Precision Medicine in Hormone Receptor-Positive Breast Cancer. Front Oncol 2018;8:144.
3. Dent R, Trudeau M, Pritchard KI, et al. Triple-negative breast cancer: clinical features and patterns of recurrence. Clin Cancer Res 2007;13(15 Pt 1):4429–34.
4. Carey LA, Perou CM, Livasy CA, et al. Race, breast cancer subtypes, and survival in the Carolina Breast Cancer Study. JAMA 2006;295(21):2492–502.
5. Moss JL, Tatalovich Z, Zhu L, et al. Triple-negative breast cancer incidence in the United States: ecological correlations with area-level sociodemographics, healthcare, and health behaviors. Breast Cancer 2021;28(1):82–91.
6. Cortazar P, Zhang L, Untch M, et al. Pathological complete response and long-term clinical benefit in breast cancer: the CTNeoBC pooled analysis. Lancet 2014;384(9938):164–72.
7. von Minckwitz G, Schneeweiss A, Loibl S, et al. Neoadjuvant carboplatin in patients with triple-negative and HER2-positive early breast cancer (GeparSixto; GBG 66): a randomised phase 2 trial. Lancet Oncol 2014;15(7):747–56.
8. Loibl S, O'Shaughnessy J, Untch M, et al. Addition of the PARP inhibitor veliparib plus carboplatin or carboplatin alone to standard neoadjuvant chemotherapy in triple-negative breast cancer (BrighTNess): a randomised, phase 3 trial. Lancet Oncol 2018;19(4):497–509.
9. Sikov WM, Berry DA, Perou CM, et al. Impact of the addition of carboplatin and/or bevacizumab to neoadjuvant once-per-week paclitaxel followed by dose-dense doxorubicin and cyclophosphamide on pathologic complete response rates in stage II to III triple-negative breast cancer: CALGB 40603 (Alliance). J Clin Oncol 2015;33(1):13–21.
10. Masuda N, Lee SJ, Ohtani S, et al. Adjuvant Capecitabine for Breast Cancer after Preoperative Chemotherapy. N Engl J Med 2017;376(22):2147–59.
11. Tutt ANJ, Garber JE, Kaufman B, et al. Adjuvant Olaparib for Patients with BRCA1- or BRCA2-Mutated Breast Cancer. N Engl J Med 2021;384(25):2394–405.
12. Rizvi NA, Hellmann MD, Snyder A, et al. Cancer immunology. Mutational landscape determines sensitivity to PD-1 blockade in non-small cell lung cancer. Science 2015;348(6230):124–8.
13. Snyder A, Makarov V, Merghoub T, et al. Genetic basis for clinical response to CTLA-4 blockade in melanoma. N Engl J Med 2014;371(23):2189–99.
14. Luen S, Virassamy B, Savas P, et al. The genomic landscape of breast cancer and its interaction with host immunity. Breast 2016;29:241–50.
15. Denkert C, von Minckwitz G, Darb-Esfahani S, et al. Tumour-infiltrating lymphocytes and prognosis in different subtypes of breast cancer: a pooled analysis of 3771 patients treated with neoadjuvant therapy. Lancet Oncol 2018;19(1):40–50.
16. Denkert C, Loibl S, Noske A, et al. Tumor-associated lymphocytes as an independent predictor of response to neoadjuvant chemotherapy in breast cancer. J Clin Oncol 2010;28(1):105–13.
17. Emens LA, Cruz C, Eder JP, et al. Long-term Clinical Outcomes and Biomarker Analyses of Atezolizumab Therapy for Patients With Metastatic Triple-Negative Breast Cancer: A Phase 1 Study. JAMA Oncol 2019;5(1):74–82.

18. Adams S, Loi S, Toppmeyer D, et al. Pembrolizumab monotherapy for previously untreated, PD-L1-positive, metastatic triple-negative breast cancer: cohort B of the phase II KEYNOTE-086 study. Ann Oncol 2019;30(3):405–11.

19. Adams S, Schmid P, Rugo HS, et al. Pembrolizumab monotherapy for previously treated metastatic triple-negative breast cancer: cohort A of the phase II KEYNOTE-086 study. Ann Oncol 2019;30(3):397–404.

20. Dirix LY, Takacs I, Jerusalem G, et al. Avelumab, an anti-PD-L1 antibody, in patients with locally advanced or metastatic breast cancer: a phase 1b JAVELIN Solid Tumor study. Breast Cancer Res Treat 2018;167(3):671–86.

21. Schmid P, Adams S, Rugo HS, et al. Atezolizumab and Nab-Paclitaxel in Advanced Triple-Negative Breast Cancer. N Engl J Med 2018;379(22):2108–21.

22. Miles D, Gligorov J, Andre F, et al. Primary results from IMpassion131, a double-blind, placebo-controlled, randomised phase III trial of first-line paclitaxel with or without atezolizumab for unresectable locally advanced/metastatic triple-negative breast cancer. Ann Oncol 2021;32(8):994–1004.

23. Cortes J, Cescon DW, Rugo HS, et al. Pembrolizumab plus chemotherapy versus placebo plus chemotherapy for previously untreated locally recurrent inoperable or metastatic triple-negative breast cancer (KEYNOTE-355): a randomised, placebo-controlled, double-blind, phase 3 clinical trial. Lancet 2020; 396(10265):1817–28.

24. Schmid P, Cortes J, Pusztai L, et al. Pembrolizumab for Early Triple-Negative Breast Cancer. N Engl J Med 2020;382(9):810–21.

25. Schmid P, Salgado R, Park YH, et al. Pembrolizumab plus chemotherapy as neoadjuvant treatment of high-risk, early-stage triple-negative breast cancer: results from the phase 1b open-label, multicohort KEYNOTE-173 study. Ann Oncol 2020; 31(5):569–81.

26. Mittendorf EA, Zhang H, Barrios CH, et al. Neoadjuvant atezolizumab in combination with sequential nab-paclitaxel and anthracycline-based chemotherapy versus placebo and chemotherapy in patients with early-stage triple-negative breast cancer (IMpassion031): a randomised, double-blind, phase 3 trial. Lancet 2020;396(10257):1090–100.

27. Loibl S, Schneeweiss A, Huober JB, et al. Durvalumab improves long-term outcome in TNBC: results from the phase II randomized GeparNUEVO study investigating neodjuvant durvalumab in addition to an anthracycline/taxane based neoadjuvant chemotherapy in early triple-negative breast cancer (TNBC). J Clin Oncol 2021;39(15_suppl):506.

28. Gianni L, Huang CS, Egle D, et al. Pathologic complete response (pCR) to neoadjuvant treatment with or without atezolizumab in triple-negative, early high-risk and locally advanced breast cancer: NeoTRIP Michelangelo randomized study. Ann Oncol 2022;33(5):534–43.

29. Nanda R, Liu MC, Yau C, et al. Effect of Pembrolizumab Plus Neoadjuvant Chemotherapy on Pathologic Complete Response in Women With Early-Stage Breast Cancer: An Analysis of the Ongoing Phase 2 Adaptively Randomized I-SPY2 Trial. JAMA Oncol 2020;6(5):676–84.

30. Boutros C, Tarhini A, Routier E, et al. Safety profiles of anti-CTLA-4 and anti-PD-1 antibodies alone and in combination. Nat Rev Clin Oncol 2016;13(8):473–86.

31. Ghisoni E, Wicky A, Bouchaab H, et al. Late-onset and long-lasting immune-related adverse events from immune checkpoint-inhibitors: An overlooked aspect in immunotherapy. Eur J Cancer 2021;149:153–64.

32. Downs-Canner S, Mittendorf E. Preoperative Immunotherapy Combined with Chemotherapy for Triple-Negative Breast Cancer: Perspective on the

KEYNOTE-522 Study. Ann Surg Oncol 2023. https://doi.org/10.1245/s10434-023-13267-z.

33. Emens LA, Adams S, Cimino-Mathews A, et al. Society for Immunotherapy of Cancer (SITC) clinical practice guideline on immunotherapy for the treatment of breast cancer. J Immunother Cancer 2021;9(8). https://doi.org/10.1136/jitc-2021-002597.

34. Friedman CF, Proverbs-Singh TA, Postow MA. Treatment of the Immune-Related Adverse Effects of Immune Checkpoint Inhibitors: A Review. JAMA Oncol 2016; 2(10):1346–53.

35. Weber JS, Yang JC, Atkins MB, et al. Toxicities of Immunotherapy for the Practitioner. J Clin Oncol 2015;33(18):2092–9.

36. Puzanov I, Diab A, Abdallah K, et al. Managing toxicities associated with immune checkpoint inhibitors: consensus recommendations from the Society for Immunotherapy of Cancer (SITC) Toxicity Management Working Group. J Immunother Cancer 2017;5(1):95.

37. Bott MJ, Cools-Lartigue J, Tan KS, et al. Safety and Feasibility of Lung Resection After Immunotherapy for Metastatic or Unresectable Tumors. Ann Thorac Surg 2018;106(1):178–83.

38. Gyorki DE, Yuan J, Mu Z, et al. Immunological insights from patients undergoing surgery on ipilimumab for metastatic melanoma. Ann Surg Oncol 2013;20(9): 3106–11.

39. Amaria RN, Reddy SM, Tawbi HA, et al. Neoadjuvant immune checkpoint blockade in high-risk resectable melanoma. Nat Med 2018;24(11):1649–54.

40. Blank CU, Rozeman EA, Fanchi LF, et al. Neoadjuvant versus adjuvant ipilimumab plus nivolumab in macroscopic stage III melanoma. Nat Med 2018;24(11): 1655–61.

41. Carthon BC, Wolchok JD, Yuan J, et al. Preoperative CTLA-4 blockade: tolerability and immune monitoring in the setting of a presurgical clinical trial. Clin Cancer Res 2010;16(10):2861–71.

42. Forde PM, Chaft JE, Smith KN, et al. Neoadjuvant PD-1 Blockade in Resectable Lung Cancer. N Engl J Med 2018;378(21):1976–86.

43. Schmid P, Cortes J, Dent R, et al. Event-free Survival with Pembrolizumab in Early Triple-Negative Breast Cancer. N Engl J Med 2022;386(6):556–67.

44. Giuliano AE, Ballman KV, McCall L, et al. Effect of Axillary Dissection vs No Axillary Dissection on 10-Year Overall Survival Among Women With Invasive Breast Cancer and Sentinel Node Metastasis: The ACOSOG Z0011 (Alliance) Randomized Clinical Trial. JAMA 2017;318(10):918–26.

45. Pilewskie M, Jochelson M, Gooch JC, et al. Is Preoperative Axillary Imaging Beneficial in Identifying Clinically Node-Negative Patients Requiring Axillary Lymph Node Dissection? J Am Coll Surg 2016;222(2):138–45.

46. Mittendorf EA, Kantor O, Weiss A, et al. Nodal Positivity in Early-Stage Triple-Negative Breast Cancer: Implications for Preoperative Immunotherapy. Ann Surg Oncol 2023;30(1):100–6.

47. González-Cao M, Moran T, Dalmau J, et al. Phase II study of durvalumab (MEDI4736) in cancer patients HIV-1-infected. J Clin Oncol 2019;37(15_suppl): 2501.

48. Uldrick TS, Goncalves PH, Abdul-Hay M, et al. Assessment of the Safety of Pembrolizumab in Patients With HIV and Advanced Cancer-A Phase 1 Study. JAMA Oncol 2019;5(9):1332–9.

49. Menzies AM, Johnson DB, Ramanujam S, et al. Anti-PD-1 therapy in patients with advanced melanoma and preexisting autoimmune disorders or major toxicity with ipilimumab. Ann Oncol 2017;28(2):368–76.
50. Abdel-Wahab N, Safa H, Abudayyeh A, et al. Checkpoint inhibitor therapy for cancer in solid organ transplantation recipients: an institutional experience and a systematic review of the literature. J Immunother Cancer 2019;7(1):106.
51. Borgers JSW, Heimovaara JH, Cardonick E, et al. Immunotherapy for cancer treatment during pregnancy. Lancet Oncol 2021;22(12):e550–61.
52. van Holstein Y, Kapiteijn E, Bastiaannet E, et al. Efficacy and Adverse Events of Immunotherapy with Checkpoint Inhibitors in Older Patients with Cancer. Drugs Aging 2019;36(10):927–38.
53. Dent R. HRQoL with neoadjuvant pembrolizumab + chemotherapy vs placebo + chemotherapy, followed by adjuvant pembrolizumab vs placebo for early-stage TNBC: results from KEYNOTE-522. ESMO Congress 2022, September 9-13, 2022 in Paris, France. Abstract 135 MO 2022.
54. Sharma P, Stecklein SR, Yoder R, et al. Clinical and biomarker results of neoadjuvant phase II study of pembrolizumab and carboplatin plus docetaxel in triple-negative breast cancer (TNBC) (NeoPACT). J Clin Oncol 2022;40(16_suppl):513.
55. Karn T, Denkert C, Weber KE, et al. Tumor mutational burden and immune infiltration as independent predictors of response to neoadjuvant immune checkpoint inhibition in early TNBC in GeparNuevo. Ann Oncol 2020;31(9):1216–22.
56. Helmink BA, Reddy SM, Gao J, et al. B cells and tertiary lymphoid structures promote immunotherapy response. Nature 2020;577(7791):549–55.
57. Petitprez F, de Reynies A, Keung EZ, et al. B cells are associated with survival and immunotherapy response in sarcoma. Nature 2020;577(7791):556–60.
58. Schott DS, Pizon M, Pachmann U, et al. Sensitive detection of PD-L1 expression on circulating epithelial tumor cells (CETCs) could be a potential biomarker to select patients for treatment with PD-1/PD-L1 inhibitors in early and metastatic solid tumors. Oncotarget 2017;8(42):72755–72.
59. Nicolazzo C, Raimondi C, Mancini M, et al. Monitoring PD-L1 positive circulating tumor cells in non-small cell lung cancer patients treated with the PD-1 inhibitor Nivolumab. Sci Rep 2016;6:31726.
60. Magbanua MJM, Wolf D, Renner D, et al. Abstract PD9-02: Personalized ctDNA as a predictive biomarker in high-risk early stage breast cancer (EBC) treated with neoadjuvant chemotherapy (NAC) with or without pembrolizumab (P). Cancer Res 2021;81(4_Supplement). PD9-02-PD9-02.
61. Ho AY, Wright JL, Blitzblau RC, et al. Optimizing Radiation Therapy to Boost Systemic Immune Responses in Breast Cancer: A Critical Review for Breast Radiation Oncologists. Int J Radiat Oncol Biol Phys 2020;108(1):227–41.
62. Vinayak S, Tolaney SM, Schwartzberg L, et al. Open-label Clinical Trial of Niraparib Combined With Pembrolizumab for Treatment of Advanced or Metastatic Triple-Negative Breast Cancer. JAMA Oncol 2019;5(8):1132–40.
63. Domchek SM, Postel-Vinay S, Im SA, et al. Olaparib and durvalumab in patients with germline BRCA-mutated metastatic breast cancer (MEDIOLA): an open-label, multicentre, phase 1/2, basket study. Lancet Oncol 2020;21(9):1155–64.
64. Ozaki Y, Mukohara T, Tsurutani J, et al. Abstract PD1-03: A multicenter phase II study evaluating the efficacy of nivolumab plus paclitaxel plus bevacizumab triple-combination therapy as a first-line treatment in patients with HER2-negative metastatic breast cancer: WJOG9917B NEWBEAT trial. Cancer Res 2020;80(4_Supplement). PD1-03-PD1-03.

Fertility and Sexual Health in Young Women with Early-Stage Breast Cancer

Marla Lipsyc-Sharf, MD[a], Ann H. Partridge, MD, MPH[b],*

KEYWORDS

- Fertility • Sexual health • Premenopausal • Breast cancer

KEY POINTS

- Fertility and sexual health are important concerns for young women with early-stage breast cancer. Optimal assessment and management of these concerns evolves throughout the care continuum from the time of diagnosis, through active treatment, and into survivorship care.
- Risk of infertility may be impacted by treatment regimens as well as patients' age, ovarian reserve, body mass index, smoking history, genetic mutations, and other factors.
- Data regarding safety of fertility preservation options as well as pregnancy after breast cancer are overall reassuring.
- Sexual health and well-being may be impacted by medications, surgery, radiation, and other physical and psychological challenges faced by patients with breast cancer.
- Treatment modalities for improving sexual health are improving and may include sexual health rehabilitation programs, medications, and other interventions.

INTRODUCTION

The incidence of breast cancer in young women is increasing, and over 10,000 young women are diagnosed annually in the United States alone.[1] Given their overall differences in developmental stage, health status, and life circumstances, young women have unique physical, mental, psychosocial, and sexual health concerns that significantly affect their oncologic and survivorship care. Initial treatment decisions, as well as care during and after treatment, can meaningfully impact patients' fertility and sexual health. Therefore, it is important to discuss and address these issues early and throughout each phase of treatment and into survivorship. Here, the authors highlight the major considerations and potential interventions related to fertility and sexual

[a] Department of Medical Oncology, Dana-Farber Cancer Institute, 450 Brookline Avenue, Yawkey 1238, Boston, MA 02215, USA; [b] Department of Medical Oncology, Dana-Farber Cancer Institute, Harvard Medical School, 450 Brookline Avenue, Dana 1608-A, Boston, MA 02215, USA
* Corresponding author.
E-mail address: Ann_Partridge@dfci.harvard.edu

Surg Oncol Clin N Am 32 (2023) 747–759
https://doi.org/10.1016/j.soc.2023.05.012

health in young women with early-stage breast cancer at each stage of their breast cancer care.

FROM THE START: PRE-THERAPY CONSIDERATIONS
Assessing Fertility Goals and Risk of Ovarian Insufficiency

Discussion of fertility considerations is important at the time of diagnosis and throughout the care continuum to ensure patients can make decisions that align with their goals, preferences, and values (**Fig. 1**). For all young women in whom systemic therapy for breast cancer is recommended, oncology teams should assess fertility goals and risk of infertility as soon as possible. Appropriate counseling regarding risks of premature menopause, infertility, and fertility preservation is important for patients' physical health and quality of life. The risk of infertility is associated with the particular medications and regimens used for systemic cancer therapy as well as the patient's age, ovarian reserve, germline genetic mutations, body mass index (BMI), and smoking history.[2] The gonadotoxicity and premature ovarian insufficiency associated with systemic therapy for breast cancer are thought to occur via multiple mechanisms including impairment of ovarian follicles, follicular activation and depletion, and/or impact on ovarian blood supply.[2,3] Discussion regarding risk of premature ovarian insufficiency is important not only for assessing risk of infertility but also for assessing risk of premature menopause, which is associated with genitourinary and vasomotor symptoms, sexual dysfunction, reduction in bone density, and other potential long-term and late effects.[4]

Medications used to treat early-stage breast cancer, including chemotherapy, endocrine therapy (ET), targeted therapy, and immunotherapy, have varying levels of evidence regarding the risk of gonadotoxicity and premature menopause and there remain several areas of uncertainty. Although most studies investigating the effect of systemic therapies assess the risk of treatment-related amenorrhea (TRA), TRA is not synonymous with infertility.[3] Some women who resume regular menstruation after cancer treatment have very poor ovarian reserve and therefore experience infertility even with normal menstrual cycles. However, many women with longer term TRA attempting pregnancy will encounter fertility challenges, and because menstrual status is a straightforward and routine assessment for both patients and providers, this

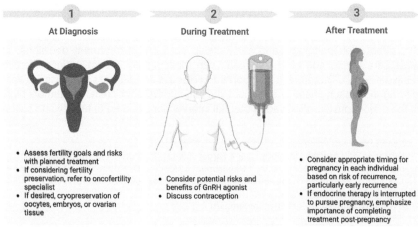

Fig. 1. Fertility considerations in young women with early-stage breast cancer. (*Created with BioRender.com.*)

continues to be used as a surrogate for ovarian function and fertility. Importantly, most young women do recover ovarian function after systemic treatment of breast cancer; over 60% of women age 40 years and younger who are treated for early-stage breast cancer resume menstruation within 1 year, and over 80% resume menstraution within 2 years after diagnosis.[5] However, given the potential for ovarian insufficiency even in the setting of continued or resumed menses, it is important to discuss these risks as early as possible.

Currently, the most common chemotherapies used for early-stage breast cancer include cyclophosphamide, taxanes, anthracyclines, and carboplatin all of which increased the risk of TRA compared with treatment without chemotherapy. This risk also depends on other factors such as age at diagnosis.[2,3] Cyclophosphamide-based regimens seem to be associated with the highest risk of TRA, conferring over twice the risk TRA compared with chemotherapy regimens without cyclophosphamide, whereas anthracyclines were shown to increase the risk of TRA by about 39%.[6] Rates of TRA with taxanes were slightly better than with anthracyclines, increasing risk of TRA by about 24%.[6] Other data show that treatment with carboplatin and a taxane may less frequently cause TRA than treatment with cyclophosphamide-based regimens.[7] Dose-dense administration of chemotherapy is not thought to affect rates of TRA.[8] Importantly, some data suggest that amenorrhea is associated with better survival outcomes regardless of chemotherapy administered or estrogen receptor (ER)-positive status. This has motivated the currently unanswered question of whether optimal ovarian suppression could simultaneously allow for de-escalation of chemotherapy, improved ovarian function, and improved survival.[9]

The impact of newer targeted therapies on TRA is less well-studied. Existing data suggest that the most common targeted agent used for early-stage breast cancer, trastuzumab (an anti-human epidermal growth factor receptor 2 [HER2] therapy), does not significantly affect rates of TRA.[10] Trastuzumab emtansine (T-DM1), which is recommended for patients with early-stage HER2-positive breast cancer found to have residual disease after neoadjuvant chemotherapy, has been associated with a lower risk of TRA than paclitaxel and trastuzumab.[11] Additional analyses including pertuzumab (another anti-HER2 therapy) suggest that this agent similarly does not confer serious gonadotoxicity.[2,5] Other targeted therapies are currently approved for patients with high-risk early-stage breast cancers, including pembrolizumab, abemaciclib, olaparib, and neratinib. Effects of these agents on rates of TRA and infertility are unclear as menopausal and fertility outcomes are generally not assessed in the pivotal trials, and many studies assessing the potential impact of these agents on ovarian function are limited to preclinical data.[12] For example, early data show that immune checkpoint inhibitors may reduce the number and quality of oocytes and impact fertility through impairment of the hypothalamic–pituitary–gonadal axis.[13,14] As new targeted agents are incorporated into standard clinical practice for the treatment of early-stage breast cancer, it is critical to study the effect of these agents on ovarian function and fertility in premenopausal patients.

For the approximately 80% of patients diagnosed with breast cancer who have ER-positive disease, ET is the cornerstone of treatment and may be prescribed for 5 to 10 years. Premenopausal women are typically treated with tamoxifen, with or without ovarian function suppression (OFS) medication (ie, gonadotropin-releasing hormone [GnRH] agonist), or an aromatase inhibitor (AI) with OFS, depending on their level of risk, preferences, and tolerance. Overall, the use of ET with chemotherapy is known to increase the risk of TRA compared with treatment with chemotherapy without ET.[15] Although tamoxifen is associated with an increased risk of TRA in premenopausal women, it likely does not impact ovarian reserve as it does not significantly affect levels of serum anti-Mullerian hormone (AMH) levels, which are indicative of ovarian reserve.[6] GnRH agonists (ie, leuprolide, goserelin, and triptorelin) are frequently used to further improve breast cancer outcomes in this setting. These medications suppress ovarian function during use, though are not thought to impair fertility, and effect on menses are generally temporary. Virtually all women under age 40 years treated with GnRH agonist alone resume menses when the treatment is stopped.[16] Data are limited regarding the effect of long-term treatment with AIs on menstrual function and fertility.[2] However, the combination of AI and OFS has been shown in recent years to improve survival over tamoxifen with or without OFS, particularly in patients with high-risk disease, so further understanding of the effect of combination GnRH agonist and AI on ovarian reserve and infertility is needed, despite a low likelihood of substantial impact given mechanisms of action.

Age is known to impact the risk of ovarian insufficiency with cancer treatment. Ovarian reserve decreases with age leading to greater risk of infertility. In the Young Women's Breast Cancer Study, a prospective cohort study of women age 40 years and younger diagnosed with breast cancer, although most patients (over 60%) resumed menses within 1 year after diagnosis, older age was associated with TRA.[5] Age more than 40 years has also been associated with TRA as has lower BMI.[3,5,15] In addition, low baseline serum AMH levels are associated with TRA and slower time to ovarian function recovery after chemotherapy.[17]

Particular consideration should be given to fertility preservation strategies for patients with germline breast cancer gene (BRCA) mutations, which affects approximately 10% of young women with breast cancer.[18] Limited available data have demonstrated lower AMH levels in women with a BRCA 1 mutation than women without germline BRCA mutation.[19] In addition to pursuing fertility preservation to mitigate the risks of infertility, women with germline BRCA mutations may elect to use assisted reproductive technology (ART), even when spontaneous conception is likely, to pursue preimplantation genetic testing to avoid passing the germline BRCA mutation to future children. All patients considering ART for any purpose should be referred to a fertility specialist for further evaluation and counseling, as existing data suggest that pregnancy and ART are safe in patients with BRCA mutations and do not confer differences in obstetrical risk or survival.[20,21]

Strategies for Fertility Preservation

Although many live births after breast cancer are the result of spontaneous pregnancies, patients who have undergone fertility preservation are more likely to become pregnant.[22] Oocyte/embryo or, less commonly, ovarian tissue cryopreservation is recommended for patients desiring fertility preservation.[23] Modern oocyte harvesting involves ovarian stimulation that can begin at any time in the menstrual cycle and lasts approximately 2 weeks.[2,3] In current practice, ovarian stimulation for fertility preservation in patients with breast cancer often includes an AI to minimize risks of rising estrogen concentrations during stimulation. Women who are intent on childbearing with a particular male partner (or using a sperm donor) may prefer to freeze embryos or both embryos and oocytes, whereas women who do not have a male partner or prefer not to freeze embryos for religious or other reasons may choose to freeze oocytes. Oocyte harvesting is typically recommended before initiation of systemic therapy.

Evidence on the safety of fertility preservation in patients with breast cancer is encouraging. Although historically there was concern that this delayed the time to cancer treatment, recent data suggest that the delay is quite short and does not impact survival.[24] Because ovarian stimulation transiently increases circulating estrogen, there has also been concern that oocyte harvesting might worsen the outcomes of patients with ER-positive breast cancers. However, fertility preservation does not seem to increase the risk of cancer recurrence or mortality, including in patients with ER-positive breast cancers.[2,3,22] Live birth rates after oocyte/embryo cryopreservation range from approximately 30% to 60%; younger age at the time of cryopreservation and a higher number of oocytes or embryos frozen are both associated with higher success rates.[2,3] For unknown reasons, a diagnosis of breast cancer is associated with worse oocyte quality compared with healthy women undergoing oocyte retrieval.[25] However, pregnancy rates overall are higher for breast cancer survivors who underwent fertility preservation than those who did not, so these strategies remain recommended for those patients who desire future biological children.[22]

Ovarian tissue cryopreservation is a less well studied and not widely available method of fertility preservation in which ovarian tissue is surgically removed, cryopreserved, and then transplanted back into the patient when conception is desired. Because ovarian stimulation is not necessary, only 2 to 3 days are needed before initiating systemic anticancer therapy. There is a theoretical risk that breast cancer metastatic to the ovaries would be reintroduced back into the patient after completion of anticancer therapy. Although there are no published accounts of this to date, ovarian tissue cryopreservation may not be the best method for patients with early-stage breast cancer with a high risk of recurrence.

The use of GnRH agonists for ovarian protection has been studied extensively. Given the ease of administration, these are often offered to premenopausal women undergoing chemotehrapy treatment for breast cancer in order to prevent ovarian insufficiency and limit the damage and depletion of ovarian follicles and therefore ovarian reserve. Although the potential mechanism of ovarian protection during cytotoxic chemotherapy is unclear and there is some controversy about the true benefits regarding GnRH for fertility preservation, several studies and meta-analyses show consistent efficacy and safety data for treatment with GnRH agonists for ovarian protection.[2,26,27] The largest meta-analysis to date studied 1231 patients receiving GnRH agonists alongside chemotherapy and found that patients receiving GnRH agonists had over 60% lower risk of premature ovarian failure and no significant difference in survival.[26] Given the uncertainty regarding efficacy for fertility outcomes, American Society of Clinical Oncology (ASCO) guidelines clearly recommend that coadministration of GnRH agonists should not be used in place of fertility preservation methods such as oocyte, embryo, or ovarian tissue cryopreservation.[23] The timing of treatment with GnRH agonist for ovarian protection may be important. Specifically, if patients undergo ovarian stimulation for oocyte or embryo cryopreservation, it is critical that GnRH agonist treatment is not started too soon after ovarian stimulation, as this can increase the risk of ovarian hyperstimulation syndrome. It is recommended that oncologists collaborate with patients' reproductive endocrinology teams to determine the earliest safe start time for GnRH agonists. Treatment with the GnRH agonist for ovarian protection is continued throughout the course of cytotoxic chemotherapy.

Surgical Considerations and Impact on Future Sexual Health

Most young women diagnosed with breast cancer have concerns about future sexual health and want information regarding how treatment may impact their sexual functioning and how to manage symptoms that arise. In initial counseling, it is important to discuss the risks and benefits of local therapy options with respect to sexual functioning. Although many young women with unilateral breast cancer are electing to have bilateral mastectomy, even in the absence of a known genetic predisposition to future breast cancer, young women treated with more extensive breast cancer surgeries have worse body image and overall sexual health than women treated with less extensive surgeries.[28,29] Specifically, women having bilateral mastectomies are at an increased risk of sexual dysfunction related to desire, excitation, lubrication, and orgasm compared with those having lumpectomy.[29] These effects were greater in women who did not undergo breast reconstruction. For women who did have breast reconstruction, autologous reconstruction was associated with improved breast satisfaction compared with implant-based or complex reconstruction.[30] Young women who have breast-conserving surgery have improved sexual functioning and better quality of life outcomes than women who underwent mastectomy with radiation. The mechanisms behind sexual dysfunction associated with mastectomy are likely multifactorial. It is possible that the loss of sensory nerves in the breast and nipple leads to loss of sexual stimulation that contributes to orgasm and libido. In addition, the impact of breast surgery on psychological health, including body image, likely affects sexual desire. As some women may value sexual health outcomes more than others, it is important to address these issues when discussing surgical planning as these risks and benefits may impact patients' decision-making.

IN THE THICK OF IT: MANAGEMENT DURING ADJUVANT TREATMENT
Assessment and Management of Sexual Health Challenges During Treatment

Many patients with breast cancer experience sexual dysfunction during treatment. Few patients report receiving any information regarding sexual health from their medical teams, and most welcome the opportunity to discuss sexual health considerations throughout the course of their treatment (**Fig. 2**). Overall, patients prefer to receive sexual health education from an oncology provider that is comfortable discussing sexuality as well as from written or online material. Assessment and discussion may include topics such as sexual desire, contraception, comfort during sexual activity,

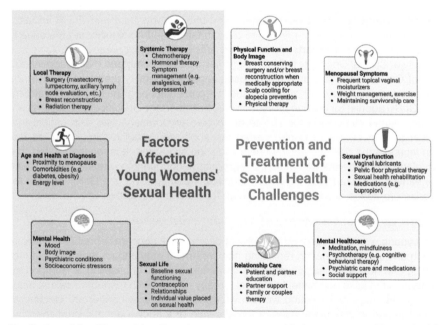

Fig. 2. Sexual health considerations in young women with breast cancer. (*Created with BioRender.com.*)

orgasm, vaginal symptoms (including discharge and/or dryness), fatigue, and relationships, among others.

Patients with breast cancer who experience TRA have significantly more sexual side effects, including worse sexual interest, body image, and vaginal pain. In addition, most women with breast cancer have ER-positive disease and receive ET, which is also associated with sexual dysfunction. In particular, treatment with AI and OFS seems to be associated with more sexual side effects than treatment with tamoxifen with or without OFS.[31] Addressing the side effects of ET is important not only for patients' sexual and overall health but also to support their adherence to breast cancer treatment.[32] For women receiving ET in whom sexual side effects are significantly impacting their quality of life, we recommend discussing the risks and benefits of de-escalation. Although AIs with OFS are likely the most effective ET for risk reduction in high-risk ER-positive breast cancer, women with moderate to severe side effects may elect to switch to tamoxifen for risk reduction associated with fewer menopausal effects.[31]

Vaginal symptoms
Vaginal dryness, irritation, itching, and dyspareunia are common factors affecting sexual health in patients with breast cancer, particularly in those with TRA. The first line of treatment for these symptoms is the use of a topical nonhormonal vaginal moisturizer (including water-based, polycarbophil, and hyaluronic formulations).[33] Nonhormonal vaginal moisturizers have been found to reduce vaginal dryness and improve dyspareunia by over 60%, and overall have been shown to reduce sexual distress.[33] In cancer survivors, frequent application has been shown to increase efficacy, so moisturizers should be applied regularly, at least three times per week.

In the general population and in patients whose breast cancers do not express hormone receptors, treatment with topical vaginal estrogen is often recommended. However, the long-term safety of vaginal estrogen in women with a history of ER-positive breast cancer is not clear. Multiple studies have found that topical estrogen does have systemic absorption, and data on how this affects breast cancer outcomes are mixed.[34] A recent large Danish cohort study found that there was overall no increased risk of recurrence or mortality for patients treated for breast cancer that subsequently received vaginal estrogen.[34] However, in the subgroup receiving AIs, there was an increased risk of recurrence. Accordingly, vaginal estrogen can be a helpful tool though is used with caution and after thorough discussion with patients. If vaginal estrogen is prescribed, consideration should be taken to prescribe the lowest effective dose and, if possible, use vaginal softgels rather than tablets to limit systemic absorption.[35]

Research is ongoing to find additional safe and effective treatments for patients with breast cancer experiencing vulvovaginal atrophy. Topical dehydroepiandrosterone has been used for vaginal symptoms in patients taking ET for breast cancer, and there was no change in estrogen concentration for patients taking AIs.[36] Monthly vaginal micro-ablative CO_2 laser therapy with experts in this modality is also a promising option under study in breast cancer survivors. Ospemifene, an oral selective ER modulator, has been shown to improve symptoms of vulvovaginal atrophy in menopausal women, though the current data in patients with breast cancer are limited. For patients specifically reporting vaginal pain with penetration during sexual intercourse, the application of topical lidocaine before vaginal penetration can improve sexual distress and sexual dysfunction. In addition, though safety in patients with breast cancer has not been ascertained, the application of testosterone cream to the vagina and clitoris is being studied for improved sexual desire and function.

The intersection of psychosocial and sexual health

There is a clear relationship between psychosocial and sexual health challenges in patients with breast cancer. Most patients report that sexual dysfunction during and after treatment negatively impacts their mental health. The converse is also true: over half of patients with breast cancer experience anxiety and depression within 5 years of diagnosis, and these also affect sexual health and function.[32] In addition, intimate relationships are strained as patients experience significant life stressors and partners assume caregiving responsibilities, which add strain to sexual relationships. Some interventions traditionally used to improve mental and psychosocial health have been shown to improve patients' sexual health. Bupropion, an antidepressant, has also been shown to improve libido and sexual function in patients receiving treatment of breast cancer.[37] However, the most efficacious interventions in this setting are education, counseling, and cognitive behavioral therapy. Mindfulness, body awareness, and sexual health rehabilitation have also been shown to significantly improve sexual function and psychological distress in young patients with breast cancer receiving OFS. Referral to a professional with expertise in sex therapy should be considered when possible.

The Intersection of Physical and Sexual Health

Some interventions to address patients' physical health and symptoms (such as the use of selective serotonin reuptake inhibitors [SSRIs] or serotonin-norepinephrine reuptake inhibitors [SNRIs] for vasomotor symptoms, neuropathic pain, or aromatase-inhibitor musculoskeletal symptoms) have been associated with impaired sexual function.[32] However, these symptoms themselves may impair sexual functioning as well, so interventions may be tried and stopped if patients do not experience net benefit. Fatigue, poor body image, weight gain, and chemotherapy-induced alopecia are all known to impair patients' sexual health. Many non-pharmacologic interventions have been shown to improve fatigue, functional impairment, and quality of life in patients with breast cancer including exercise programs, cognitive behavioral therapy, acupuncture, acupressure, yoga, mindfulness, and martial arts.[32] There are also several efficacious interventions for weight loss in patients with breast cancer, and these include a combination of physical activity, nutritional changes, and behavioral therapy.[32] To prevent hair loss, scalp cooling systems are increasingly used by patients with breast cancer. Existing data suggest that this is a safe intervention, and efficacy for prevention of alopecia varies by chemotherapy regimen. Communicating these evidence-based strategies to patients is important for increasing utilization of these interventions that improve patients' health and well-being.

Contraception and Pregnancy During Adjuvant Treatment

Young women with breast cancer often have significant concerns about their fertility. For some, this may even affect their treatment choices or adherence.[38] Patients' desire for future pregnancy should inform providers' recommendations. In general, it is recommended that nonpregnant premenopausal women use contraception to avoid conceiving during active treatment of breast cancer. Contraception is an essential part of sexual health for women who do not desire current pregnancy or are receiving teratogenic medications. Chemotherapy administration during first trimester may impair healthy fetal development, and tamoxifen is a known teratogen. In women desiring future pregnancy, adjuvant zoledronic acid, a bisphosphonate that has been shown to improve disease-free survival in some patients with early-stage breast cancer, is generally avoided due to the long skeletal half-life and data suggesting adverse effects on pregnancy and neonatal outcomes. It is important for oncology providers to discuss contraception with their patients, as some patients may incorrectly assume that they are infertile during or after treatment and therefore decide not to use contraception. Hormonal oral contraceptives or intrauterine devices (IUDs) are avoided in patients with ER-positive breast cancers. Safe and effective methods of contraception include copper IUDs, barrier contraceptives, or sterilization of patients or their sexual partners.

Most data on the safety and success rates of pregnancy after breast cancer have focused on patients who have completed active adjuvant therapy. However, given the long duration of adjuvant ET, the recently reported POSITIVE trial was designed to assess the safety of temporary interruption of ET to attempt pregnancy in patients with a history of early-stage ER-positive breast cancer.[39,40] In this study, patients who received between 18 and 30 months of adjuvant ET stopped treatment, and 3 months later, attempted pregnancy. Patients remained off ET for up to 2 years during attempted conception, pregnancy, delivery, and, in some women, breastfeeding, with resumption of ET after this time to complete 5 to 10 years of adjuvant treatment. The initial trial results suggest that this strategy of interruption of ET does not compromise early breast cancer outcomes, and 43% of women used ART during trial participation.[39]

LIFE AFTER TREATMENT: POST-THERAPY CONSIDERATIONS
Fertility, pregnancy, and sexual health after breast cancer treatment

Although patients with breast cancer who underwent fertility preservation before treatment are ultimately more likely to become pregnant, pregnancy rates in these patients are lower than in women who have not had breast cancer.[22,41] This is likely multifactorial due to competing risks including disease recurrence, as well as infertility from systemic cancer therapies and increased age as pregnancy is delayed to allow for completion of systemic therapy. A large meta-analysis of over 8 million women showed that pregnant women with a history of breast cancer, especially those who received chemotherapy, have a higher risk of Cesarean Section, preterm birth, and low birth weight infants compared with the general population.[41] Interestingly, even after adjusting for confounders and clinicopathologic risk factors, breast cancer survivors with subsequent pregnancy had improved survival compared with breast cancer survivors without pregnancy. Importantly, patients with a history of ER-positive breast cancers who had a subsequent pregnancy did not have significantly different survival than those with no subsequent pregnancy.

The optimal interval between completion of breast cancer treatment and conception is not clear and may be individualized for each patient. Factors to consider include which treatments the patient received, their breast cancer biology and risk of recurrence, family planning goals, and their general health and well-being. Women who conceive within a year of completing chemotherapy are at an increased risk of preterm birth, so it is often recommended that most patients delay conception until at least 1 year after chemotherapy administration.[42] Patients receiving tamoxifen, a known teratogen, are generally advised wait at least 3 months after stopping before attempting conception, and the US FDA recommends waiting 9 months after tamoxifen based on animal data. It is unclear how long patients should delay conception after receiving AIs or targeted therapies. Women with ER-negative breast cancers have the highest risk of recurrence within the first 3 years after treatment, so many of these patients choose to delay pregnancy until after this interval. However, for patients with hormone receptor-positive breast cancers, the risk of recurrence persists for decades. The timing of pregnancy in these patients will likely depend on age and other clinicopathologic risk factors, whether ET will need to be interrupted, and patient desires and values.

The importance of sexual health care persists even after concluding active therapy for breast cancer. Treatment with chemotherapy and ET has been associated with lower rates of sexual activity and function long after the completion of therapy. Ongoing care of breast cancer survivors to manage sexual health challenges is essential to comprehensive long-term survivorship care.

CLINICS CARE POINTS

- It is critical to assess and address fertility and sexual health considerations at diagnosis and through survivorship.
- Future fertility interest and risk should be considered with all patients, and those interested should be referred to an infertility specialist for discussion and management of fertility preservation.
- Recommendations regarding timing of pregnancy should involve shared decision-making based on individual patient factors and available data.
- Patients should be counseled about the effects of cancer treatment on sexual health outcomes including libido, vaginal dryness and dyspareunia, and body image, as well as strategies for prevention and management of impairment.

FUNDING

Lipsyc-Sharf M., is supported by the Terri Brodeur Breast Cancer Foundation. Partridge A.H. is supported by Susan G. Komen and the Breast Cancer Research Foundation.

DISCLOSURES

AHP: Authorship for UpToDate. MLS: Honoraria from MJH Life Sciences.

REFERENCES

1. American Cancer Society, Breast Cancer Facts and Figures 2019-2020. Available at: https://www.cancer.org/content/dam/cancer-org/research/cancer-facts-and-statistics/breast-cancer-facts-and-figures/breast-cancer-facts-and-figures-2019-2020.pdf Accessed March 20, 2022.
2. Martelli V, Latocca MM, Ruelle T, et al. Comparing the Gonadotoxicity of Multiple Breast Cancer Regimens: Important Understanding for Managing Breast Cancer in Pre-Menopausal Women. Breast Cancer 2021;13:341–51. Dove Med Press.
3. Yildiz S, Bildik G, Benlioglu C, et al. Breast cancer treatment and ovarian function. Reprod Biomed Online 2022. https://doi.org/10.1016/j.rbmo.2022.09.014.
4. Rocca WA, Gazzuola-Rocca L, Smith CY, et al. Accelerated Accumulation of Multimorbidity After Bilateral Oophorectomy: A Population-Based Cohort Study. Mayo Clin Proc 2016;91(11):1577–89.
5. Poorvu PD, Hu J, Zheng Y, et al. Treatment-related amenorrhea in a modern, prospective cohort study of young women with breast cancer. NPJ Breast Cancer 2021;7(1):99.

6. Zhao J, Liu J, Chen K, et al. What lies behind chemotherapy-induced amenorrhea for breast cancer patients: a meta-analysis. Breast Cancer Res Treat 2014; 145(1):113–28.

7. Gast KC, Cathcart-Rake EJ, Norman AD, et al. Regimen-Specific Rates of Chemotherapy-Related Amenorrhea in Breast Cancer Survivors. JNCI Cancer Spectr 2019;3(4). https://doi.org/10.1093/jncics/pkz081.

8. Lambertini M, Ceppi M, Cognetti F, et al. Dose-dense adjuvant chemotherapy in premenopausal breast cancer patients: A pooled analysis of the MIG1 and GIM2 phase III studies. Eur J Cancer 2017;71:34–42.

9. Swain SM, Jeong J-H, Geyer CE, et al. Longer Therapy, Iatrogenic Amenorrhea, and Survival in Early Breast Cancer. N Engl J Med 2010;362(22):2053–65.

10. Lambertini M, Campbell C, Bines J, et al. Adjuvant Anti-HER2 Therapy, Treatment-Related Amenorrhea, and Survival in Premenopausal HER2-Positive Early Breast Cancer Patients. J Natl Cancer Inst 2019;111(1):86–94.

11. Ruddy KJ, Trippa L, Hu J, et al. Abstract P2-13-02: Chemotherapy-related amenorrhea (CRA) after adjuvant trastuzumab emtansine (T-DM1) compared to paclitaxel in combination with trastuzumab (TH) (TBCRC033: ATEMPT trial). Cancer Res 2020;80(4_Supplement). https://doi.org/10.1158/1538-7445.SABCS19-P2-13-02.

12. Cui W, Francis PA, Loi S, et al. Assessment of Ovarian Function in Phase III (Neo) Adjuvant Breast Cancer Clinical Trials: A Systematic Evaluation. J Natl Cancer Inst 2021;113(12):1770–8.

13. Winship AL, Alesi LR, Sant S, et al. Checkpoint inhibitor immunotherapy diminishes oocyte number and quality in mice. Nature Cancer 2022;3(8):1–13.

14. Garutti M, Lambertini M, Puglisi F. Checkpoint inhibitors, fertility, pregnancy, and sexual life: a systematic review. ESMO Open 2021;6(5):100276.

15. Lee S, Kil WJ, Chun M, et al. Chemotherapy-related amenorrhea in premenopausal women with breast cancer. Menopause 2009;16(1):98–103.

16. Bernhard J, Zahrieh D, Castiglione-Gertsch M, et al. Adjuvant Chemotherapy Followed By Goserelin Compared With Either Modality Alone: The Impact on Amenorrhea, Hot Flashes, and Quality of Life in Premenopausal Patients—The International Breast Cancer Study Group Trial VIII. J Clin Oncol 2007;25(3):263–70.

17. Su HC, Haunschild C, Chung K, et al. Prechemotherapy antimullerian hormone, age, and body size predict timing of return of ovarian function in young breast cancer patients. Cancer 2014;120(23):3691–8.

18. Guzmán-Arocho YD, Rosenberg SM, Garber JE, et al. Clinicopathological features and BRCA1 and BRCA2 mutation status in a prospective cohort of young women with breast cancer. Br J Cancer 2022;126(2):302–9.

19. Turan V, Lambertini M, Lee DY, et al. Association of Germline BRCA Pathogenic Variants With Diminished Ovarian Reserve: A Meta-Analysis of Individual Patient-Level Data. J Clin Oncol 2021;39(18):2016–24.

20. Condorelli M, Bruzzone M, Ceppi M, et al. Safety of assisted reproductive techniques in young women harboring germline pathogenic variants in BRCA1/2 with a pregnancy after prior history of breast cancer. ESMO Open 2021;6(6):100300.

21. Lambertini M, Ameye L, Hamy A-S, et al. Pregnancy After Breast Cancer in Patients With Germline BRCA Mutations. J Clin Oncol 2020;38(26):3012–23.

22. Wang Y, Tesch ME, Lim C, et al. Risk of recurrence and pregnancy outcomes in young women with breast cancer who do and do not undergo fertility preservation. Breast Cancer Res Treat 2022;195(2):201–8.

23. Oktay K, Harvey BE, Partridge AH, et al. Fertility Preservation in Patients With Cancer: ASCO Clinical Practice Guideline Update. J Clin Oncol 2018;36(19): 1994–2001.

24. Greer AC, Lanes A, Poorvu PD, et al. The impact of fertility preservation on the timing of breast cancer treatment, recurrence, and survival. Cancer 2021; 127(20):3872–80.

25. Fabiani C, Guarino A, Meneghini C, et al. Oocyte Quality Assessment in Breast Cancer: Implications for Fertility Preservation. Cancers 2022;14(22). https://doi.org/10.3390/cancers14225718.

26. Lambertini M, Ceppi M, Poggio F, et al. Ovarian suppression using luteinizing hormone-releasing hormone agonists during chemotherapy to preserve ovarian function and fertility of breast cancer patients: a meta-analysis of randomized studies. Ann Oncol 2015;26(12):2408–19.

27. Lambertini M, Moore HCF, Leonard RCF, et al. Gonadotropin-Releasing Hormone Agonists During Chemotherapy for Preservation of Ovarian Function and Fertility in Premenopausal Patients With Early Breast Cancer: A Systematic Review and Meta-Analysis of Individual Patient-Level Data. J Clin Oncol 2018;36(19):1981–90.

28. Rosenberg SM, Dominici LS, Gelber S, et al. Association of Breast Cancer Surgery With Quality of Life and Psychosocial Well-being in Young Breast Cancer Survivors. JAMA Surg 2020;155(11):1035–42.

29. Cobo-Cuenca AI, Martín-Espinosa NM, Sampietro-Crespo A, et al. Sexual dysfunction in Spanish women with breast cancer. PLoS One 2018;13(8):e0203151.

30. Dominici L, Hu J, Zheng Y, et al. Association of Local Therapy With Quality-of-Life Outcomes in Young Women With Breast Cancer. JAMA Surgery 2021;156(10): e213758.

31. Saha P, Regan MM, Pagani O, et al. Treatment Efficacy, Adherence, and Quality of Life Among Women Younger Than 35 Years in the International Breast Cancer Study Group TEXT and SOFT Adjuvant Endocrine Therapy Trials. J Clin Oncol 2017;35(27):3113–22.

32. Franzoi MA, Agostinetto E, Perachino M, et al. Evidence-based approaches for the management of side-effects of adjuvant endocrine therapy in patients with breast cancer. Lancet Oncol 2021;22(7):e303–13.

33. Loprinzi CL, Abu-Ghazaleh S, Sloan JA, et al. Phase III randomized double-blind study to evaluate the efficacy of a polycarbophil-based vaginal moisturizer in women with breast cancer. J Clin Oncol 1997;15(3):969–73.

34. Cold S, Cold F, Jensen M-B, et al. Systemic or Vaginal Hormone Therapy After Early Breast Cancer: A Danish Observational Cohort Study. JNCI: Journal of the National Cancer Institute 2022;114(10):1347–54.

35. Santen RJ, Mirkin S, Bernick B, et al. Systemic estradiol levels with low-dose vaginal estrogens. Menopause 2020;27(3):361–70.

36. Barton DL, Shuster LT, Dockter T, et al. Systemic and local effects of vaginal dehydroepiandrosterone (DHEA): NCCTG N10C1 (Alliance). Support Care Cancer 2018;26(4):1335–43.

37. Mathias C, Cardeal Mendes CM, Pondé de Sena E, et al. An open-label, fixed-dose study of bupropion effect on sexual function scores in women treated for breast cancer. Ann Oncol 2006;17(12):1792–6.

38. Sella T, Poorvu PD, Ruddy KJ, et al. Impact of fertility concerns on endocrine therapy decisions in young breast cancer survivors. Cancer 2021;127(16):2888–94.

39. Partridge AH NS, Ruggeri M, et al. GS4-09 Pregnancy Outcome and Safety of Interrupting Therapy for women with endocrine responsIVE breast cancer: Primary Results from the POSITIVE Trial (IBCSG 48-14/BIG 8-13).

40. Partridge AH, Niman SM, Ruggeri M, et al. Interrupting Endocrine Therapy to Attempt Pregnancy after Breast Cancer. N Engl J Med 2023;388(18):1645–56.
41. Lambertini M, Blondeaux E, Bruzzone M, et al. Pregnancy After Breast Cancer: A Systematic Review and Meta-Analysis. J Clin Oncol 2021;39(29):3293–305.
42. Hartnett KP, Mertens AC, Kramer MR, et al. Pregnancy after cancer: Does timing of conception affect infant health? Cancer 2018;124(22):4401–7.

Prepectoral Versus Subpectoral Implant-Based Reconstruction

How Do We Choose?

Perri S. Vingan, BS[1], Minji Kim, BS[1], Danielle Rochlin, MD,
Robert J. Allen Jr, MD, Jonas A. Nelson, MD, MPH*

KEYWORDS

• Prepectoral • Subpectoral • Implant • Breast reconstruction • Breast cancer

KEY POINTS

- Reconstructive options for patients undergoing implant-based breast reconstruction include one- or two-staged procedures and prepectoral or subpectoral implant placement.
- Patient-reported outcomes between prepectoral and subpectoral patients are similar, but patients with subpectoral reconstruction may experience more pain postoperatively than patients with preoperative reconstruction.
- Preoperatively, patients with risk factors for wound healing problems and/or impaired mastectomy skin flap perfusion should not be considered good candidates for prepectoral reconstruction; these include peripheral vascular disease, poorly controlled diabetes, active or recent smoking, obesity, connective tissue disorders, and preoperative radiation.
- Prepectoral device placement must be evaluated intraoperatively following the mastectomy, as skin flap perfusion may be the most critical factor in the final decision, ultimately dictating whether prepectoral implant placement is possible.

INTRODUCTION

Implant-based reconstruction (IBBR) is the most common form of breast reconstruction performed in the United States.[1] There is much heterogeneity in this practice, with changing popularity in the placement of implants underneath or on top of the pectoralis major muscle, as well as differing opinions on the use of acellular dermal matrices (ADM). Reconstructive procedures are constantly evolving, and with advances in both

Plastic and Reconstructive Surgery Service, Department of Surgery, Memorial Sloan Kettering Cancer Center, 1275 York Avenue, New York, NY 10065, USA
[1] Co-first author.
* Corresponding author.
E-mail address: nelsonj1@mskcc.org

Surg Oncol Clin N Am 32 (2023) 761–776
https://doi.org/10.1016/j.soc.2023.05.007
1055-3207/23/© 2023 Elsevier Inc. All rights reserved.
surgonc.theclinics.com

technique and technology, surgeons are able to focus on improving both clinical and quality-of-life outcomes for patients. This article aims to review developments in prosthetic breast reconstruction and provide recommendations to help providers choose the best approach for each of their patients.

A BRIEF HISTORY OF PROSTHETIC BREAST RECONSTRUCTION
Why Implant-Based Reconstruction?

Breast reconstruction results in better quality of life compared with no breast reconstruction.[2] When it comes to surgical modality, however, there is ongoing debate on the superiority of autologous or IBBR.[2–6] In order to achieve predictable, positive outcomes for any surgical procedure, surgeons must determine which patients are the best candidates by appreciating the likelihood of complications based on their medical history and goals. Patients that are traditionally good candidates for autologous breast reconstruction are those with excess abdominal tissue, or those whose prior surgery or radiation left them with insufficient or nonpliable chest wall tissue to confidently sustain an implant. Patients with serious comorbid conditions are generally not well suited for autologous reconstruction. Relative to autologous reconstruction, the best candidates for IBBR are those who do not have enough adipose tissue for free flap reconstruction, have small-to-moderate size breasts (although the spectrum of suitable breast sizes for IBBR has expanded with advances in technique), and those who desire ease of recovery. Patients who are obese or have larger breasts have been found to be at greater risk for complications after IBBR.[7–12] In addition, although patients who are medically complex should optimize their health before undergoing surgery (ie, those with risk factors for problematic wound healing like smokers and diabetics), these patients are better suited for implant-based than autologous reconstruction.[13–16] In breast reconstruction, there are many preference-based nuances; nevertheless, it is important that providers use evidenced-based guidelines to complement patient preferences.

Prepectoral Versus Subpectoral and Advances in Technique

Early descriptions of IBBR involved placement of the implant in the prepectoral (ie, subcutaneous or subglandular) plane.[17–19] This approach was ultimately dismissed due to a pronounced risk of complications that included implant malposition, palpability, wrinkling, and exposure in the setting of mastectomy skin flap breakdown.[20–22] Subsequently, submuscular implant coverage was popularized. This change in implant placement seemingly addressed the issues associated with the subcutaneous technique, lowering rates of capsular contracture, exposure, infection, and displacement of the implant.[23,24] With the advent of biologic materials like ADM, surgeons were able to adjust previous subpectoral techniques, leading to the partial submuscular or dual-plane approach.[25,26] Subpectoral techniques remained predominant for more than 4 decades; however, these are associated with a higher incidence of pain and animation deformity, which negatively impacted patient outcomes and satisfaction.[27–30]

Owing to the use of ADM and indocyanine green (ICG) angiography, as well as improved implant design and fat grafting, we have again seen a shift in practice with the revival of prepectoral breast reconstruction in the last half decade (Fig. 1).[31–35] Adequate mastectomy skin flap perfusion is a prerequisite for prepectoral implant placement. Methods to assess mastectomy skin viability were previously limited to checking for dermal bleeding and palpating flap thickness; however, ICG angiography has provided a more robust method of visualizing skin flap perfusion.[36] Placement of implants on top of the pectoralis muscle decreases the morbidity

Fig. 1. A brief history of prosthetic breast reconstruction. (*From* Chopra S, Al-Ishaq Z, Vidya R. The Journey of Prepectoral Breast Reconstruction through Time. *World J Plast Surg.* 2021;10(2):3-13. https://doi.org/10.29252/wjps.10.2.3.)

associated with muscle dissection, affording patients decreased pain in the postoperative period and fewer issues with animation deformity.[25,28,32,37–44]

Cost is also an important factor when considering implant plane. Patients undergoing two-stage prepectoral IBBR require fewer clinic visits before the final reconstruction and face a more expeditious timeline to final reconstruction than their subpectoral counterparts.[24,45,46] Although indirect costs may be minimized from these aforementioned factors, prepectoral breast reconstruction is usually compounded by the use of ADM or other materials that increase surgical expenses.[47] Synthetic meshes are, however, becoming increasingly popular alternatives to ADM and are less expensive.

One Versus Two-Stage Implant-Based Reconstruction

Prosthetic breast reconstruction can be completed using a single-stage (direct-to-implant [DTI]) or two-stage (tissue expander [TE]) approach. Regardless of the approach, the device can be placed prepectorally or subpectorally. Less-aggressive mastectomies in the setting of improvements in neoadjuvant and adjuvant therapies and changing oncologic indications have allowed for greater preservation of the breast skin envelope, permitting DTI reconstructions.[48]

When comparing single-stage reconstructions by plane of implant insertion, Manrique and colleagues found that there were no significant differences in complications or satisfaction scores between subpectoral and prepectoral placement.[49] Another study comparing short-term outcomes found no significant differences in early postoperative pain by plane of implant insertion; a majority of the cohort was made up of DTI patients.[50] Opposingly, Caputo and colleagues' case series revealed prepectoral DTI patients had decreased pain and upper-limb functional impairment in the immediate postoperative period relative to dual-plane DTI patients.[51] Other studies echo these conclusions.[52,53] A meta-analysis found that prepectoral reconstruction was more commonly performed as a single-stage than as a two-stage procedure.[54] This may be because both prepectoral and DTI reconstructions require robust mastectomy flaps. Interestingly, a study by King and colleagues found that single-stage procedures are associated with decreased odds of prosthesis failure.[55] It is possible that the collinearity between implant plane and staging of the reconstruction can explain why prepectoral placement is associated with fewer prosthesis failures.

When comparing 2-stage procedures by plane of implant insertion, our group found that prepectoral TE patients had lower postoperative pain in the short term.[56] At our institution, we have ongoing efforts looking at long-term clinical and patient-reported outcomes in prepectoral and subpectoral TE patients.

CHOOSING A PLANE

Overall, compared to its inaugural use, prepectoral breast reconstruction has successfully reintegrated into the repertoire of many plastic surgeons due to advances in technique and materials. This then begs the question, what patient-specific and intraoperative factors would make a surgeon choose prepectoral over subpectoral implant placement? Aspects of a patient's lifestyle, state of health, breast size, and mastectomy skin flap quality all influence this choice.

Obesity is a factor that increases complications in IBBR overall. Regardless of the plane of placement, the odds of a complication after IBBR increase by 7% for every point increase in body mass index (BMI), and physicians report better esthetics in patients with a BMI less than 25 than in those with higher BMI.[57] Higher BMI can increase the chance of prosthesis loss in IBBR patients and increase the hospital length of stay and operative times for all breast reconstruction patients.[11,58,59] Studies suggest, however, that there are greater rates of implant exposure and asymmetry in patients with higher BMI undergoing prepectoral reconstruction than similar patients undergoing subpectoral reconstruction.[57] Overall, patients with higher BMI planning to undergo IBBR need to be counseled about their increased risk for complications and the possibility of lower satisfaction, and they should be made aware that they may benefit from subpectoral implant placement.[60]

Despite the genetic interplay between BMI and breast size, breast size itself may influence outcomes in breast reconstruction.[61,62] Patients with larger breasts may benefit from subpectoral placement, as more severe rippling deformities may occur with prepectoral implants in this group.[43] Regardless of the implant plane, since increased mastectomy weight is associated with increased complication rates, patients with larger breasts need to be counseled thoroughly.[55,62,63] Due to the animation deformity associated with submuscular implant placement, patients who are more physically active with their chest muscles (ie, patients who regularly weight train or participate in high-intensity-type workouts) may also be better suited for prepectoral reconstruction.

Of the critical intraoperative characteristics that determine success in prepectoral breast reconstruction, the quality and thickness of the mastectomy skin flap are the most important ones.[64] For patients with a more robust skin flap, prepectoral implant placement is acceptable and encouraged. However, for those with thinner skin, patients may benefit from alternative techniques using muscular coverage or more ADM coverage. A preoperative evaluation can be performed, examining the patient or imaging for a simple assessment of flap thickness. However, intraoperative evaluation using ICG is more thorough and reliable.[65] If vascularity of the skin flap is determined to be suboptimal, subpectoral reconstruction is preferred over prepectoral reconstruction.[43]

Tumor proximity to the pectoralis muscle is another factor that may determine the optimal prosthesis plane. If a tumor is too close to the pectoralis muscle or if the tumor is more than 3 cm, subpectoral reconstruction is favored.[43,66] Before surgery, imaging can be reviewed to assess tumor size and location. In breast cancer patients, prevention of recurrence is paramount. Although breast reconstruction does not adversely affect the likelihood or detection of relapse, identification of recurrence is easier when the pectoralis muscle is displaced in front of a prosthesis (**Fig. 2**).[43,66,67] In such situations where a tumor is close to the chest wall, discussion between the oncologic surgeon and reconstructive surgeon is critical. This should not be viewed as an absolute contraindication, but one for suggested intraoperative consideration.

ACELLULAR DERMAL MATRICES

ADMs are tissues engineered from human or animal cadaveric materials, which serve to provide additional soft-tissue coverage and structural support in plastic surgical procedures.[68–70] In breast reconstruction, ADM was first used to supplement partial submuscular implant placement.[68]

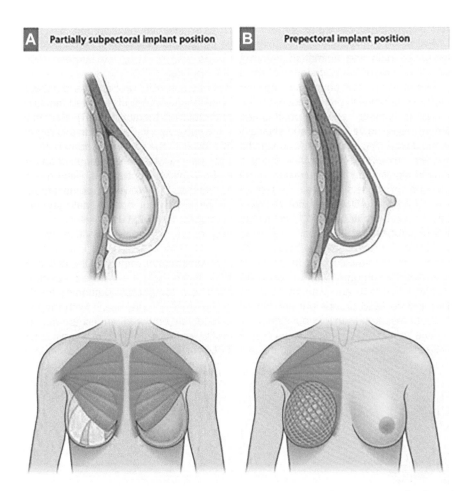

Fig. 2. IBBR with ADM. (*A*) Subpectoral TE/implant placement with ADM as an inferolateral sling. (*B*) Prepectoral TE/implant placement with anterior prosthesis coverage by ADM. ADM, acellular dermal matrices; IBBR, implant-based reconstruction; TE, tissue expander. (*Adapted from* Weinzierl A, Schmauss D, Brucato D, Harder Y. Implant-Based Breast Reconstruction after Mastectomy, from the Subpectoral to the Prepectoral Approach: An Evidence-Based Change of Mind? Journal of Clinical Medicine. 2022; 11(11):3079. https://doi.org/10.3390/jcm11113079.)

ADM-assisted subpectoral reconstruction helps to limit the inferior lateral musculofascial dissection involved in total submuscular reconstruction while still providing adequate implant coverage and bolstering implant positioning and breast contour.[68] Several studies have cited advantages afforded by ADM use in patients with partial submuscular implant coverage, including added definition to the lateral breast margin and inframammary fold, support for optimal device position, and reduced rates of capsular contracture.[71–75] Specifically for patients undergoing two-stage reconstruction, ADM allows for increased fill volume during the operation, and ultimately, a shorter time to optimal expansion.[26,72,74,76] As the revival of prepectoral reconstruction is still quite young, we do not yet have substantial long-term results about ADM in this population. In this case, when ADM is used, it is implanted for anterior or even full prosthesis coverage, rather than just as an inferolateral sling (**Fig. 3**).[74,77,78] ADM-assisted prepectoral IBBR provides the benefits of prepectoral reconstruction (decreased pain and animation deformity) while also granting the surgeon more discrete control of the boundaries of the implant pocket.[77,79,80]

There is also no true consensus regarding the effect of ADM on clinical and patient-reported outcomes in breast reconstruction. One longitudinal study showed the utility of ADM in patients requiring postmastectomy radiation therapy (PMRT). Radiation compromises the vascularity and elasticity of the subjected tissues, but in this report, the incidence of explantation was significantly lower in the patients who had ADM-assisted procedures.[81] Another study found that ADM-assisted reconstructions required significantly fewer revision surgeries for capsular contracture, likely due to additional prosthesis covered by biological material.[82,83] However, some studies have found that ADM does not decrease reoperations, nor does it yield superior patient-reported outcomes.[84–86] In fact, some suggest that ADM use in either prepectoral or subpectoral IBBR can lead to increased risk of seroma, infection, wound dehiscence, or reconstructive failure.[82,86–88]

Few outcome studies exist for prepectoral reconstruction without ADM, and even fewer directly compare ADM to no ADM.[89,90] Of those that do compare prepectoral reconstruction with and without ADM, results show comparable outcomes for the ADM and no ADM groups but are limited by the small sample size.[90] With the lack of robust research in this population, more adequately powered studies are needed to refine indications for ADM use in prepectoral breast reconstruction patients. While the literature does not suggest that the use of ADM in IBBR is unsafe, larger studies on

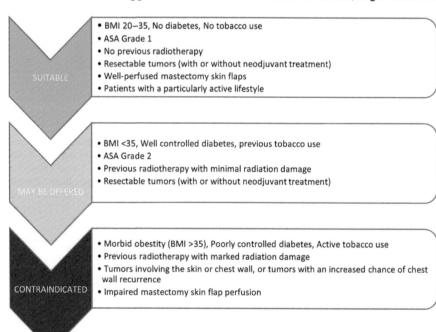

Fig. 3. Patient selection for prepectoral breast reconstruction. (*Adapted from* Vidya R, Berna G, Sbitany H, et al. Prepectoral implant-based breast reconstruction: a joint consensus guide from UK, European and USA breast and plastic reconstructive surgeons. *Ecancermedicalscience.* 2019;13:927. Published 2019 May 7. https://doi.org/10.3332/ecancer.2019.927.)

the subject are warranted, especially as trends in breast reconstructive techniques change. The use of ADM is a continued area of research and one of the most important questions within prepectoral reconstruction currently, with no current consensus.

INDOCYANINE GREEN ANGIOGRAPHY

Favorable tissue perfusion is critical for successful outcomes in breast reconstruction. When a skin flap has poor blood flow, the surgeon must be mindful to resect enough specimen to avoid perfusion-related complications, while also preserving enough to achieve an aesthetically optimal result. With the evolution of trends in breast reconstruction, techniques that accurately measure perfusion have been the subject of much research.[64,91–96] Technological advances have been made to minimize perfusion-related complications, including implementation of ICG angiography and the adoption of the SPY intraoperative perfusion assessment system (Stryker, Kalamazoo, MI).

ICG is an injectable dye used to assess tissue vascularization.[97] At our institution, ICG is given by an anesthesiologist, after which a laser is used to excite the molecules, leading to fluorescence that can be captured using the camera on the SPY system.[98] In addition to its tool as a real-time perfusion measurement, ICG angiography has been used to predict mastectomy skin flap necrosis and perfusion-related complications in both implant and autologous breast reconstruction.[99] Moreover the use of the SPY system may contribute to reduced frequency and severity of perfusion-related complications in postmastectomy patients.[36,93,100]

This objective measure detects ischemic skin and helps prognosticate other nonviable tissue, supplementing clinical judgment in the operating room. As prepectoral IBBR patients are unique, given the lack of vascularized tissue between their mastectomy skin and their implant, the adoption of ICG and SPY into clinical practice provides an adjunct objective criterion to help determine candidates for prepectoral versus subpectoral reconstruction.

CLINICAL OUTCOMES

Clinical and esthetic outcomes vary based on implant pocket; however, even prior to the recovery period, patients undergoing prepectoral IBBR benefit from decreased time under anesthesia compared with subpectoral patients.[45] The most common complications following prepectoral reconstruction include rippling of the skin overlying the prosthesis, seroma, and skin flap necrosis.[54] Rippling is due to inadequate soft-tissue coverage over the implant and can be worsened with subcutaneous placement of the implant. It can be mitigated with ADM, fat grafting, and overfilling the pocket (placing an implant larger than the TE previously in place).[55] Patients with subpectoral reconstruction are more frequently affected by animation deformity, postoperative pain, and capsular contracture.[31,55,101]

In patients who undergo PMRT, rates of capsular contracture increase three-fold when comparing subpectoral to prepectoral.[102] Studies have also shown that a pocket exchange from subpectoral to prepectoral is effective in addressing animation deformity associated with a prior subpectoral implant procedure.[103] When comparing the two approaches, studies have found that placement of implants in the prepectoral plane results in lower rates of prosthesis failure and unplanned reoperations but higher rates of seroma and rippling deformities than subpectoral reconstruction.[24,43,54,55,66,101,104,105] Subpectoral reconstruction patients tend to require more revision procedures than prepectoral patients (this includes soft-tissue rearrangement, fat grafting, and nipple reconstruction).[53]

PATIENT-REPORTED OUTCOMES AND POSTOPERATIVE PAIN

Patient-reported outcome measures (PROMs) are an important consideration in choice of implant plane. In a meta-analysis of prepectoral reconstruction, the average composite BREAST-Q score was 72.6 ± 9.7, which is higher than the majority of the "normative" values that exist, with the exception of physical well-being of the chest.[54,106] Most existing studies have found no significant differences in the BREAST-Q scores between single-stage prepectoral versus subpectoral reconstruction.[49] Interestingly, Le and colleagues found that among DTI patients, those who had subpectoral implants had higher sexual well-being than those who had prepectoral implants.[107]

For two-stage IBBR patients, Walia and colleagues found that there were no significant differences between subpectoral and prepectoral groups for any domain of the BREAST-Q.[25] A propensity-matched analysis in the same surgical population also found that there were no significant differences between the groups for physical well-being of the chest.[56] In addition to using BREAST-Q, Walia and colleagues used RAND-36 Physical Health and Mental Health surveys to compare outcomes among TE patients.[25] The authors found that physical health was lower in the prepectoral TE group than that in the subpectoral TE group; however, mental health between the groups was comparable. Lastly, Lee and colleagues compared PROMs among DTI patients using the visual analog scale (VAS) and Disabilities of the Arm, Shoulder, and Hand (DASH) questionnaire.[108] The VAS aims to assess pain intensity during shoulder abduction motion, and DASH assesses abilities of the shoulder function; for both, higher score means worse pain, and thus, worse quality of life. The authors found that prepectoral patients had lower scores on both surveys than subpectoral patients at 2 weeks postoperatively, suggesting that subpectoral placement is associated with more pain.

Although breast reconstruction offers patients improved quality of life, patients may experience postoperative pain following reconstructive surgery.[109,110] In addition, patients who are younger, undergo bilateral procedures, have comorbid anxiety or depression, have IBBR (vs autologous reconstruction or no reconstruction), or are afflicted by more severe preoperative pain are more likely to have more severe acute postoperative pain.[38,111,112] In addition to the PROM studies on pain discussed above, a comprehensive examination of the literature found that most authors report significantly lower patient-reported pain in prepectoral patient groups than subpectoral comparators.[25,43,46,113–116] Studies have also found that prepectoral placement is associated with decreased postoperative ketorolac use and decreased inpatient opioid use postoperatively.[56,117] This is unsurprising since the morbidity produced by muscular manipulation was an integral part of the shift back to prepectoral reconstruction.

Current literature indicates that patients may experience similar quality of life and satisfaction whether they opt for prepectoral or subpectoral placement. Unfortunately, most of the reports on this subject are short-term studies. Our research group is currently investigating differences in long-term clinical and patient-reported outcomes by implant pocket in two-stage IBBR patients. It is possible that our data may show differences exist in the long term.

QUESTIONS LEFT TO BE ANSWERED

Comprehensive examinations of clinical, patient-reported, and functional outcomes after prepectoral and subpectoral breast reconstruction are currently underway or are planned to begin as randomized clinical trials (ClinicalTrials.gov Identifiers:

NCT03959709, NCT04874402, NCT05527769, NCT04293146, NCT04842240, NCT04477538). One of these studies (NCT03959709) compares single-stage IBBR patients by plane of implant placement, while another (NCT04874402) compares two-stage reconstruction patients. Some of these additional studies examining pain and functional outcomes may contribute to optimization of postoperative pain management for these patients. In addition, at our institution, there is active investigation into the benefits and drawbacks of ADM use in prepectoral breast reconstruction (ClinicalTrials.gov Identifier: NCT05316324).

SUMMARY AND CLINICS CARE POINTS

Choosing the plane of dissection is a staged process with important clinical decision points both preoperatively and intraoperatively. Preoperatively, patients with risk factors for wound healing problems and/or impaired mastectomy skin flap perfusion should not be considered candidates for prepectoral reconstruction; these risk factors include peripheral vascular disease, poorly controlled diabetes, active or recent smoking, obesity, connective tissue disorders, and preoperative radiation.[35] Although preoperative radiation is a contraindication to prepectoral placement, PMRT may favor prepectoral placement due to evidence of a similar complication profile with less capsular contracture than subpectoral placement in this population.[35,118]

The candidacy of patients who are thought to be appropriate for prepectoral placement must be reevaluated intraoperatively following the mastectomy, as perfusion of the mastectomy skin flap will ultimately dictate whether planned prepectoral implant placement may proceed. If the mastectomy skin flap shows signs of poor perfusion in areas that cannot be excised (eg, not at the flap margin), either by clinical assessment of dermal bleeding and flap thickness or via ICG angiography, prepectoral placement is not advised due to increased risk of infection and exposure if the mastectomy skin becomes nonviable. Although beyond the scope of this chapter, this principle also extends to DTI reconstruction; if mastectomy skin flap perfusion is questionable, the device should not be placed directly under the skin (ie, prepectoral) or in a manner that places pressure on the skin (ie, DTI) to minimize complications and allow the skin to revascularize.

DISCLOSURE

The authors have nothing to disclose.

REFERENCES

1. Surgeons ASoP. Plastic Surgery Statistics Report. Available at: https://www.plasticsurgery.org/documents/News/Statistics/2020/plastic-surgery-statistics-full-report-2020.pdf. Accessed February 17, 2023.
2. Broyles JM, Balk EM, Adam GP, et al. Implant-based versus Autologous Reconstruction after Mastectomy for Breast Cancer: A Systematic Review and Meta-analysis. Plast Reconstr Surg Glob Open 2022;10(3):e4180.
3. Polanco TO, Shamsunder MG, Parikh RP, et al. Quality-of-Life Outcomes in Autologous and Implant-Based Breast Reconstruction Patients Following Post-Mastectomy Radiation to the Tissue Expander: A Propensity Matched Preliminary Analysis. Plast Reconstr Surg 2023. https://doi.org/10.1097/PRS.0000000000010249.
4. Asaad M, Mitchell D, Murphy B, et al. Surgical Outcomes of Implant versus Autologous Breast Reconstruction in Patients with Previous Breast-Conserving Surgery and Radiotherapy. Plast Reconstr Surg 2023;151(2):190e–9e.

5. Halani SH, Jones K, Liu Y, et al. Reconstructive Burnout after Mastectomy: Implications for Patient Selection. Plast Reconstr Surg 2023;151(1):13e–9e.
6. Sawyer JD, Franke J, Scaife S, et al. Autologous Breast Reconstruction is Associated with Lower 90-day Readmission Rates. Plast Reconstr Surg Glob Open 2022;10(2):e4112.
7. Thompson PW, Carlson GW. Chap 59: Breast reconstruction: prosthetic techniques. In: Chung KC, editor. Grabb and Smith's plastic surgery. 8th edition. Philadelphia, PA: Wolters Kluwer; 2020. p. 2076–110.
8. Huo J, Smith BD, Giordano SH, et al. A comparison of patient-centered economic and clinical outcomes of post-mastectomy breast reconstruction between obese and non-obese patients. Breast 2016;30:118–24.
9. Woerdeman LA, Hage JJ, Hofland MM, et al. A prospective assessment of surgical risk factors in 400 cases of skin-sparing mastectomy and immediate breast reconstruction with implants to establish selection criteria. Plast Reconstr Surg 2007;119(2):455–63.
10. Blok YL, van Lierop E, Plat VD, et al. Implant Loss and Associated Risk Factors following Implant-based Breast Reconstructions. Plast Reconstr Surg Glob Open 2021;9(7):e3708.
11. Fischer JP, Nelson JA, Serletti JM, et al. Peri-operative risk factors associated with early tissue expander (TE) loss following immediate breast reconstruction (IBR): a review of 9305 patients from the 2005-2010 ACS-NSQIP datasets. J Plast Reconstr Aesthet Surg 2013;66(11):1504–12.
12. McCarthy CM, Mehrara BJ, Riedel E, et al. Predicting complications following expander/implant breast reconstruction: an outcomes analysis based on preoperative clinical risk. Plast Reconstr Surg 2008;121(6):1886–92.
13. Goodwin SJ, McCarthy CM, Pusic AL, et al. Complications in smokers after postmastectomy tissue expander/implant breast reconstruction. Ann Plast Surg 2005;55(1):16–9, discussion 19-20.
14. Coon D, Tuffaha S, Christensen J, et al. Plastic surgery and smoking: a prospective analysis of incidence, compliance, and complications. Plast Reconstr Surg 2013;131(2):385–91.
15. Hart A, Funderburk CD, Chu CK, et al. The Impact of Diabetes Mellitus on Wound Healing in Breast Reconstruction. Ann Plast Surg 2017;78(3):260–3.
16. Nahabedian MY. Implant-based breast reconstruction: Strategies to achieve optimal outcomes and minimize complications. J Surg Oncol 2016;113(8):895–905.
17. Glatt BS, Afifi G, Noone RB. Long-term follow-up of a sponge breast implant and review of the literature. Ann Plast Surg 1999;42(2):196–201.
18. Snyderman RK, Guthrie RH. Reconstruction of the female breast following radical mastectomy. Plast Reconstr Surg 1971;47(6):565–7.
19. Rebowe RE, Allred LJ, Nahabedian MY. The Evolution from Subcutaneous to Prepectoral Prosthetic Breast Reconstruction. Plast Reconstr Surg Glob Open 2018;6(6):e1797.
20. Schlenker JD, Bueno RA, Ricketson G, et al. Loss of silicone implants after subcutaneous mastectomy and reconstruction. Plast Reconstr Surg 1978;62(6):853–61.
21. Frey JD, Salibian AA, Karp NS, et al. Implant-Based Breast Reconstruction: Hot Topics, Controversies, and New Directions. Plast Reconstr Surg 2019;143(2):404e–16e.

22. Gruber RP, Kahn RA, Lash H, et al. Breast reconstruction following mastectomy: a comparison of submuscular and subcutaneous techniques. Plast Reconstr Surg 1981;67(3):312–7.
23. Sbitany H. Pre-pectoral breast reconstruction: a less invasive option. Gland Surg 2019;8(1):1–2.
24. Plachinski SJ, Boehm LM, Adamson KA, et al. Comparative Analysis of Prepectoral versus Subpectoral Implant-based Breast Reconstruction. Plast Reconstr Surg Glob Open 2021;9(7):e3709.
25. Walia GS, Aston J, Bello R, et al. Prepectoral Versus Subpectoral Tissue Expander Placement: A Clinical and Quality of Life Outcomes Study. Plast Reconstr Surg Glob Open 2018;6(4):e1731.
26. Sbitany H, Sandeen SN, Amalfi AN, et al. Acellular dermis-assisted prosthetic breast reconstruction versus complete submuscular coverage: a head-to-head comparison of outcomes. Plast Reconstr Surg 2009;124(6):1735–40.
27. Smith L. Where will your breast implants be placed?. Available at: https://www.plasticsurgery.org/news/blog/where-will-your-breast-implants-be-placed   Accessed February 17, 2023.
28. Dyrberg DL, Bille C, Koudahl V, et al. Evaluation of Breast Animation Deformity following Pre- and Subpectoral Direct-to-Implant Breast Reconstruction: A Randomized Controlled Trial. Arch Plast Surg 2022;49(5):587–95.
29. Fracol M, Feld LN, Chiu WK, et al. An overview of animation deformity in prosthetic breast reconstruction. Gland Surg 2019;8(1):95–101.
30. Kim JYS, Qiu CS, Chiu WK, et al. A Quantitative Analysis of Animation Deformity in Prosthetic Breast Reconstruction. Plast Reconstr Surg 2019;144(2):291–301.
31. Li Y, Xu G, Yu N, et al. Prepectoral Versus Subpectoral Implant-Based Breast Reconstruction: A Meta-analysis. Ann Plast Surg 2020;85(4):437–47.
32. Sbitany H, Piper M, Lentz R. Prepectoral Breast Reconstruction: A Safe Alternative to Submuscular Prosthetic Reconstruction following Nipple-Sparing Mastectomy. Plast Reconstr Surg 2017;140(3):432–43.
33. Sigalove S, Maxwell GP, Sigalove NM, et al. Prepectoral Implant-Based Breast Reconstruction: Rationale, Indications, and Preliminary Results. Plast Reconstr Surg 2017;139(2):287–94.
34. Goodreau AM, Driscoll CR, Nye A, et al. Revising Prepectoral Breast Reconstruction. Plast Reconstr Surg 2022;149(3):579–84.
35. Graziano FD, Lu J, Sbitany H. Prepectoral Breast Reconstruction. Clin Plast Surg 2023;50(2):235–42.
36. Duggal CS, Madni T, Losken A. An outcome analysis of intraoperative angiography for postmastectomy breast reconstruction. Aesthet Surg J 2014;34(1):61–5.
37. Holland M, Su P, Piper M, et al. Prepectoral Breast Reconstruction Reduces Opioid Consumption and Pain After Mastectomy: A Head-to-Head Comparison With Submuscular Reconstruction. Ann Plast Surg 2022;89(5):492–9.
38. Wallace MS, Wallace AM, Lee J, et al. Pain after breast surgery: a survey of 282 women. Pain 1996;66(2–3):195–205.
39. Bozzuto LM, Bartholomew AJ, Tung S, et al. Decreased postoperative pain and opioid use following prepectoral versus subpectoral breast reconstruction after mastectomy: A retrospective cohort study: Pain after pre- versus subpectoral reconstruction. J Plast Reconstr Aesthet Surg 2021;74(8):1763–9.
40. Marks JM, Farmer RL, Afifi AM. Current Trends in Prepectoral Breast Reconstruction: A Survey of American Society of Plastic Surgeons Members. Plast Reconstr Surg Glob Open 2020;8(8):e3060.

41. Becker H, Fregosi N. The Impact of Animation Deformity on Quality of Life in Post-Mastectomy Reconstruction Patients. Aesthet Surg J 2017;37(5):531–6.

42. Kobraei EM, Cauley R, Gadd M, et al. Avoiding Breast Animation Deformity with Pectoralis-Sparing Subcutaneous Direct-to-Implant Breast Reconstruction. Plast Reconstr Surg Glob Open 2016;4(5):e708.

43. Yang JY, Kim CW, Lee JW, et al. Considerations for patient selection: Prepectoral versus subpectoral implant-based breast reconstruction. Arch Plast Surg 2019; 46(6):550–7.

44. Samra F, Sobti N, Nelson JA, et al. Frontiers in Oncologic Reconstruction. Plast Reconstr Surg Glob Open. Jun 2019;7(6):e2181.

45. Kraenzlin F, Darrach H, Khavanin N, et al. Tissue Expander-Based Breast Reconstruction in the Prepectoral Versus Subpectoral Plane: An Analysis of Short-Term Outcomes. Ann Plast Surg 2021;86(1):19–23.

46. Wormer BA, Valmadrid AC, Ganesh Kumar N, et al. Reducing Expansion Visits in Immediate Implant-Based Breast Reconstruction: A Comparative Study of Prepectoral and Subpectoral Expander Placement. Plast Reconstr Surg 2019; 144(2):276–86.

47. de Blacam C, Momoh AO, Colakoglu S, et al. Cost analysis of implant-based breast reconstruction with acellular dermal matrix. Ann Plast Surg 2012;69(5): 516–20.

48. Cil TD, McCready D. Modern Approaches to the Surgical Management of Malignant Breast Disease: The Role of Breast Conservation, Complete Mastectomy, Skin- and Nipple-Sparing Mastectomy. Clin Plast Surg 2018;45(1):1–11.

49. Manrique OJ, Kapoor T, Banuelos J, et al. Single-Stage Direct-to-Implant Breast Reconstruction: A Comparison Between Subpectoral Versus Prepectoral Implant Placement. Ann Plast Surg 2020;84(4):361–5.

50. Baker BG, Irri R, MacCallum V, et al. A Prospective Comparison of Short-Term Outcomes of Subpectoral and Prepectoral Strattice-Based Immediate Breast Reconstruction. Plast Reconstr Surg 2018;141(5):1077–84.

51. Caputo GG, Zingaretti N, Kiprianidis I, et al. Quality of Life and Early Functional Evaluation in Direct-to-Implant Breast Reconstruction After Mastectomy: A Comparative Study Between Prepectoral Versus Dual-Plane Reconstruction. Clin Breast Cancer 2021;21(4):344–51.

52. Franceschini G, Scardina L, Di Leone A, et al. Immediate Prosthetic Breast Reconstruction after Nipple-Sparing Mastectomy: Traditional Subpectoral Technique versus Direct-to-Implant Prepectoral Reconstruction without Acellular Dermal Matrix. J Pers Med 2021;11(2). https://doi.org/10.3390/jpm11020153.

53. Mirhaidari SJ, Azouz V, Wagner DS. Prepectoral Versus Subpectoral Direct to Implant Immediate Breast Reconstruction. Ann Plast Surg 2020;84(3):263–70.

54. Abbate O, Rosado N, Sobti N, et al. Meta-analysis of prepectoral implant-based breast reconstruction: guide to patient selection and current outcomes. Breast Cancer Res Treat 2020;182(3):543–54.

55. King CA, Bartholomew AJ, Sosin M, et al. A Critical Appraisal of Late Complications of Prepectoral versus Subpectoral Breast Reconstruction Following Nipple-Sparing Mastectomy. Ann Surg Oncol 2021;28(13):9150–8.

56. Nelson JA, Shamsunder MG, Vorstenbosch J, et al. Prepectoral and Subpectoral Tissue Expander-Based Breast Reconstruction: A Propensity-Matched Analysis of 90-Day Clinical and Health-Related Quality-of-Life Outcomes. Plast Reconstr Surg 2022;149(4):607e–16e.

57. Walker NJ, Park JG, Maus JC, et al. Prepectoral Versus Subpectoral Breast Reconstruction in High-Body Mass Index Patients. Ann Plast Surg 2021;87(2): 136–43.

58. Fischer JP, Nelson JA, Kovach SJ, et al. Impact of obesity on outcomes in breast reconstruction: analysis of 15,937 patients from the ACS-NSQIP datasets. J Am Coll Surg 2013;217(4):656–64.

59. Panayi AC, Agha RA, Sieber BA, et al. Impact of Obesity on Outcomes in Breast Reconstruction: A Systematic Review and Meta-Analysis. J Reconstr Microsurg 2018;34(5):363–75.

60. Srinivasa DR, Clemens MW, Qi J, et al. Obesity and Breast Reconstruction: Complications and Patient-Reported Outcomes in a Multicenter, Prospective Study. Plast Reconstr Surg 2020;145(3):481e–90e.

61. Ooi BNS, Loh H, Ho PJ, et al. The genetic interplay between body mass index, breast size and breast cancer risk: a Mendelian randomization analysis. Int J Epidemiol 2019;48(3):781–94.

62. Duggal CS, Grudziak J, Metcalfe DB, et al. The effects of breast size in unilateral postmastectomy breast reconstruction. Ann Plast Surg 2013;70(5):506–12.

63. Davies K, Allan L, Roblin P, et al. Factors affecting post-operative complications following skin sparing mastectomy with immediate breast reconstruction. Breast 2011;20(1):21–5.

64. Lauritzen E, Damsgaard TE. Use of Indocyanine Green Angiography decreases the risk of complications in autologous- and implant-based breast reconstruction: A systematic review and meta-analysis. J Plast Reconstr Aes 2021;74(8): 1703–17.

65. Frey JD, Salibian AA, Choi M, et al. Mastectomy Flap Thickness and Complications in Nipple-Sparing Mastectomy: Objective Evaluation using Magnetic Resonance Imaging. Plast Reconstr Surg Glob Open 2017;5(8):e1439.

66. Salibian AA, Frey JD, Karp NS. Strategies and considerations in selecting between subpectoral and prepectoral breast reconstruction. Gland Surg 2019; 8(1):11–8.

67. Brett EA, Aitzetmuller MM, Sauter MA, et al. Breast cancer recurrence after reconstruction: know thine enemy. Oncotarget 2018;9(45):27895–906.

68. Margulies IG, Salzberg CA. The use of acellular dermal matrix in breast reconstruction: evolution of techniques over 2 decades. Gland Surgery 2019; 8(1):3–10.

69. Mihalecko J, Bohac M, Danisovic L, et al. Acellular Dermal Matrix in Plastic and Reconstructive Surgery. Physiol Res 2022;71(Suppl 1):S51–7.

70. Fosnot J, Kovach SJ, Serletti JM. Acellular Dermal Matrix: General Principles for the Plastic Surgeon. Aesthetic Surgery Journal 2011;31(7):5s–12s.

71. Bindingnavele V, Gaon M, Ota KS, et al. Use of acellular cadaveric dermis and tissue expansion in postmastectomy breast reconstruction. J Plast Reconstr Aesthet Surg 2007;60(11):1214–8.

72. Sbitany H, Langstein HN. Acellular dermal matrix in primary breast reconstruction. Aesthet Surg J 2011;31(7 Suppl):30S–7S.

73. Nahabedian MY. Acellular Dermal Matrices in Primary Breast Reconstruction: Principles, Concepts, and Indications. Plast Reconstr SurgSurgery 2012; 130(5):44s–53s.

74. Luo J, Moss WD, Pires GR, et al. A Nationwide Analysis Evaluating the Safety of Using Acellular Dermal Matrix with Tissue Expander-Based Breast Reconstruction. Arch Plast Surg 2022;49(6):716–23.

75. Gravina PR, Pettit RW, Davis MJ, et al. Evidence for the Use of Acellular Dermal Matrix in Implant-Based Breast Reconstruction. Semin Plast Surg 2019;33(4): 229–35.

76. Collis GN, TerKonda SP, Waldorf JC, et al. Acellular dermal matrix slings in tissue expander breast reconstruction: are there substantial benefits? Ann Plast Surg 2012;68(5):425–8.

77. Scheflan M, Allweis TM, Ben Yehuda D, et al. Meshed Acellular Dermal Matrix in Immediate Prepectoral Implant-based Breast Reconstruction. Plast Reconstr Surg Glob Open 2020;8(11):e3265.

78. Onesti MG, Di Taranto G, Ribuffo D, et al. ADM-assisted prepectoral breast reconstruction and skin reduction mastectomy: Expanding the indications for subcutaneous reconstruction. J Plast Reconstr Aesthet Surg 2020;73(4): 673–80.

79. Wazir U, Mokbel K. The Evolving Role of Pre-pectoral ADM-assisted Approach in Implant-based Immediate Breast Reconstruction Following Conservative Mastectomy: An Overview of the Literature and Description of Technique. In Vivo 2018;32(6):1477–80.

80. Sbitany H. Important Considerations for Performing Prepectoral Breast Reconstruction. Plast Reconstr Surg 2017;140(6):7s–13s.

81. Craig ES, Clemens MW, Koshy JC, et al. Outcomes of Acellular Dermal Matrix for Immediate Tissue Expander Reconstruction with Radiotherapy: A Retrospective Cohort Study. Aesthet Surg J 2019;39(3):279–88.

82. Wilson RL, Kirwan CC, Johnson RK, et al. Breast Reconstruction Outcomes With and without StratticE (BROWSE)- Long-term outcomes of a multi-centre study comparing Strattice TM immediate implant breast reconstruction with submuscular implant reconstruction. Plast Reconstr Surg 2023. https://doi.org/10.1097/PRS.0000000000010157.

83. Basu CB, Leong M, Hicks MJ. Acellular cadaveric dermis decreases the inflammatory response in capsule formation in reconstructive breast surgery. Plast Reconstr Surg 2010;126(6):1842–7.

84. Lohmander F, Lagergren J, Johansson H, et al. Effect of Immediate Implant-Based Breast Reconstruction After Mastectomy With and Without Acellular Dermal Matrix Among Women With Breast Cancer: A Randomized Clinical Trial. JAMA Netw Open 2021;4(10):e2127806.

85. Hong HK, Kim YH, Lee JS, et al. Prepectoral breast reconstruction with complete anterior implant coverage using a single, large, square-shaped acellular dermal matrix. Bmc Surg 2022;22(1). https://doi.org/10.1186/s12893-022-01683-z.

86. Ganesh Kumar N, Berlin NL, Kim HM, et al. Development of an evidence-based approach to the use of acellular dermal matrix in immediate expander-implant-based breast reconstruction. J Plast Reconstr Aesthet Surg 2021;74(1):30–40.

87. Antony AK, McCarthy CM, Cordeiro PG, et al. Acellular human dermis implantation in 153 immediate two-stage tissue expander breast reconstructions: determining the incidence and significant predictors of complications. Plast Reconstr Surg 2010;125(6):1606–14.

88. Mangialardi ML, Salgarello M, Cacciatore P, et al. Complication Rate of Prepectoral Implant-based Breast Reconstruction Using Human Acellular Dermal Matrices. Plast Reconstr Surg Glob Open 2020;8(12):e3235.

89. Singla A, Singla A, Lai E, et al. Subcutaneously Placed Breast Implants after a Skin-Sparing Mastectomy: Do We Always Need ADM? Plast Reconstr Surg Glob Open 2017;5(7):e1371.

90. Salibian AA, Bekisz JM, Kussie HC, et al. Do We Need Support in Prepectoral Breast Reconstruction? Comparing Outcomes with and without ADM. Plast Reconstr Surg Glob Open 2021;9(8):e3745.

91. Khavanin N, Qiu C, Darrach H, et al. Intraoperative Perfusion Assessment in Mastectomy Skin Flaps: How Close are We to Preventing Complications? Journal of Reconstructive Microsurgery 2019;35(7):471–8.

92. Munabi NCO, Olorunnipa OB, Goltsman D, et al. The ability of intra-operative perfusion mapping with laser-assisted indocyanine green angiography to predict mastectomy flap necrosis in breast reconstruction: A prospective trial. J Plast Reconstr Aes 2014;67(4):449–55.

93. Liu EH, Zhu SL, Hu J, et al. Intraoperative SPY Reduces Post-mastectomy Skin Flap Complications: A Systematic Review and Meta-Analysis. Plast Reconstr Surg Glob Open 2019;7(4):e2060.

94. Pagliara D, Schiavone L, Garganese G, et al. Predicting Mastectomy Skin Flap Necrosis: A Systematic Review of Preoperative and Intraoperative Assessment Techniques. Clin Breast Cancer 2023. https://doi.org/10.1016/j.clbc.2022.12.021.

95. Lauritzen E, Bredgaard R, Bonde C, et al. Indocyanine green angiography in breast reconstruction: a narrative review. Annals of Breast Surgery 2021;6.

96. Burnier P, Niddam J, Bosc R, et al. Indocyanine green applications in plastic surgery: A review of the literature. J Plast Reconstr Aesthet Surg 2017;70(6):814–27.

97. Jones GE, King VA, Yoo A, et al. Use of New Technologies in Implant-Based Breast Reconstruction. Semin Plast Surg 2019;33(4):258–63.

98. Johnson AC, Colakoglu S, Chong TW, et al. Indocyanine Green Angiography in Breast Reconstruction: Utility, Limitations, and Search for Standardization. Plast Reconstr Surg Glob Open 2020;8(3):e2694.

99. Phillips BT, Lanier ST, Conkling N, et al. Intraoperative Perfusion Techniques Can Accurately Predict Mastectomy Skin Flap Necrosis in Breast Reconstruction: Results of a Prospective Trial. Plast Reconstr Surg 2012;129(5):778e–88e.

100. Sood M, Glat P. Potential of the SPY intraoperative perfusion assessment system to reduce ischemic complications in immediate postmastectomy breast reconstruction. Ann Surg Innov Res 2013;7(1):9.

101. Ostapenko E, Nixdorf L, Devyatko Y, et al. Prepectoral Versus Subpectoral Implant-Based Breast Reconstruction: A Systemic Review and Meta-analysis. Ann Surg Oncol 2023;30(1):126–36.

102. Sinnott CJ, Persing SM, Pronovost M, et al. Impact of Postmastectomy Radiation Therapy in Prepectoral Versus Subpectoral Implant-Based Breast Reconstruction. Ann Surg Oncol 2018;25(10):2899–908.

103. Lentz R, Alcon A, Sbitany H. Correction of animation deformity with subpectoral to prepectoral implant exchange. Gland Surg 2019;8(1):75–81.

104. Manrique OJ, Banuelos J, Abu-Ghname A, et al. Surgical Outcomes of Prepectoral Versus Subpectoral Implant-based Breast Reconstruction in Young Women. Plast Reconstr Surg Glob Open 2019;7(3):e2119.

105. Escandon JM, Sweitzer K, Christiano JG, et al. Subpectoral versus prepectoral two-stage breast reconstruction: A propensity score-matched analysis of 30-day morbidity and long-term outcomes. J Plast Reconstr Aesthet Surg 2023;76:76–87.

106. Mundy LR, Homa K, Klassen AF, et al. Breast Cancer and Reconstruction: Normative Data for Interpreting the BREAST-Q. Plast Reconstr Surg 2017;139(5):1046e–55e.

107. Le NK, Persing S, Dinis J, et al. A Comparison of BREAST-Q Scores between Prepectoral and Subpectoral Direct-to-Implant Breast Reconstruction. Plastic and Reconstructive Surgery 2021;148(5):708e–14e.

108. Lee JS, Park E, Lee JH, et al. A prospective comparison study of early functional outcomes after implant-based breast reconstruction: subpectoral versus prepectoral technique. Ann Palliat Med 2021;10(3):2520–9.

109. Atisha D, Alderman AK, Lowery JC, et al. Prospective analysis of long-term psychosocial outcomes in breast reconstruction: two-year postoperative results from the Michigan Breast Reconstruction Outcomes Study. Ann Surg 2008; 247(6):1019–28.

110. Shiraishi M, Sowa Y, Tsuge I, et al. Long-Term Patient Satisfaction and Quality of Life Following Breast Reconstruction Using the BREAST-Q: A Prospective Cohort Study. Front Oncol 2022;12:815498.

111. Gassman AA, Yoon AP, Maxhimer JB, et al. Comparison of postoperative pain control in autologous abdominal free flap versus implant-based breast reconstructions. Plast Reconstr Surg 2015;135(2):356–67.

112. Kulkarni AR, Pusic AL, Hamill JB, et al. Factors Associated with Acute Postoperative Pain Following Breast Reconstruction. JPRAS Open 2017;11:1–13.

113. Campbell CA, Losken A. Understanding the Evidence and Improving Outcomes with Implant-Based Prepectoral Breast Reconstruction. Plast Reconstr Surg 2021;148(3):437e–50e.

114. Schaeffer CV, Dassoulas KR, Thuman J, et al. Early Functional Outcomes After Prepectoral Breast Reconstruction A Case-Matched Cohort Study. Ann Plas Surg 2019;82:S399–403.

115. Cattelani L, Polotto S, Arcuri MF, et al. One-Step Prepectoral Breast Reconstruction With Dermal Matrix-Covered Implant Compared to Submuscular Implantation: Functional and Cost Evaluation. Clin Breast Cancer 2018;18(4):E703–11.

116. Zhu L, Mohan AT, Abdelsattar JM, et al. Comparison of subcutaneous versus submuscular expander placement in the first stage of immediate breast reconstruction. J Plast Reconstr Aes 2016;69(4):E77–86.

117. Darrach H, Kraenzlin FS, Khavanin N, et al. Pectoral placement of tissue expanders affects inpatient opioid use. Breast J 2021;27(2):126–33.

118. Sigalove S. Prepectoral breast reconstruction and radiotherapy-a closer look. Gland Surg 2019;8(1):67–74.

Incorporating Value-Based Decisions in Breast Cancer Treatment Algorithms

Ton Wang, MD, MS[a], Lesly A. Dossett, MD, MPH[b,c],*

KEYWORDS

- Breast cancer • De-implementation • Overtreatment • Value in health care
- Cancer care continuum

KEY POINTS

- Patients with early-stage breast cancer have an excellent prognosis and are at risk of overtreatment.
- There are many evidence-based opportunities to improve value across the breast cancer care continuum, requiring thoughtful approaches to breast cancer screening, diagnostics, surgical oncology, medical oncology, and radiation oncology.
- Value-based decisions in breast cancer care offer the opportunity to improve patient outcomes while minimizing the risks associated with low-value services.

INTRODUCTION: DEFINING "VALUE" IN BREAST CANCER CARE

Value in health care is measured by improvements in patient health outcomes relative to the cost of achieving that result.[1] This definition is centered around the patient, with the expectation that health-care services rendered provide a measurable benefit. While the goal of achieving high-value care is often mistaken for pure cost-saving efforts, the emphasis is on the delivery of appropriate but not excessive or potentially harmful care.

The United States spends $760 to 935 billion annually on health-care waste.[2] A significant and avoidable sector of waste is low-value care, defined as unnecessary tests, procedures, medications, or other services resulting in increased health-care expenditures without a clinically meaningful benefit. This issue is particularly important in cancer care which was estimated in 2019 to cost Americans over $21 billion annually in out-of-pocket costs and lost wages.[3] Of all cancer types, the costs associated with breast cancer diagnosis and survivorship is the greatest, with risks of financial toxicity present long after the initial diagnosis.[4,5]

[a] Department of Surgery, Cedars-Sinai Medical Center, Los Angeles, CA, USA; [b] Department of Surgery, University of Michigan, Ann Arbor, MI, USA; [c] Institute for Healthcare Policy and Innovation, University of Michigan, 1500 East Medical Center Drive, Ann Arbor, MI 48109, USA
* Corresponding author.
E-mail address: ldossett@umich.edu

Surg Oncol Clin N Am 32 (2023) 777–797
https://doi.org/10.1016/j.soc.2023.05.008
1055-3207/23/© 2023 Elsevier Inc. All rights reserved.

surgonc.theclinics.com

There are numerous opportunities to improve value in breast cancer care. The delivery of high-value care requires balancing patient preferences with evidence-based practice to develop a high-value approach. This review summarizes the current literature and recommends strategies to avoid overtreatment throughout the breast cancer care continuum with the goal of improving patient outcomes while minimizing the risks associated with low-value services.

IMPROVING VALUE-BASED DECISIONS IN SCREENING AND DIAGNOSTICS
Genetic Testing

Although most breast cancers are sporadic, approximately 5% to 10% are associated with a heritable syndrome.[6] The implications of diagnosing a pathogenic mutation have evolved with the introduction of new breast cancer therapies. Consequently, identifying high-penetrance mutations (BRCA1, BRCA2, CDH1, PALB2, PTEN, and TP53) has the potential to affect screening, surgical, and medical decision-making for patients and their family members. However, the potential benefits of genetic testing must be balanced against the overall low prevalence of high-penetrance pathogenic or likely variants (PGVs) and the potential consequences associated with identifying nonactionable mutations or variants of unknown significance (VUS).

Proponents of multigene panel testing for all breast cancer patients argue clear utility in identifying high-penetrance PGVs. In a prospective study of newly diagnosed breast cancer patients, results from genetic testing changed clinical management in more than 75% of patients.[7] While the majority of these changes were risk-reducing strategies such as high-risk screening, chemoprevention, or specialist referrals, patients with PGVs were also found to have alterations in surgical and chemotherapy strategies for their primary breast cancer. Notably, this study found similar numbers of PGVs and subsequent changes in clinical management in patients who both did and did not meet National Comprehensive Cancer Network (NCCN) screening guidelines. This is consistent with studies showing that traditional screening strategies relying on family history, patient age, or other risk factors miss up to 50% of all potentially actionable genetic mutations.[8,9]

While it was previously difficult to directly link genetic testing to improved patient survival, the OlympiA trial demonstrated improved progression-free survival with the Poly ADP-ribose polymerase (PARP) inhibitor Olaparib for germline BRCA1/2 patients with early-stage breast cancer.[10] This trial was particularly groundbreaking for utilizing targeted therapy in the adjuvant setting rather than in metastatic disease, underscoring a need to identify patients with actionable mutations earlier in their clinical course. In addition, the potential impact of diagnosing a PGV is not limited to a patient's initial breast cancer treatment. Patients with high-penetrance mutations for breast cancer are known to be at risk of other cancer types and should be counseled on the need for risk-reducing surgeries (eg, bilateral salpingo-oophorectomy for patients with BRCA1/2 mutations or total gastrectomy for patients with CDH1 mutations) and modified screening protocols for other cancer types.[11] Finally, the identification of a PGV in a breast cancer patient can trigger cascade genetic testing, in which relatives of an index patient are offered genetic testing. Although cascade testing is infrequently implemented, it is a cost-effective cancer-prevention strategy with the potential to exponentially impact surveillance and management strategies of at-risk individuals.[12]

Despite the potential advantages, there are several risks of universal multigene panel testing. Pretest and posttest genetic counseling provides patients with detailed risk assessments and has been shown to improve accuracy of risk perception and decrease cancer-related worry, anxiety, and depression.[13] As a result, candidates for genetic testing should be referred for appropriate counseling. The expanding indications for genetic testing have led to a national shortage of trained genetic counselors; estimates suggest there is only 1 genetic counselor per 300,000 people in the United States.[14] A fully implemented universal multigene panel testing strategy would exacerbate this issue and result in many patients who do not receive appropriate counseling about the implications of their testing results. Some strategies to expand the reach of genetic counseling include telemedicine visits, web-based patient education platforms, and specialized training of selected medical providers to serve as genetic counselor extenders.[15]

The costs of genetic testing have decreased significantly, and contemporary analyses suggest that a universal testing strategy can be cost-effective.[16] However, the costs of genetic testing are not limited to the test itself, and the indirect costs associated with identifying PGVs in low- to moderate-penetrance genes or VUS must be considered. In studies of multigene panel testing, up to 50% of patients can be found to have a VUS.[8] The identification of mutations for which guidelines do not support a change in breast cancer management has been shown to result in overtreatment, unindicated high-risk surveillance, and patient anxiety, all of which are costly and potentially harmful.[17] In one study of patients with BRCA1/2 VUS, nearly 40% of patients without a diagnosis of breast cancer received prophylactic bilateral mastectomies. In follow-up, 22% of patients underwent reclassification of their VUS, with 95% of reclassifications as benign.[18] Similarly, while current guidelines support bilateral mastectomy in patients with high-penetrance mutations, best practice for management of moderate-penetrance genes such as ATM and CHEK2 (2- to 4-fold increased risk of breast cancer) are less clear. Despite a lack of evidence to support prophylactic surgery in these patients, studies suggest nearly a third of patients without breast cancer and half of patients with breast cancer who have mutations in moderate-penetrance genes receive bilateral mastectomies, equivalent to that of patients with high-penetrance mutations.[19,20]

Breast Magnetic Resonance Imaging for Screening in Women at Average Risk

Breast magnetic resonance imaging (MRI) has emerged as an important imaging adjunct for patients because of its high sensitivity for cancer detection (95% vs 55% for mammogram).[21] Meta-analyses demonstrate that MRI can increase identification of additional malignancies, with the finding of a synchronous ipsilateral or contralateral cancer in up to 16% and 4% of patients, respectively.[22,23] While the role of MRI for breast cancer screening in high-risk patients (defined as >20% lifetime breast cancer risk) is well-established and cost-effective, population-based studies suggest more than 80% of patients undergoing screening breast MRI are patients at average risk.[24,25]

A potential reason why breast MRI utilization has increased dramatically in the last two decades is conflicting evidence as to whether breast MRI is a better screening tool in patients with dense breasts. Legislation in the United States requires patients to be notified if they have heterogeneously or extremely dense breasts; however, this includes nearly 50% of women in the age range of 40 to 74 years.[26] The DENSE trial in the Netherlands was the first randomized, controlled trial to specifically evaluate the role of breast MRI as an adjunct in patients with extremely dense breasts and normal screening mammograms.[27] Although this study demonstrated breast MRI results in increased detection of breast cancer over mammography alone, the variable sensitivity of breast MRI resulted in a false-positive rate of 8%.

Breast MRI is a costly study with an average payment of $1200, compared to $350 for diagnostic mammography, $130 for tomosynthesis, and $130 for ultrasound.[28] Abbreviated breast MRI has been proposed as a solution to decrease the time of image acquisition, study reading time, and subsequent cost of breast MRI to increase its value as a screening tool.[29] Abbreviated breast MRI, which relies on rapid protocols capturing the very early postcontrast phase, has equal sensitivity and specificity to traditional breast MRI in detecting breast cancer at a fraction of the time and cost. However, breast MRI is associated with significant care cascades that must be considered before widespread implementation of screening MRI. Studies have consistently demonstrated that receipt of breast MRI is an independent risk factor for surgical overtreatment with unilateral and contralateral mastectomy.[30,31] In addition, breast MRI recipients have significantly greater mammary and extramammary cascade events including additional imaging, procedures, clinic visits, hospitalizations, and new diagnoses with higher total and out-of-pocket spending.[32]

Screening in Asymptomatic Patients with a Limited Life Expectancy

None of the randomized controlled trials that established the efficacy of screening mammography included patients older than 74 years, and thus the value of breast cancer screening in elderly patients is unknown.[33] For breast cancer screening, meta-analyses demonstrate a lag-time of approximately 10 years to prevent 1 death per 1000 people screened, suggesting minimal utility of breast cancer screening in patients with a limited life expectancy.[34] Consequently, national guidelines recommend cessation of routine screening mammography in patients with a less than a 5- to 10-year life expectancy. Despite these recommendations, studies show that up to 53% of women with a high 9-year mortality risk receive screening mammography.[35]

The harms associated with breast cancer screening in women with limited life expectancy result from care cascades associated with a false-positive result and overdiagnosis of in-situ or low-risk carcinomas. Estimates suggest that over a 10-year screening period, 20% of women aged ≥75 years will experience a false-positive mammogram, which can result in additional imaging, unnecessary biopsies, and significant anxiety and distress.[36] In addition, women with a limited life expectancy are at high risk of overdiagnosis for low-risk breast cancers that may have never become symptomatic or otherwise impacted their quality of life.

The reasons for persistent breast cancer screening despite limited life-expectancy are multifactorial. Obtaining an annual mammogram as part of routine health care is an entrenched habit developed over several decades, and physician recommendation for screening cessation is insufficient to influence patient behavior.[37,38] This is supported by studies showing that among individuals who recall having had a discussion about screening cessation with their physician, 40% plan to continue cancer screening.[39] At least some patient hesitancy to trust recommendations for screening cessation is related to poor accuracy of clinician and patient survival predictions, with studies showing both groups overestimate life expectancy.[40,41] This bias is compounded by a tendency to overestimate the benefits and underestimate the risks of receiving a particular medical intervention.[42,43] Some strategies to deimplement breast cancer screening in older women with limited life expectancies include the incorporation of validated life-expectancy calculators, decision-aids, and reframing screening cessation from "taking something away" from patients to "redistributing health-care priorities".[44,45]

IMPROVING VALUE-BASED DECISIONS IN BREAST SURGICAL ONCOLOGY
Utilization of Outpatient Mastectomy and Enhanced Recovery After Surgery Protocols

The safety of outpatient mastectomy in patients undergoing bilateral mastectomies, modified radical mastectomy, and immediate implant-based breast reconstruction is well established, with systematic reviews showing no difference in major or minor complications, including rates of hematoma, seroma, reoperations, or readmissions for patients undergoing same-day unilateral or bilateral mastectomy with or without implant-based immediate reconstruction.[46] Outpatient surgery offers many benefits to health-care systems including significant cost savings and the opportunity to increase inpatient capacity for other admissions, an advantage that was notable during the COVID-19 pandemic.[47] In addition to financial benefits, outpatient surgery is associated with improved patient satisfaction, decreased opioid usage, decreased anxiety, and improved time to independence.[47,48]

Although same-day mastectomy has been shown to be feasible for over 20 years, only approximately 20% of mastectomies nationally are performed as outpatient procedures.[49] Unlike many other cancer operations such as pancreatectomies that are largely centralized in major medical centers, breast cancer operations are decentralized and therefore subject to significant variations in performance patterns. A recent study of facilities across the state of Michigan demonstrated that only 16% of mastectomies without reconstruction were performed as an outpatient procedure, and 23% of patients were admitted for 2 days or more.[50] These variations in practice patterns accounted for a nearly 2-fold difference in 30- and 90-day episode cost.

A commonly cited barrier to same-day mastectomy is the concern about inadequate pain control in the outpatient setting. This concern has largely been addressed through protocols for multimodal pain management based on Enhanced Recovery After Surgery principles.[51,52] There are several instances in which institutional implementation of outpatient protocols for same-day mastectomy with or without reconstruction have been highly successful. A notable example is the Kaiser Permanente Northern California group which instituted a pilot project across 21 medical centers to implement same-day unilateral or bilateral mastectomy with or without immediate breast reconstruction over a 6-month time period.[53] The protocol included preoperative patient education, multimodal analgesia, and a defined postoperative care plan and was highly successful, increasing same-day mastectomy rates from 16% to 75%.

De-escalation of Axillary Surgery in Breast Cancer Patients

Lymphedema occurs in 20% of patients after axillary lymph node dissection (ALND), with the risk doubling when combined with adjuvant chemotherapy or radiotherapy.[54,55] While the risks associated with ALND are well-accepted, long-term studies demonstrate that up to 5% of patients undergoing sentinel lymph node biopsy (SLNB) also develop lymphedema.[54] Long-term consequences of lymphedema include infectious complications, frequent utilization of outpatient medical services, significantly restricted mobility, reduced quality of life, and decreased psychosocial well-being.[56,57] In addition, lymphedema is a leading cause of financial toxicity in breast cancer survivors, accounting for decreased ability to return to work and up to 112% higher out-of-pocket costs up to 10 years after breast cancer diagnosis.[5,58] As a result, de-escalation of axillary surgery in appropriate circumstances has the potential to significantly improve long-term outcomes for breast cancer survivors.

Current evidence supports the de-escalation of axillary surgery in three circumstances. The first is avoiding ALND in patients with limited nodal disease who are undergoing breast-conserving surgery (BCS) with adjuvant radiotherapy. This recommendation is based on results from the ACOSOG Z0011 trial which demonstrated no improvement in disease-free or overall survival with completion ALND for patients with 1 to 2 positive sentinel lymph nodes.[59] The second is avoiding upfront ALND without attempting SLNB in patients with previously positive axillary lymph nodes who become clinically node negative (cN0) following neoadjuvant chemotherapy. This is based on the SENTINA and ACOSOG Z1071 trials which demonstrated the feasibility and accuracy of SLNB for axillary staging in these patients.[60,61] The final is avoiding routine SLNB in cN0 women ≥70 years old with estrogen-receptor-positive (ER+), HER2-negative (HER2−) early-stage breast cancer. This is based on the CALGB 9343 trial which demonstrated no improvement in breast-cancer-specific or overall survival with nodal staging.[62]

Current national trends suggest appropriate omission of completion ALND for patients undergoing BCS is excellent, with recent studies showing only 14% of patients who are potential candidates for omission of ALND receiving this procedure.[63] Similarly, national rates of SLNB in clinically node-positive patients who become cN0 following neoadjuvant chemotherapy have increased significantly from 30% in 2012 to 50% in 2015 following dissemination of clinical trial results, and the current rate of SLNB is likely much higher.[64] However, SLNB in older women with low-risk, cN0 breast cancer continues to be performed at high rates, with estimates suggesting that up to 87% of patients who are eligible of SLNB omission continue to receive this procedure.[63] In addition to the risk for lymphedema and other surgical complications associated with SLNB in women ≥70 years old, axillary staging at the time of breast cancer resection is associated with a 65% increase in 90-day episode cost and increased likelihood of care cascades, including a nearly 2-fold increase in postoperative radiotherapy for women who may have been candidates for omission of both axillary staging and radiotherapy.[65]

Potential patient-level barriers to the deimplementation of SLNB in older patients include a desire to know their pathological axillary status for "peace of mind," the perception they are healthier than average patient and more likely to benefit from additional therapies, and concern that age-based guidelines are discriminatory.[66] Some strategies to reduce low-value SLNB at the patient level include emphasizing the excellent prognosis associated with early-stage, ER+ breast cancer; educating patients on the risks of overtreatment; and improved decision-making tools such as decision aids.[66–68] Potential provider-level barriers to the deimplementation of SLNB in older patients with early-stage breast cancer include the belief that it is a low-risk procedure that adds minimal time to an operation and the misperception that the result of the biopsy will change adjuvant chemotherapy or radiotherapy recommendations.[69] However, the results of RxPONDER and supporting retrospective studies have increasingly emphasized that nodal status does not predict tumor biology and that recurrence scores based on genomic tests such as Oncotype Dx and Mammaprint more accurately predict benefit from adjuvant therapies.[70,71]

Contralateral Prophylactic Mastectomy in Average-Risk Patients with Unilateral Breast Cancer

The utilization of contralateral prophylactic mastectomy (CPM) has increased over the last two decades, with a greater proportion of patients electing for bilateral mastectomy after a diagnosis of breast cancer without a clear indication. Recent estimates suggesting that bilateral mastectomies comprise 10% to 13% of all breast cancer procedures and 28% to 30% of all mastectomy cases.[72] Notably, this trend includes patients with early stage or in situ breast cancers who would otherwise be excellent candidates for breast conservation therapy.[73]

The single greatest factor contributing to widespread utilization of CPM is the increasing availability of breast reconstruction.[73,74] In one analysis of women with unilateral breast cancer, 46% of patients who received CPM underwent breast reconstruction compared with 17% of patients who received unilateral mastectomy.[74] Compared with unilateral mastectomy, bilateral mastectomy with breast reconstruction is known to be an independent risk factor for major and minor postoperative complications including wound complications, need for reoperation, flap loss for patients undergoing autologous reconstruction, and longer length of stay.[75,76] In addition, despite more extensive oncologic surgery and potential history of radiation to the therapeutic side, the risk associated with a postoperative complication after bilateral mastectomy has been shown to be equivalent between the therapeutic and prophylactic side, with nearly 20% of patients experiencing a complication on the prophylactic breast.[77]

Unsurprisingly, CPM is associated with significantly higher costs than unilateral mastectomy during the index oncologic procedure and additional reconstructive procedures, particularly given the average patient requires 2 to 3 operations to complete breast reconstruction.[78–80] Cost-effectiveness studies have attempted to justify CPM given the potential savings associated with cessation of life-long screening surveillance.[81] However, the literature suggests many patients continue to receive non-evidence-based imaging surveillance following bilateral mastectomy.[82] Importantly, the financial burden of CPM is not limited to costs to the health-care system; compared with BCS, patients undergoing bilateral mastectomy report higher incurred debt, altered employment, and financial toxicity.[83]

The reasons for the increased popularity and high utilization of CPM are complex. Multiple studies have shown the decision for bilateral mastectomy to be preference sensitiveness and that patient-level factors driving an increase in CPM rates include a desire for "peace of mind," the misperception that a more intensive surgery will improve survival, and potential for improved symmetry.[84,85] No single strategy for the deimplementation of CPM exists. However, current evidence suggests definite gaps in patient preoperative education; studies suggest patients have poor understanding of the risks of bilateral mastectomy including increased postoperative complications, loss of skin and nipple sensation, and financial toxicity while simultaneously overestimating the oncologic benefit.[86,87]

IMPROVING VALUE-BASED DECISIONS IN MEDICAL ONCOLOGY
Routine Staging of Asymptomatic Patients at Low Risk of Metastatic Breast Cancer

National organizations advise against routine staging with CT, positron emission tomography (PET), or bone scans for asymptomatic patients with early-stage breast cancer based on evidence that only 0.2% and 1.2% of patients with stage I or II breast cancer, respectively, are found to have distant metastases on preoperative staging.[88] However, the risk of false-positive results or incidental findings associated with unnecessary diagnostic testing is costly and can result in harmful care cascades. Despite these recommendations, routine staging scans remain prevalent. In one study evaluating the utilization of staging chest CTs in patients with clinical stage I or II breast, 11% of stage I breast cancer patients and 36% of stage II breast cancer patients underwent a staging chest CT.[89] Although 23% of stage I patients were found to have pulmonary nodules, only 1% of all patients had pulmonary metastases. However, the finding of a pulmonary nodule resulted in an average of 2.3 follow-up CTs, with some patients followed up for several years with up to 16 additional CT scans.

Efforts from Choosing Wisely and American Society of Clinical Oncology to reduce unnecessary staging for patients diagnosed with early-stage breast cancer have had a modest impact, with time-series analyses of national data showing a 16% decline in imaging overutilization following the release of guidelines to avoid routine staging scans.[90] Similarly, state-wide registries have shown a significant decrease over time in utilization of staging scans for patients with stage 0-IIA breast cancer, but not stage IIB.[91] Greater deimplementation of routine staging for asymptomatic, early-stage breast cancer patients will require more than published guidelines; although studies suggest over 80% of physicians treating breast cancer are aware of guidelines recommending against routine staging, they are not influenced to order less imaging.[92] While this finding has been attributed to patient preferences, studies evaluating physician-level variation associated with overutilization found the odds of a patient receiving staging scans were 3-fold higher if the ordering physician's prior patient also received scans, suggesting provider-driven overutilization.[93]

Personalized Decision-Making for Adjuvant Chemotherapy

While the development of novel chemotherapeutic agents has resulted in improved survival for breast cancer patients, an equally ground-breaking advance has been the ability to leverage genomic testing to identify patients who can safely omit adjuvant chemotherapy. The TAILORx and RxPONDER trials demonstrated the utility of the 21-gene Oncotype Dx recurrence score in predicting the absolute benefit of adjuvant chemotherapy in patients with ER+/HER2− disease, shifting this decision from one that was largely based on anatomical staging to one based on tumor biology.[70,94] As a result, there has been a decrease in national rates of chemotherapy utilization, with one study showing a decline from 27% in 2013 to 14% in 2015 among patients with stage I-II ER+/HER2− disease and a decline from 81% to 64% among patients with node-positive disease.[95] This decrease in adjuvant chemotherapy administration has occurred concurrently with increased utilization of recurrence score tests.[96]

The routine incorporation of genomic tests into practice offers a key opportunity for improving value in breast cancer care. The benefit of this personalized approach is greatest in older patients who are the most vulnerable to the toxicities of chemotherapy. Simulations suggest older patients with hormone receptor (HR) positive breast cancer may experience negative quality-adjusted life-years if they receive chemotherapy compared with endocrine therapy alone.[97] Before RxPONDER, postmenopausal patients with node-positive disease would likely have been considered to be at high risk and recommended adjuvant chemotherapy. However, incorporating recurrence risk scores into the decision-making algorithm has significantly improved the likelihood that an individual patient will benefit from adjuvant chemotherapy.

IMPROVING VALUE-BASED DECISIONS IN RADIATION ONCOLOGY
Radiotherapy Omission in Older Patients with Low-Risk Breast Cancer

Although all breast cancer patients have traditionally been treated with the same combination of therapies, modern evidence suggests older women are more likely to be diagnosed with ER+ breast cancers with favorable tumor biology.[98] These tumors are associated with an excellent long-term prognosis, and the probability of a woman aged ≥70 years dying from breast cancer is less than 1%.[99] As a result, substantial evidence exists to support the de-escalation of certain adjuvant therapies, including radiotherapy, in this low-risk population.

There are two key trials supporting radiotherapy omission for older women with small, ER+ breast cancers. The CALGB 9343 trial randomized cN0 breast cancer patients aged ≥70 years with ER+ tumors ≤2 cm to endocrine therapy alone or whole-breast radiotherapy and endocrine therapy.[62] This was followed by the PRIME II trial, which randomized pathologically node-negative breast cancer patients aged ≥65 years with ER+ tumors ≤3 cm to endocrine therapy alone or whole-breast radiotherapy and endocrine therapy.[100] The findings from both trials confirmed an expected higher rate of locoregional recurrence for the cohorts treated without radiotherapy, but no difference in rates of salvage mastectomy, distant metastases, or breast-cancer-specific and overall survival. In fact, the 10-year breast-cancer-specific survival in the CALGB 9343 trial was >97%, regardless of radiotherapy receipt. These findings have led to additional efforts to expand the indications for adjuvant radiotherapy omission; the preliminary results of the LUMINA trial suggest patients aged ≥55 years with stage I, low- to intermediate-grade luminal A tumors receiving endocrine therapy can safely omit adjuvant radiotherapy after BCS with a 5-year local recurrence rate of only 2.3%.[101]

While the improvement in locoregional recurrence is often cited to justify adjuvant radiotherapy in this low-risk population, it is notable that the locoregional recurrence rate at 10 years in both CALGB 9343 and PRIME II, was 10%, which is within the accepted range for locoregional recurrence following breast cancer treatment.[62,100] In addition, the modern rate of locoregional recurrence is likely lower than reported in these trials, given these trials used tamoxifen for endocrine therapy rather than the more efficacious aromatase inhibitors typically used today.[102]

Importantly, women aged ≥70 years with cN0, stage I ER+ breast cancer should not be required to undergo SLNB to be considered for omission of adjuvant radiotherapy. CALGB 9343 did not require pathological confirmation of negative nodal status as an inclusion criterion.[62] This trial predated widespread utilization of SLNB, and two-thirds of patients did not undergo any axillary staging given the morbidity of ALND for staging purposes. This is further supported by retrospective studies suggesting adjuvant radiotherapy does not improve survival even in patients with pathologically node-positive lymph nodes if they receive endocrine therapy.[103]

Despite the strong data supporting the safety of radiotherapy omission in cN0 breast cancer patients aged ≥70 years with stage I ER+ tumors, up to 65% of patients eligible for omission continue to receive adjuvant radiotherapy after BCS, a trend that has remained stable since 2005 when the NCCN guidelines were updated to allow for radiotherapy omission in this low-risk population.[104] The overutilization of radiotherapy is costly; the estimated cost of radiotherapy ranges from $5300 per patient for accelerated partial-beam irradiation (APBI) to $13,000 for whole-breast radiation.[65,105] In addition to the financial consequences, older patients are at higher risk of experiencing significant decreases in quality of life with adjuvant radiotherapy, which is supported by studies showing that older women heavily consider the frequency of appointments required for radiotherapy and its impact on their caregivers.[66,106] While there are likely some patient-level factors contributing to the persistent utilization of radiotherapy in older women with low-risk breast cancer, studies have shown that if given the choice, most patients would decline radiotherapy.[66,107] Rather, the decision is heavily influenced by provider recommendations and a tendency for both patients and providers to overestimate the potential benefit of radiotherapy in improving locoregional recurrence rates.[106,108]

Shorter Radiation Therapy Schedules in Appropriate Patients

The original studies supporting adjuvant whole-breast irradiation following BCS used a conventional fractionation schedule delivering 1.8 to 2 Gy per fraction over 5 to 7 weeks. Since that time, multiple trials have demonstrated the efficacy of hypofractionation of whole-breast irradiation, which delivers a higher dose per fraction over 3 to 4 weeks, at providing equivalent locoregional control, cosmesis, and potentially reduced acute toxicities. In addition to improved patient convenience, hypofractionation is significantly cheaper.[109] Although the initial American Society for Radiation Oncology (ASTRO) guidelines in 2011 endorsed hypofractionation only for patients aged ≥50 years with pT1-2N0 tumors, updated guidelines in 2018 expanded the indications to recommend hypofractionated whole-breast irradiation delivered in 15 to 16 fractions as the preferred regimen for all breast cancer patients, regardless of age or tumor characteristics.

Despite the significant advantages of hypofractionated regimens, adoption in the United States has been slow, with studies showing conventional fractionation remains the most common method of delivery, with under 40% of patients receiving hypofractionation.[110] This contrasts significantly with the relatively quick adoption of hypofractionation schedules internationally, with shorter radiotherapy schedules the current standard of care in Canada and the United Kingdom.[110] Although there are relatively little data on national practice patterns over the last few years, there is some evidence that the resource-limited environment of the COVID-19 pandemic may have encouraged more widespread adoption of hypofractionation in the United States.[111]

Similarly, APBI offers another opportunity to personalize adjuvant radiotherapy for a subset of patients with low-risk tumor features. While randomized trials comparing APBI techniques via brachytherapy, external beam, or intraoperative radiation have demonstrated noninferiority when compared with whole-breast radiotherapy, APBI has been associated with poorer long-term cosmetic outcomes and worse long-term locoregional control for patients with higher-risk tumor features.[112,113] However, APBI is associated with significant cost savings compared with whole-breast irradiation, the shorter treatment schedule is more convenient for patients, and patients who are reluctant to accept adjuvant radiotherapy due to the concern for side effects may find APBI acceptable. As a result, ASTRO allows for APBI as an alternative to whole-breast irradiation following BCS in patients aged ≥50 years with Tis-T1 breast cancer and negative margins.[114]

IMPROVING VALUE-BASED DECISIONS IN POSTCANCER SURVEILLANCE
Breast Cancer Surveillance Recommendations for Detecting Locoregional Recurrence

Current national guidelines recommend annual mammography for locoregional surveillance for patients undergoing BCS. The recommendation for when to obtain the first mammogram after surgery differs, with some organizations suggesting that the first mammogram be obtained 6 months after surgery to establish a baseline and confirm removal of the imaging abnormality.[115] Although some institutions routinely perform semi-annual mammography for the first 2 to 5 years after BCS because of the higher risk of locoregional recurrence in the early postoperative years, there are no data to suggest this improves detection of locoregional recurrence compared with annual mammography.[116]

For patients undergoing mastectomy with or without reconstruction, there is some controversy about the appropriateness of imaging surveillance, with most national guidelines recommending against any routine imaging. An exception is the American College of Radiology, which states that surveillance mammography with or without digital breast tomosynthesis may be appropriate for patients undergoing mastectomy with tissue-based reconstruction.[117] No studies have demonstrated the cost-effectiveness of routine postmastectomy surveillance with mammography, breast ultrasound, or breast MRI when compared with clinical breast exam alone. A recent systematic review and meta-analysis demonstrated low yield of imaging surveillance following mastectomy with or with reconstruction, with an overall pooled cancer detection rate ranging from 1.9 per 1000 examinations for mammography to 5.2 per 1000 examinations for MRI.[82] For all imaging modalities, the rates of imaging-detected cancers were lower than the overall cancer detection rates, suggesting most cancers were clinically detected on physical exam.

Breast Cancer Surveillance Recommendations for Detecting Distant Recurrence

To date, there is no evidence that early detection of breast cancer metastasis improves breast-cancer-specific or overall survival.[118] Consequently, national guidelines recommend against routine imaging or laboratory testing for asymptomatic patients treated with a curative intent.[119] While it is notable these recommendations are based on older studies that predate current imaging techniques, improved understanding of tumor biology, and modern systemic therapies, an updated Cochrane review in 2016 again did not support routine surveillance imaging.[120] A recent study evaluating outcomes of patients with recurrent disease detected on surveillance imaging versus symptoms showed a potential survival benefit with detection of recurrence on imaging for patients with high-risk tumor subtypes (HER2+, triple negative breast cancers), but no benefit for patients with ER+, HER2− breast cancers.[121]

Utilization of surveillance imaging such as PET-CT scans and radionuclide bone scans vary widely among providers. In addition to being costly and associated with false-positive findings, these studies are frequently no better than physical exam alone. For example, most bony metastases are diagnosed based on symptoms rather than imaging.[122] Similarly, tumor markers such as CA 1503, CA 27.29, CEA, and "liquid biopsies" have not been shown to be sensitive nor specific and can lead to either false reassurance or significant anxiety if elevated without an imaging correlate.[123] Despite the lack of utility, tumor markers continue to be used at high rates by providers, with recent surveys suggesting over 40% of oncologists routinely order tumor marker testing.[124] One study found that 42% of patients aged 65 years and older with stage I-III breast cancer received at least 1 tumor marker test within 2 years of diagnosis.[125] Tumor marker testing was associated with increased receipt of advanced imaging and subsequent biopsy. In addition, patients who underwent tumor marker testing had significantly increased overall cost of care by 35% in the first 12 months after diagnosis and by 28% in months 13 to 24 after diagnosis.

SUMMARY

In conclusion, breast cancer treatment has evolved significantly in the last few decades with an increasing emphasis on tailoring treatment recommendations based on tumor biology. With this has come a natural de-escalation of care for patients with favorable tumor characteristics, with multiple clinical trials in surgical, medical, and radiation oncology supporting the safety of omitting previously routine care in selected patients. The ability to personalize cancer therapies based on a patient's tumor biology offers a key opportunity to ensure that patients receive high-value services across the breast cancer care continuum.

CLINICS CARE POINTS

Recommendations	
Screening and diagnostics	
Genetic testing	There is significant variability in recommendations from major organizations on which patients genetic testing should be ordered.
	National Comprehensive Cancer Network (NCCN) guidelines are the most restrictive and suggest testing for high-penetrance breast cancer susceptibility genes under limited

	circumstances based on patient age, tumor type, family history, and probability models. American Society of Clinical Oncology (ASCO) guidelines recommend genetic testing be offered to individuals with a personal or family history with features suggestive of a genetic cancer susceptibility gene if the results will influence management of the patient or at-risk family members. ASCO recommends that all genetic testing be accompanied by pretest and posttest counseling.
	The American Society of Breast Surgeons (ASBrS) has advocated for genetic testing in all individuals diagnosed with breast cancer.
Breast magnetic resonance imaging (MRI) for breast cancer screening in average-risk women	NCCN, ASBrS, and American College of Surgeons (ACS) agree that breast MRI should not be used for routine breast cancer screening in average-risk women.
	Indications for screening breast MRI include: • Screening in patients at high risk for breast cancer, defined as a high-risk germline genetic mutation, a history of chest wall irradiation, or >20-25% lifetime risk of breast cancer based on a probability model. • As a diagnostic adjunct to mammography after weighing the risks vs benefits.
Breast cancer screening cessation in asymptomatic women with limited life expectancy	ASBrS and ACS recommend cessation of screening mammography in women with a less than 5–10 y life expectancy, even among women with a personal history of breast cancer.
	The United States Preventive Services Task Force (USPSTF) recommends breast cancer screening for patients up to the age of 74 years. For patients aged ≥75 y, USPSTF concludes that there is insufficient evidence to assess the risks vs benefits of continued screening.
Breast surgical oncology	
Breast surgery in the outpatient setting	Unilateral and bilateral mastectomy with or without immediate reconstruction is safe in the outpatient setting and should be performed concurrently with the implementation of an Enhanced Recovery After Surgery (ERAS) protocol.
	An appropriate ERAS protocol should include: • Preoperative education to set expectations for the patient and their family. • Multimodal analgesia in the preoperative and postoperative setting to limit opioid utilization and improve likelihood of discharge from the recovery suite. • A plan for close postoperative follow-up.
De-escalation of axillary surgery	Current evidence supports de-escalation of axillary surgery in three circumstances:

	1. Avoid axillary lymph node dissection (ALND) in patients with cT1-T2, cN0 invasive breast cancer with 1–2 positive lymph nodes who are undergoing breast-conserving surgery (BCS) with adjuvant radiotherapy.
	2. Avoid ALND without first performing sentinel lymph node biopsy (SLNB) in patients with previously clinically node-positive breast cancer who become cN0 following neoadjuvant chemotherapy.
	3. Avoid SLNB in cN0 women aged $\geq$70 years with ER+, HER2− early-stage breast cancer.
Contralateral prophylactic mastectomy	Major organizations including ASBrS recommend against bilateral mastectomy for patients with unilateral breast cancer at average risk of contralateral breast cancer. Patients who strongly desire this procedure should be fully educated on the lack of survival benefit associated with contralateral prophylactic mastectomy, increased postoperative risks of bilateral surgery, higher potential for financial toxicity, and uncertainty regarding long-term patient-reported outcomes.
Breast medical oncology	
Staging for patients with early-stage breast cancer	<1% of patients with early-stage breast cancer have metastatic disease at diagnosis. ASCO and NCCN recommend against routine staging for asymptomatic patients with stage 0-II breast cancer.
Personalizing recommendations for adjuvant chemotherapy	Patients with ER+/HER2− breast cancer should be considered for genomic tests such as Oncotype Dx to evaluate recurrence risk and potential benefit associated with chemotherapy administration. Patients who are not candidates for or who would decline chemotherapy regardless of genomic test results should not undergo testing.
Breast radiation oncology	
Radiotherapy in older patients with low-risk breast cancer	NCCN guidelines allow for omission of adjuvant radiotherapy in women aged $\geq$70 years with pT1, cN0, ER+, HER2− breast cancer who plan to receive adjuvant endocrine therapy.
	Patients should be informed of the potential for radiotherapy omission prior to decision-making for BCS vs mastectomy, as this may encourage patients to undergo BCS rather than mastectomy.
	The decision to omit SLNB should be independent of the decision to omit radiotherapy in eligible patients.
Shorter adjuvant radiotherapy schedules	ASTRO guidelines support hypofractionation rather than conventional fractionation as the standard of care for all breast cancer patients requiring adjuvant whole breast irradiation.
	ASTRO guidelines support accelerated partial-beam irradiation (APBI) as an acceptable alternative to whole breast irradiation in

	patients $\geq$ 50 y with T1 invasive breast cancer and negative margins. APBI can also be considered in patients with low-risk ductal carcinoma in situ (DCIS), defined as screen-detected, low to intermediate nuclear grade, $\leq$ 2.5 cm, and resected with negative margins $\geq$ 3 mm.
Post-breast-cancer surveillance	
Detection of locoregional recurrence	NCCN and ASCO guidelines recommend asymptomatic patients receive routine surveillance with annual mammography, with the first mammogram obtained between 6 and 12 months after breast conserving therapy for breast cancer. Following mastectomy with or without reconstruction for breast cancer, annual clinical breast exam without any routine imaging is sufficient for surveillance of asymptomatic patients.
Detection of distant recurrence	NCCN and ASCO guidelines recommend against routine surveillance imaging and laboratory markers in asymptomatic patients following breast cancer treatment with curative intent.

DISCLOSURES

The authors have nothing to disclose.

REFERENCES

1. Porter ME. What is value in health care? N Engl J Med 2010;363(26):2477–81.
2. Shrank WH, Rogstad TL, Parekh N. Waste in the US Health Care System: Estimated Costs and Potential for Savings. JAMA 2019;322(15):1501–9.
3. Yabroff KR, Mariotto A, Tangka F, et al. Annual report to the nation on the status of cancer, Part 2: patient economic burden associated with cancer care. J Natl Cancer Inst 2021;113(12):1670–82.
4. Mariotto AB, Enewold L, Zhao J, et al. Medical Care Costs Associated with Cancer Survivorship in the United States. Cancer Epidemiol Biomarkers Prev 2020; 29(7):1304–12.
5. Dean LT, Moss SL, Ransome Y, et al. "It still affects our economic situation": long-term economic burden of breast cancer and lymphedema. Support Care Cancer 2019;27(5):1697–708.
6. Tung N, Lin NU, Kidd J, et al. Frequency of Germline Mutations in 25 Cancer Susceptibility Genes in a Sequential Series of Patients With Breast Cancer. J Clin Oncol 2016;34(13):1460–8.
7. Whitworth PW, Beitsch PD, Patel R, et al. Clinical Utility of Universal Germline Genetic Testing for Patients With Breast Cancer. JAMA Netw Open 2022;5(9):e2232787.
8. Beitsch PD, Whitworth PW, Hughes K, et al. Underdiagnosis of Hereditary Breast Cancer: Are Genetic Testing Guidelines a Tool or an Obstacle? J Clin Oncol 2019;37(6):453–60.
9. Yadav S, Hu C, Hart SN, et al. Evaluation of Germline Genetic Testing Criteria in a Hospital-Based Series of Women With Breast Cancer. J Clin Oncol 2020; 38(13):1409–18.

10. Tutt ANJ, Garber JE, Kaufman B, et al. Adjuvant Olaparib for Patients with BRCA1- or BRCA2-Mutated Breast Cancer. N Engl J Med 2021;384(25):2394–405.

11. National Comprehensive Cancer Network. Genetic/Familial High-Risk Assessment: Breast, Ovarian, and Pancreatic (Version 1.2023). Available at: https://www.nccn.org/professionals/physician_gls/pdf/genetics_bop.pdf. Published 2022. Accessed December 29, 2022.

12. Roberts MC, Dotson WD, DeVore CS, et al. Delivery Of Cascade Screening For Hereditary Conditions: A Scoping Review Of The Literature. Health Aff 2018; 37(5):801–8.

13. Nelson HD, Pappas M, Zakher B, et al. Risk assessment, genetic counseling, and genetic testing for BRCA-related cancer in women: a systematic review to update the U.S. Preventive Services Task Force recommendation. Ann Intern Med 2014;160(4):255–66.

14. Raspa M, Moultrie R, Toth D, et al. Barriers and Facilitators to Genetic Service Delivery Models: Scoping Review. Interact J Med Res 2021;10(1):e23523.

15. Kinney AY, Steffen LE, Brumbach BH, et al. Randomized Noninferiority Trial of Telephone Delivery of BRCA1/2 Genetic Counseling Compared With In-Person Counseling: 1-Year Follow-Up. J Clin Oncol 2016;34(24):2914–24.

16. Sun L, Brentnall A, Patel S, et al. A Cost-effectiveness Analysis of Multigene Testing for All Patients With Breast Cancer. JAMA Oncol 2019;5(12):1718–30.

17. Murphy BL, Yi M, Arun BK, et al. Contralateral Risk-Reducing Mastectomy in Breast Cancer Patients Who Undergo Multigene Panel Testing. Ann Surg Oncol 2020;27(12):4613–21.

18. Welsh JL, Hoskin TL, Day CN, et al. Clinical Decision-Making in Patients with Variant of Uncertain Significance in BRCA1 or BRCA2 Genes. Ann Surg Oncol 2017;24(10):3067–72.

19. Reid S, Roberson ML, Koehler K, et al. Receipt of Bilateral Mastectomy Among Women With Hereditary Breast Cancer. JAMA Oncol 2022;9(1):143–5.

20. Comeaux JG, Culver JO, Lee JE, et al. Risk-reducing mastectomy decisions among women with mutations in high- and moderate- penetrance breast cancer susceptibility genes. Mol Genet Genomic Med 2022;10(10):e2031.

21. Aristokli N, Polycarpou I, Themistocleous SC, et al. Comparison of the diagnostic performance of Magnetic Resonance Imaging (MRI), ultrasound and mammography for detection of breast cancer based on tumor type, breast density and patient's history: A review. Radiography 2022;28(3):848–56.

22. Houssami N, Ciatto S, Macaskill P, et al. Accuracy and surgical impact of magnetic resonance imaging in breast cancer staging: systematic review and meta-analysis in detection of multifocal and multicentric cancer. J Clin Oncol 2008; 26(19):3248–58.

23. Brennan ME, Houssami N, Lord S, et al. Magnetic resonance imaging screening of the contralateral breast in women with newly diagnosed breast cancer: systematic review and meta-analysis of incremental cancer detection and impact on surgical management. J Clin Oncol 2009;27(33):5640–9.

24. Taneja C, Edelsberg J, Weycker D, et al. Cost effectiveness of breast cancer screening with contrast-enhanced MRI in high-risk women. J Am Coll Radiol 2009;6(3):171–9.

25. Stout NK, Nekhlyudov L, Li L, et al. Rapid increase in breast magnetic resonance imaging use: trends from 2000 to 2011. JAMA Intern Med 2014;174(1): 114–21.

26. Kerlikowske K, Miglioretti DL, Vachon CM. Discussions of Dense Breasts, Breast Cancer Risk, and Screening Choices in 2019. JAMA 2019;322(1):69–70.

27. Bakker MF, de Lange SV, Pijnappel RM, et al. Supplemental MRI Screening for Women with Extremely Dense Breast Tissue. N Engl J Med 2019;381(22): 2091–102.

28. Vlahiotis A, Griffin B, Stavros AT, et al. Analysis of utilization patterns and associated costs of the breast imaging and diagnostic procedures after screening mammography. Clinicoecon Outcomes Res 2018;10:157–67.

29. Tollens F, Baltzer PAT, Dietzel M, et al. Economic potential of abbreviated breast MRI for screening women with dense breast tissue for breast cancer. Eur Radiol 2022;32(11):7409–19.

30. Pettit K, Swatske ME, Gao F, et al. The Impact of Breast MRI on Surgical Decision-Making: Are Patients at Risk for Mastectomy? J Surg Oncol 2009;100(7):553–8.

31. Kuritzky AM, Lee MC. Long-term impact of staging breast magnetic resonance imaging-a risk for overtreatment? Transl Cancer Res 2017;6:S476–8.

32. Ganguli I, Keating NL, Thakore N, et al. Downstream Mammary and Extramammary Cascade Services and Spending Following Screening Breast Magnetic Resonance Imaging vs Mammography Among Commercially Insured Women. JAMA Netw Open 2022;5(4):e227234.

33. Chen TH, Yen AM, Fann JC, et al. Clarifying the debate on population-based screening for breast cancer with mammography: A systematic review of randomized controlled trials on mammography with Bayesian meta-analysis and causal model. Medicine (Baltim) 2017;96(3):e5684.

34. Lee SJ, Boscardin WJ, Stijacic-Cenzer I, et al. Time lag to benefit after screening for breast and colorectal cancer: meta-analysis of survival data from the United States, Sweden, United Kingdom, and Denmark. Bmj-Brit Med J 2013;346:e8441.

35. Royce TJ, Hendrix LH, Stokes WA, et al. Cancer screening rates in individuals with different life expectancies. JAMA Intern Med 2014;174(10):1558–65.

36. Walter LC, Schonberg MA. Screening Mammography in Older Women A Review. Jama-J Am Med Assoc 2014;311(13):1336–47.

37. Torke AM, Schwartz PH, Holtz LR, et al. Older adults and forgoing cancer screening: "I think it would be strange". JAMA Intern Med 2013;173(7):526–31.

38. Housten AJ, Pappadis MR, Krishnan S, et al. Resistance to discontinuing breast cancer screening in older women: A qualitative study. Psycho Oncol 2018;27(6): 1635–41.

39. Kotwal AA, Walter LC, Lee SJ, et al. Are We Choosing Wisely? Older Adults' Cancer Screening Intentions and Recalled Discussions with Physicians About Stopping. J Gen Intern Med 2019;34(8):1538–45.

40. White N, Reid F, Harris A, et al. A Systematic Review of Predictions of Survival in Palliative Care: How Accurate Are Clinicians and Who Are the Experts? PLoS One 2016;11(8):e0161407.

41. Allen LA, Yager JE, Funk MJ, et al. Discordance between patient-predicted and model-predicted life expectancy among ambulatory patients with heart failure. JAMA 2008;299(21):2533–42.

42. Hoffmann TC, Del Mar C. Patients' expectations of the benefits and harms of treatments, screening, and tests: a systematic review. JAMA Intern Med 2015; 175(2):274–86.

43. Hoffmann TC, Del Mar C. Clinicians' Expectations of the Benefits and Harms of Treatments, Screening, and Tests: A Systematic Review. JAMA Intern Med 2017; 177(3):407–19.

44. Schoenborn NL, Boyd CM, Lee SJ, et al. Communicating About Stopping Cancer Screening: Comparing Clinicians' and Older Adults' Perspectives. Gerontol 2019;59(Suppl 1):S67–76.

45. Schoenborn NL, Bowman TL 2nd, Cayea D, et al. Primary Care Practitioners' Views on Incorporating Long-term Prognosis in the Care of Older Adults. JAMA Intern Med 2016;176(5):671–8.
46. Marxen T, Shauly O, Losken A. The Safety of Same-day Discharge after Immediate Alloplastic Breast Reconstruction: A Systematic Review. Plast Reconstr Surg Glob Open 2022;10(7):e4448.
47. Specht MC, Kelly BN, Tomczyk E, et al. One-Year Experience of Same-Day Mastectomy and Breast Reconstruction Protocol. Ann Surg Oncol 2022;29(9): 5711–9.
48. Marla S, Stallard S. Systematic review of day surgery for breast cancer. Int J Surg 2009;7(4):318–23.
49. Sibia US, Klune JR, Turcotte JJ, et al. Hospital-Based Same-Day Compared to Overnight-Stay Mastectomy: An American College of Surgeons National Surgical Quality Improvement Program Analysis. Ochsner J 2022;22(2):139–45.
50. Hughes TM, Ellsworth B, Berlin NL, et al. Statewide Episode Spending Variation of Mastectomy for Breast Cancer. J Am Coll Surg 2022;234(1):14–23.
51. Jogerst K, Thomas O, Kosiorek HE, et al. Same-Day Discharge After Mastectomy: Breast Cancer Surgery in the Era of ERAS((R)). Ann Surg Oncol 2020; 27(9):3436–45.
52. Offodile AC 2nd, Gu C, Boukovalas S, et al. Enhanced recovery after surgery (ERAS) pathways in breast reconstruction: systematic review and meta-analysis of the literature. Breast Cancer Res Treat 2019;173(1):65–77.
53. Vuong B, Graff-Baker AN, Yanagisawa M, et al. Implementation of a Postmastectomy Home Recovery Program in a Large, Integrated Health Care Delivery System. Ann Surg Oncol 2019;26(10):3178–84.
54. DiSipio T, Rye S, Newman B, et al. Incidence of unilateral arm lymphoedema after breast cancer: a systematic review and meta-analysis. Lancet Oncol 2013; 14(6):500–15.
55. Kwan JYY, Famiyeh P, Su J, et al. Development and Validation of a Risk Model for Breast Cancer-Related Lymphedema. JAMA Netw Open 2020;3(11):e2024373.
56. Shih YC, Xu Y, Cormier JN, et al. Incidence, treatment costs, and complications of lymphedema after breast cancer among women of working age: a 2-year follow-up study. J Clin Oncol 2009;27(12):2007–14.
57. Jorgensen MG, Toyserkani NM, Hansen FG, et al. The impact of lymphedema on health-related quality of life up to 10 years after breast cancer treatment. NPJ Breast Cancer 2021;7(1):70.
58. Boyages J, Kalfa S, Xu Y, et al. Worse and worse off: the impact of lymphedema on work and career after breast cancer. SpringerPlus 2016;5:657.
59. Giuliano AE, Ballman KV, McCall L, et al. Effect of Axillary Dissection vs No Axillary Dissection on 10-Year Overall Survival Among Women With Invasive Breast Cancer and Sentinel Node Metastasis: The ACOSOG Z0011 (Alliance) Randomized Clinical Trial. JAMA 2017;318(10):918–26.
60. Kuehn T, Bauerfeind I, Fehm T, et al. Sentinel-lymph-node biopsy in patients with breast cancer before and after neoadjuvant chemotherapy (SENTINA): a prospective, multicentre cohort study. Lancet Oncol 2013;14(7):609–18.
61. Boughey JC, Suman VJ, Mittendorf EA, et al. Sentinel lymph node surgery after neoadjuvant chemotherapy in patients with node-positive breast cancer: the ACOSOG Z1071 (Alliance) clinical trial. JAMA 2013;310(14):1455–61.
62. Hughes KS, Schnaper LA, Bellon JR, et al. Lumpectomy plus tamoxifen with or without irradiation in women age 70 years or older with early breast cancer: long-term follow-up of CALGB 9343. J Clin Oncol 2013;31(19):2382–7.

63. Wang T, Bredbeck BC, Sinco B, et al. Variations in Persistent Use of Low-Value Breast Cancer Surgery. JAMA Surg 2021;156(4):353–62.

64. Wong SM, Weiss A, Mittendorf EA, et al. Surgical Management of the Axilla in Clinically Node-Positive Patients Receiving Neoadjuvant Chemotherapy: A National Cancer Database Analysis. Ann Surg Oncol 2019;26(11):3517–25.

65. Bredbeck BC, Baskin AS, Wang T, et al. Incremental Spending Associated with Low-Value Treatments in Older Women with Breast Cancer. Ann Surg Oncol 2022;29(2):1051–9.

66. Wang T, Mott N, Miller J, et al. Patient Perspectives on De-Escalation of Breast Cancer Treatment Options in Older Women with Hormone-Receptor Positive Breast Cancer: A Qualitative Study. JAMA Netw Open 2020;3(9):e2017129. Under Review.

67. Baskin A, Wang T, Hawley ST, et al. Gaps in Breast Cancer Treatment Information for Older Women. Ann Surg Oncol 2020;28(2):950–7. Manuscript in progress.

68. Schonberg MA, Freedman RA, Recht AR, et al. Developing a patient decision aid for women aged 70 and older with early stage, estrogen receptor positive, HER2 negative, breast cancer. J Geriatr Oncol 2019;10(6):980–6.

69. Smith ME, Vitous CA, Hughes TM, et al. Barriers and Facilitators to De-Implementation of the Choosing Wisely((R)) Guidelines for Low-Value Breast Cancer Surgery. Ann Surg Oncol 2020;27(8):2653–63.

70. Kalinsky K, Barlow WE, Gralow JR, et al. 21-Gene Assay to Inform Chemotherapy Benefit in Node-Positive Breast Cancer. N Engl J Med 2021;385(25):2336–47.

71. Bello DM, Russell C, McCullough D, et al. Lymph Node Status in Breast Cancer Does Not Predict Tumor Biology. Ann Surg Oncol 2018;25(10):2884–9.

72. Wang T, Baskin AS, Dossett LA. Deimplementation of the Choosing Wisely Recommendations for Low-Value Breast Cancer Surgery: A Systematic Review. JAMA Surg 2020;155(8):759–70.

73. Baskin AS, Wang T, Bredbeck BC, et al. Trends in Contralateral Prophylactic Mastectomy Utilization for Small Unilateral Breast Cancer. J Surg Res 2021;262:71–84.

74. Agarwal S, Kidwell KM, Kraft CT, et al. Defining the relationship between patient decisions to undergo breast reconstruction and contralateral prophylactic mastectomy. Plast Reconstr Surg 2015;135(3):661–70.

75. Osman F, Saleh F, Jackson TD, et al. Increased postoperative complications in bilateral mastectomy patients compared to unilateral mastectomy: an analysis of the NSQIP database. Ann Surg Oncol 2013;20(10):3212–7.

76. Momoh AO, Cohen WA, Kidwell KM, et al. Tradeoffs Associated With Contralateral Prophylactic Mastectomy in Women Choosing Breast Reconstruction: Results of a Prospective Multicenter Cohort. Ann Surg 2017;266(1):158–64.

77. Sergesketter AR, Marks C, Broadwater G, et al. A Comparison of Complications in Therapeutic versus Contralateral Prophylactic Mastectomy Reconstruction: A Paired Analysis. Plast Reconstr Surg 2022;149(5):1037–47.

78. Boughey JC, Schilz SR, Van Houten HK, et al. Contralateral Prophylactic Mastectomy with Immediate Breast Reconstruction Increases Healthcare Utilization and Cost. Ann Surg Oncol 2017;24(10):2957–64.

79. Billig JI, Duncan A, Zhong L, et al. The Cost of Contralateral Prophylactic Mastectomy in Women with Unilateral Breast Cancer. Plast Reconstr Surg 2018; 141(5):1094–102.

80. Eom JS, Kobayashi MR, Paydar K, et al. The number of operations required for completing breast reconstruction. Plast Reconstr Surg Glob Open 2014;2(10): e242.

81. Zendejas B, Moriarty JP, O'Byrne J, et al. Cost-effectiveness of contralateral pro-phylactic mastectomy versus routine surveillance in patients with unilateral breast cancer. J Clin Oncol 2011;29(22):2993–3000.

82. Smith D, Sepehr S, Karakatsanis A, et al. Yield of Surveillance Imaging After Mastectomy With or Without Reconstruction for Patients With Prior Breast Cancer: A Systematic Review and Meta-analysis. JAMA Netw Open 2022;5(12): e2244212.

83. Greenup RA, Rushing C, Fish L, et al. Financial Costs and Burden Related to Decisions for Breast Cancer Surgery. J Oncol Pract 2019;15(8):e666–76.

84. Buchanan PJ, Abdulghani M, Waljee JF, et al. An Analysis of the Decisions Made for Contralateral Prophylactic Mastectomy and Breast Reconstruction. Plast Reconstr Surg 2016;138(1):29–40.

85. Sando IC, Billig JI, Ambani SW, et al. An Evaluation of the Choice for Contralateral Prophylactic Mastectomy and Patient Concerns About Recurrence in a Reconstructed Cohort. Ann Plast Surg 2018;80(4):333–8.

86. Offodile AC 2nd, Hwang ES, Greenup RA. Contralateral Prophylactic Mastectomy in the Era of Financial Toxicity: An Additional Point for Concern? Ann Surg 2020;271(5):817–8.

87. Rosenberg SM, Tracy MS, Meyer ME, et al. Perceptions, knowledge, and satisfaction with contralateral prophylactic mastectomy among young women with breast cancer: a cross-sectional survey. Ann Intern Med 2013;159(6):373–81.

88. Brennan ME, Houssami N. Evaluation of the evidence on staging imaging for detection of asymptomatic distant metastases in newly diagnosed breast cancer. Breast 2012;21(2):112–23.

89. Dull B, Linkugel A, Margenthaler JA, et al. Overuse of Chest CT in Patients With Stage I and II Breast Cancer: An Opportunity to Increase Guidelines Compliance at an NCCN Member Institution. J Natl Compr Canc Netw 2017;15(6): 783–9.

90. Baltz AP, Siegel ER, Kamal AH, et al. Clinical Impact of ASCO Choosing Wisely Guidelines on Staging Imaging for Early-Stage Breast Cancers: A Time Series Analysis Using SEER-Medicare Data. JCO Oncol Pract 2022;19(2):e274–85.

91. Henry NL, Braun TM, Breslin TM, et al. Variation in the use of advanced imaging at the time of breast cancer diagnosis in a statewide registry. Cancer 2017; 123(15):2975–83.

92. Simos D, Hutton B, Graham ID, et al. Imaging for metastatic disease in patients with newly diagnosed breast cancer: are doctor's perceptions in keeping with the guidelines? J Eval Clin Pract 2015;21(1):67–73.

93. Lipitz-Snyderman A, Sima CS, Atoria CL, et al. Physician-Driven Variation in Nonrecommended Services Among Older Adults Diagnosed With Cancer. JAMA Intern Med 2016;176(10):1541–8.

94. Sparano JA, Gray RJ, Makower DF, et al. Adjuvant Chemotherapy Guided by a 21-Gene Expression Assay in Breast Cancer. N Engl J Med 2018;379(2):111–21.

95. Kurian AW, Bondarenko I, Jagsi R, et al. Recent Trends in Chemotherapy Use and Oncologists' Treatment Recommendations for Early-Stage Breast Cancer. J Natl Cancer Inst 2018;110(5):493–500.

96. Schaafsma E, Zhang B, Schaafsma M, et al. Impact of Oncotype DX testing on ER+ breast cancer treatment and survival in the first decade of use. Breast Cancer Res 2021;23(1):74.

97. Chandler Y, Jayasekera JC, Schechter CB, et al. Simulation of Chemotherapy Effects in Older Breast Cancer Patients With High Recurrence Scores. J Natl Cancer Inst 2020;112(6):574–81.

98. Van Herck Y, Feyaerts A, Alibhai S, et al. Is cancer biology different in older patients? Lancet Healthy Longev 2021;2(10):e663–77.

99. Giaquinto AN, Sung H, Miller KD, et al. Breast Cancer Statistics, 2022. CA Cancer J Clin 2022;72(6):524–41.

100. Kunkler IH, Williams LJ, Jack WJL, et al. Breast-Conserving Surgery with or without Irradiation in Early Breast Cancer. N Engl J Med 2023;388(7):585–94.

101. Whelan T, Smith S, Nielsen T, et al. LUMINA: A prospective trial omitting radiotherapy (RT) following breast conserving surgery (BCS) in T1N0 luminal A breast cancer (BC). J Clin Oncol 2022;40(17).

102. Early Breast Cancer Trialists' Collaborative G. Aromatase inhibitors versus tamoxifen in early breast cancer: patient-level meta-analysis of the randomised trials. Lancet 2015;386(10001):1341–52.

103. McKevitt E, Cheifetz R, DeVries K, et al. Sentinel Node Biopsy Should Not be Routine in Older Patients with ER-Positive HER2-Negative Breast Cancer Who Are Willing and Able to Take Hormone Therapy. Ann Surg Oncol 2021;28(11): 5950–7.

104. Taylor LJ, Steiman JS, Anderson B, et al. Does persistent use of radiation in women > 70 years of age with early-stage breast cancer reflect tailored patient-centered care? Breast Cancer Res Treat 2020;180(3):801–7.

105. Greenup RA, Camp MS, Taghian AG, et al. Cost comparison of radiation treatment options after lumpectomy for breast cancer. Ann Surg Oncol 2012;19(10): 3275–81.

106. Shumway DA, Griffith KA, Hawley ST, et al. Patient views and correlates of radiotherapy omission in a population-based sample of older women with favorable-prognosis breast cancer. Cancer 2018;124(13):2714–23.

107. Dossett LA, Mott NM, Bredbeck BC, et al. Using Tailored Messages to Target Overuse of Low-Value Breast Cancer Care in Older Women. J Surg Res 2022; 270:503–12.

108. Shumway DA, Griffith KA, Sabel MS, et al. Surgeon and Radiation Oncologist Views on Omission of Adjuvant Radiotherapy for Older Women with Early-Stage Breast Cancer. Ann Surg Oncol 2017;24(12):3518–26.

109. Bekelman JE, Sylwestrzak G, Barron J, et al. Uptake and costs of hypofractionated vs conventional whole breast irradiation after breast conserving surgery in the United States, 2008-2013. JAMA 2014;312(23):2542–50.

110. Kang MM, Hasan Y, Waller J, et al. Has Hypofractionated Whole-Breast Radiation Therapy Become the Standard of Care in the United States? An Updated Report from National Cancer Database. Clin Breast Cancer 2022;22(1):e8–20.

111. Knowlton CA. Breast Cancer Management During the COVID-19 Pandemic: the Radiation Oncology Perspective. Curr Breast Cancer Rep 2022;14(1):8–16.

112. Vicini FA, Cecchini RS, White JR, et al. Long-term primary results of accelerated partial breast irradiation after breast-conserving surgery for early-stage breast cancer: a randomised, phase 3, equivalence trial. Lancet 2019;394(10215): 2155–64.

113. Whelan TJ, Julian JA, Berrang TS, et al. External beam accelerated partial breast irradiation versus whole breast irradiation after breast conserving surgery in women with ductal carcinoma in situ and node-negative breast cancer (RAPID): a randomised controlled trial. Lancet 2019;394(10215):2165–72.

114. Correa C, Harris EE, Leonardi MC, et al. Accelerated Partial Breast Irradiation: Executive summary for the update of an ASTRO Evidence-Based Consensus Statement. Pract Radiat Oncol 2017;7(2):73–9.

115. Lam DL, Houssami N, Lee JM. Imaging Surveillance After Primary Breast Cancer Treatment. AJR Am J Roentgenol 2017;208(3):676–86.
116. McNaul D, Darke M, Garg M, et al. An evaluation of post-lumpectomy recurrence rates: is follow-up every 6 months for 2 years needed? J Surg Oncol 2013;107(6):597–601.
117. Expert Panel on Breast I, Heller SL, Lourenco AP, et al. ACR Appropriateness Criteria(R) Imaging After Mastectomy and Breast Reconstruction. J Am Coll Radiol 2020;17(11S):S403–14.
118. Cheun JH, Jung J, Lee ES, et al. Intensity of metastasis screening and survival outcomes in patients with breast cancer. Sci Rep 2021;11(1):2851.
119. NCCN Clinical Practice Guidelines in Oncology: Breast Cancer Version 4.2023. Available at: https://www.nccn.org/professionals/physician_gls/pdf/breast_blocks.pdf. Published 2023. Accessed March 23, 2023.
120. Moschetti I, Cinquini M, Lambertini M, et al. Follow-up strategies for women treated for early breast cancer. Cochrane Database Syst Rev 2016;2016(5):CD001768.
121. Schumacher JR, Neuman HB, Yu M, et al. Surveillance Imaging vs Symptomatic Recurrence Detection and Survival in Stage II-III Breast Cancer (AFT-01). J Natl Cancer Inst 2022;114(10):1371–9.
122. Wickerham L, Fisher B, Cronin W. The efficacy of bone scanning in the follow-up of patients with operable breast cancer. Breast Cancer Res Treat 1984;4(4):303–7.
123. Harris L, Fritsche H, Mennel R, et al. American Society of Clinical Oncology 2007 update of recommendations for the use of tumor markers in breast cancer. J Clin Oncol 2007;25(33):5287–312.
124. Hahn EE, Munoz-Plaza C, Wang J, et al. Anxiety, Culture, and Expectations: Oncologist-Perceived Factors Associated With Use of Nonrecommended Serum Tumor Marker Tests for Surveillance of Early-Stage Breast Cancer. J Oncol Pract 2017;13(1):e77–90.
125. Ramsey SD, Henry NL, Gralow JR, et al. Tumor marker usage and medical care costs among older early-stage breast cancer survivors. J Clin Oncol 2015;33(2):149–55.

Addressing Inequalities in Breast Cancer Care Delivery

Leisha C. Elmore, MD, MPHS[a,b],
Oluwadamilola M. Fayanju, MD, MA, MPHS[b],*

KEYWORDS

- Health equity • Health disparities • Breast cancer

KEY POINTS

- The etiology of health disparities is multifactorial and driven in large part by challenges in access to care, differential receipt of guideline-concordant care, and limited enrollment of diverse patients in clinical trials that serve as the foundation for treatment development.
- Black women diagnosed with breast cancer have a mortality rate that is 40% higher than White women. Hispanic ethnicity is associated with increased likelihood of not receiving guideline-concordant breast cancer treatment.
- Aggregate reporting of Asian American, Native Hawaiians, and Other Pacific Islanders limits subgroup analysis that may reveal within-group disparities.
- Intentional dismantling of structural barriers to equitable care requires intervention at the societal, health system, institution, and provider level.

INTRODUCTION/HISTORY/DEFINITIONS/BACKGROUND
Epidemiology of Breast Cancer

Breast cancer is the most common cancer diagnosed among women in the United States and much of the world. One in eight US women will develop breast cancer in their lifetime. Although overall incidence for breast cancer has been stable for decades, these rates fail to capture the nuance within subpopulations. When we look at trends in incidence over time, there are notable differences by race and ethnicity. Historically, incidence rates were higher among White women than Black women, but these rates have now converged and are now comparable. Incidence rates are notably lower for American Indian/Alaska Natives, Hispanic, and Asian/Pacific Islander

[a] Department of Surgery, Penn Presbyterian Medical Center, University of Pennsylvania, Perelman School of Medicine, 51 North 39th Street, 266 Wright Sanders, Philadelphia, PA 19104, USA; [b] Division of Breast Surgery, Department of Surgery, Hospital of the University of Pennsylvania, 3400 Spruce Street, Silverstein 4, Philadelphia, PA 19104, USA
* Corresponding author.
E-mail address: Oluwadamilola.fayanju@pennmedicine.upenn.edu
Twitter: @DrLolaFayanju (L.C.E.)

Surg Oncol Clin N Am 32 (2023) 799–810
https://doi.org/10.1016/j.soc.2023.05.009
1055-3207/23/© 2023 Elsevier Inc. All rights reserved.

women, but they are increasing most significantly among Asian/Pacific Islander and American Indian/Alaska Native women.[1]

Despite the relatively stable incidence of breast cancer in the general population, mortality has declined by approximately 40% since 1975 owing to improvements in early detection, a better understanding of tumor biology, the development of targeted therapies, and improved treatment algorithms. However, this improvement in mortality has not been equally realized by all patients. In fact, in 2021, breast cancer became the leading cause of cancer death in Black women, surpassing lung cancer. Furthermore, Black women have the highest breast cancer death rate of all racial/ethnic groups, and a mortality rate that has been 40% higher than their White peers in recent years.[2] Of note, despite the rising incidence of breast cancer in the Asian/Pacific Islander population, mortality in this group remains the lowest of all racial and ethnic groups.[1]

When systemic differences emerge in any health outcome, interrogation of these differences requires an examination of how much they represent variations driven by nonmodifiable factors versus targets that are amenable to change. For example, with regard to breast cancer incidence, we know that certain factors are associated with a higher incidence; female sex is a predisposing factor, and breast cancer incidence increases steadily with age, making both biological sex and age nonmodifiable risk factors. Conversely, unequal access to care or treatment serves as potentially modifiable forces in disparate health outcomes.

Understanding Health Equity

To provide a foundation for the remainder of this article, it is important to understand the definition of the terms health disparity and health equity.

The Office of Disease Prevention and Health Promotion defines a *health disparity* as a *"… health difference that is closely linked with social, economic, and/or environmental disadvantage. Health disparities adversely affect groups of people who have systematically experienced greater obstacles to health based on their racial or ethnic group; religion; socioeconomic status; gender; age; mental health; cognitive, sensory, or physical disability; sexual orientation or gender identity; geographic location; or other characteristics historically linked to discrimination or exclusion."*[3] The key component of this definition is that the health difference disproportionally affects a historically marginalized population.

The Centers for Disease Control defines *health equity* as *"the state in which everyone has a fair and just opportunity to attain their highest level of health. Achieving this requires ongoing societal efforts to (1) Address historical and contemporary injustices (2) Overcome economic, social and other obstacles to health and (3) eliminate preventable health disparities."*[4] This definition highlights that many of the driving forces behind health inequities are the result of long-standing, systemic biases that must be dismantled. Promoting health equity does not simply mean providing the *same* care to everyone, but rather may ultimately involve allotting extra resources to elevate certain individuals to an appropriate standard of care.

Limitations in Data Reporting

The striking difference in breast cancer mortality in Black women relative to their peers represents a health disparity rooted in inequitable care at both the health system and societal levels. Although most of the existing data surrounding disparities address this pervasive and long-standing racial inequity, poor outcomes among Black women are not the only opportunity for improvement in care delivery.

In many studies on breast cancer, Asian Americans, Native Hawaiians, and Other Pacific Islanders are reported in aggregate and limit the ability to appreciate nuance within subpopulations.[5,6] This phenomenon is also true in reporting for Hispanic ethnicity, where more frequent use of disaggregated data could reveal within-group disparities along racial dimensions.[7] Furthermore, most of our data on breast cancer exclude male patients, limiting our ability to understand differences in biology, treatment response, and outcomes by sex. Finally, limited collection and availability of data on self-reported sexual orientation and gender identity in health care settings hinder attempts to quantify and mitigate disparities in access and outcome known to exist in the lesbian, gay, bisexual, transgender, queer or questioning and more (LGBTQ) community.[8]

In the remainder of this article, the authors describe the landscape of health disparities in breast cancer care delivery with a focus on racial/ethnic disparities.

Biological Differences

Black women are more likely to present with triple-negative breast cancer (TNBC), a subtype known to be more aggressive with fewer targeted therapy options and poorer disease-free and overall survival as compared with other variants. TNBC represents 21% of new breast cancer diagnoses in Black women, compared with 10% in White, Asian/Pacific Islander and 12% in Hispanic and American Indian/Alaska Native.[1]

The field of oncologic anthropology, coined by Dr Lisa Newman and Dr Linda Kaljee, studies how population migration can affect breast cancer epidemiology.[9] African American women have a combination of African, European, and indigenous ancestry as a result of their ancestors' passage to the Americas via the trans-Atlantic slave trade. An analysis of breast cancer in Africa demonstrated TNBC in 53.2% of Ghanaian/West African women. The evaluation of slave trade routes demonstrates that West Africans were predominantly routed to North America, and this understanding has prompted increased interrogation of how genetic ancestry originating in West Africa might affect rates of TNBC among African American women.[10]

The African American Breast Cancer Epidemiology and Risk Consortium, which is a collaboration of four breast cancer research programs, conducted an analysis of 3629 cases in Black women with 4648 control patients. In this analysis, they identified a novel gene (3q26.21) for estrogen receptor negative breast cancer among Black women.[11]

This work supports that there are biological contributors to variation in the epidemiology of TNBC. However, the vast majority of breast cancer, even for Black women, is hormone receptor (HR) positive, and much of the racial disparity in survival observed among Black women after breast cancer diagnosis is due to worse outcomes among those with HR-positive disease.[12] Furthermore, among women with TNBC, Black–White differences in outcome are less pronounced and can, in large part, be attributed to differential, and likely inequitable, receipt of surgery and chemotherapy.[13] Thus, although higher incidence of TNBC contributes to worse mortality among Black women relative to other groups to racial disparities in breast cancer outcomes, it is not the sole driver.

In the remainder of this article, the authors explores largely modifiable factors driving disparate and unequal breast cancer outcomes and discuss ways they can work toward a collective goal of promoting equitable health care for individuals with breast cancer.

DISCUSSION
Access to Care

Access to high-quality medical care optimizes health outcomes. Concomitantly, for many patients, the lack of access serves as a significant barrier and is a contributor to disparities in health outcomes. Below, the authors explore ways in which limited access to care impacts breast cancer outcomes.

- *Insurance Coverage, Screening, and Early Detection*
- The percentage of uninsured individuals in the United States has decreased since the passage of the Affordable Care Act in 2010, but disparities in coverage still exist. The individuals of American Indian and Alaska Natives have the highest uninsured rates, followed by Hispanic, Native Hawaiian, Pacific Islander, and Black individuals. However, Asian Americans have the lowest uninsured rates,[14] again highlighting the importance of disaggregating Asians and Pacific Islanders in research.
- Insurance coverage is associated with access to primary care providers and likelihood of receiving screening mammography. Individuals who are underinsured and uninsured are less likely to receive screening mammography, are more likely to be screened at lower resource and nonaccredited facilities, and are less likely to be screened with tomosynthesis, that is, 3D mammography. Furthermore, there is evidence that underinsured and uninsured individuals experience longer delays in follow-up of abnormal results.[15] The early detection is associated with improved survival outcomes for women diagnosed with breast cancer. Thus, challenges with access to care, in part because of disparate rates of insurance coverage, are a barrier to equitable health outcomes.
- Even with insurance, a diagnosis of cancer is associated with a significant financial burden to patients. The cost of treatment and resultant financial toxicity affect treatment decisions, adherence to recommended therapy, and posttreatment surveillance.[16] Furthermore, likelihood of experiencing financial toxicity after breast cancer diagnosis is increased among women of color.[17]
- *Treatment Location*
- Many patients do not live near health care facilities that provide screening services, and likewise, access to specialty care is not universally accessible. As a result, differential proximity to high-quality treatment facilities also facilitates disparity among patients with breast cancer with regard to stage at diagnosis and time to treatment.[18] In a study from Detroit, living in areas with greater Black segregation and limited mammography access was associated with a higher risk of advanced stage breast cancer diagnoses.[19] In a study of patients in Chicago, Black and Hispanic patients were more likely to be treated at facilities that are not accredited by the National Consortium of Breast Centers or deemed a Breast Imaging Center of Excellence by the American College of Radiology.[20] This finding was also corroborated by a Surveillance, Epidemiology, and End Results (SEER) analysis of 51,878 women undergoing breast surgery, which demonstrated that Black women were more likely to be treated at lower volume and lower quality hospitals. Black, Hispanic, and Asian patients with breast cancer were also more likely to receive care at hospitals with a higher proportion of Medicaid patients.[18] Treatment facility choice is multifactorial but in part reflects referral patterns and spatial accessibility. Elevating care in areas serving minority patients should be a public health mission and could significantly mitigate geography-related disparities in breast cancer care and outcomes.

Breast Cancer Treatment

The implementation of new technology and treatment options often reach low-resource populations at a slower rate, thereby transiently or permanently exacerbating disparities in health outcomes. Even with access to guideline-concordant care, there is evidence of systematic differences in receipt of treatment based on patient factors, such as weight, race, and ethnicity. Here, the authors briefly explore disparities in care delivery.

- *Chemotherapy*
- Chemotherapy represents a critical element in the treatment of locally advanced breast cancer and is also increasingly used in earlier stage triple-negative and HER2-positive breast cancer. The role of systemic therapy is to prolong disease-free intervals and overall survival. In select patients, systemic therapy in the neoadjuvant setting can also facilitate downstaging, thereby enabling patients to receive less extensive, less morbid locoregional treatment (ie, surgery and radiation) to the breast and axilla.
- In a study evaluating chemotherapy dosing over a 12-year period, data demonstrated that Black women were more likely to receive lower relative dose intensity compared with White women.[21] In a contemporary systematic review and meta-analysis, findings of dose intensity differences were not noted, but Black women were more likely to experiences delays in initiating therapy greater than 90 days. Furthermore, Black women with early-stage disease who were eligible for chemotherapy were significantly more likely to discontinue chemotherapy.[22] Hispanic ethnicity has also been associated with delays in time to chemotherapy.[23,24] Delays in initiating adjuvant chemotherapy are associated with worse clinical outcomes, particularly when delays are greater than 90 days.[23] Taken together, this suggests that there are both patient and provider factors that impact chemotherapy utilization and represent modifiable targets driving inequities in breast cancer care delivery.
- *Surgery*
- Surgical treatment of breast cancer represents a mainstay of curative intent therapy. Black women are more likely to experience postoperative complications and have longer length of stay compared with White women.[25,26] Hispanic women have also been shown to have higher rates of postoperative complications.[25,27] Finally, Black and Hispanic women have overall higher body mass index (BMIs) and more comorbid medical conditions that place them at higher surgical risk than White peers, and these factors are also believed to contribute to their lower rates of postmastectomy reconstruction. Although preoperative optimization and comanagement with primary care and subspecialty providers are critical, there is often limited time for medical optimization due to the need to provide timely cancer care and prevent compromise to cancer outcomes. Improvement in surgical outcomes is in part dependent on addressing disparities in health outcomes that occur before an individual's breast cancer diagnosis and requires interventions aimed at the level of primary care.
- *Radiation*
- Adjuvant radiation therapy is a critical element in the treatment of many people with breast cancer and it facilitates improvements in local regional control. Although contemporary literature supports select indications for omission of radiotherapy, adjuvant radiation has been the long-standing standard of care after partial mastectomy. Radiation is also indicated after mastectomy in select patients with locally advanced disease.
- Black women are less likely than White women to receive adjuvant radiation.[28–31] In an analysis of the SEER database over 17 years, non-Hispanic Black and Hispanic patients were less likely to receive radiation than White patients, a finding most pronounced with receipt of postmastectomy radiation therapy.[30]

Significant racial disparities in utilization of radiation after breast conservation have also been reported.[31] Treatment at a facility that is less likely to administer a treatment modality will result in lower utilization of that service. In a population-based analysis, Black women were less likely than White women to receive care at high-quality hospitals, defined as being in the top quartile for rates of radiation after breast-conserving surgery.[32]

- *Endocrine Therapy*
- In HR-positive breast cancer, adjuvant endocrine therapy for patients without contraindications is recommended to reduce the risk of breast cancer recurrence. Despite this recommendation, non-initiation, nonadherence, and nonpersistence in the use of endocrine therapy are seen across all racial and ethnic groups. However, Black race and Hispanic ethnicity, as well as having low income, has been associated with especially low rates of adherence to endocrine therapy. Reasons cited include concerns about side effects, cost, and perceived patient-provider communication.[33]
- *Challenges during Survivorship*
- The early detection of breast cancer recurrence can influence clinical outcomes. Although there are no established guidelines for survivorship management, surveillance mammography is critical in women with intact breast tissue after treatment. In a systematic review and meta-analysis over a 20-year period, Black, Hispanic, and Asian American women were less likely to receive timely surveillance mammography compared with White women.[34]
- Obesity has been associated with as much as a 35% to 40% increased risk of breast cancer recurrence and with worse overall survival.[35] Rates of obesity are higher in Black women and in women of Hispanic ethnicity.[36] Targeted interventions to promote healthy weight may represent an actionable intervention, though patients may find weight loss hard to prioritize in the midst of and immediately following treatment of breast cancer.[37] Data suggest, however, that there is a much bigger public health crisis. Black and Hispanic children are twice as likely to be obese by the age of 7 years as White children are, highlighting the need for large-scale public health interventions targeting obesity in communities of color.[38,39]

Research and Clinical Trials

Although the early detection is critical and has been a major contributor to improvements in breast cancer outcomes, research and clinical trials have resulted in marked improvement in treatment approaches for women diagnosed with breast cancer. Clinical trials have provided the foundation for de-escalation of surgical management, targeted therapy for HER2-positive breast cancer, and treatment algorithms for TNBC, which represent just a few of the myriad examples of ways that care has been advanced by research.

In many clinical trials, there has been a fundamental lack of racial/ethnic and gender representation. An analysis of cell lines from two major suppliers used for preclinical and clinical trials—the American Type Culture Collection (ATCC) and European Collection of Authenticated Cell Cultures (ECACC)—was conducted to analyze representation of women of African ancestry compared with women of European ancestry. Women of European ancestry represented 80% of the ATCC cell lines and 94% of the ECACC cell lines.[40] Enrollment in clinical trials, while limited across all demographics, is also reported to be lowest in Black, Hispanic, and Asian/Pacific Islander patients, a finding that is also observed among surgical trials of patients with breast cancer.[41,42]

Patients of color are less likely to be treated at institutions where there is access to clinical trials. In addition, stringent trial exclusion criteria related to Eastern cooperative oncology group (ECOG) performance scores and the absence of particular comorbidities further decrease participation of minoritized patients, given higher chronic disease burdens in these groups.[42] Even with geographic access, limited voluntary participation in clinically trials is in part rooted in mistrust within communities of color resulting from episodes of exploitation. The US Public Health Service Syphilis Study at Tuskegee is one well-known example.[43] Black men were enrolled in an observational study of syphilis but not provided informed consent about their participation or even told about their diagnosis. Furthermore, even after treatment with penicillin became available, these men were not provided care for their diagnosis. Another well-known example is displayed in the development of HeLa cells. Henrietta Lacks was a Black mother who ultimately succumbed to cervical cancer. Cells obtained from her cervix were used without her knowledge or consent and ultimately served as the foundation for therapeutic development across a range of diseases. Furthermore, beginning in 1946, the US government conducted experiments in which over 5000 Guatemalan citizens were intentionally infected with bacteria that cause sexually transmitted infections without their informed consent.[44] Many remained untreated into the 2010s. Although these historical examples have helped fuel generations of mistrust toward the health care system, ongoing systemic racism as well as microaggression and macroaggression toward patients and communities of color persist and affect both enrollment in clinical trials and collective impressions about the institution of medicine as a whole.

In a literature review assessing minority participation in clinical trials by Clark and colleagues, five key themes emerged as barriers to enrollment in clinical trials: mistrust, lack of comfort with clinical trial process, lack of information about clinical trials, time and resource constraints associated with clinical trial participation, and lack of clinical trial awareness.[45] Understanding and overcoming these barriers are critical in encouraging diverse participation in clinical trials. Of note, a major reason many patients of color cite for nonparticipation is a failure of health care providers to ask whether they were interested. The Just Ask! program developed by Nadine Barrett, PhD, and available through the Association of Community Cancer Centers and American Cancer Society is an educational program aimed at improving the ability of investigators and research teams recruit diverse clinical trial participants.[46]

Exclusion of male patients has limited our understanding of breast cancer in patients of male sex.[47] Although male breast cancer represents only 1% of all newly diagnosed breast cancer, men typically present with advanced disease and are more likely to die from breast cancer than women are. Furthermore, treatment of men diagnosed with breast cancer is often extrapolated from trials that exclude men. Given the low prevalence of breast cancer in men, accruing a sufficient number of patients to conduct an adequately powered analysis represents a challenge to the medical community that can potentially be enhanced through targeted enrollment outreach and community engagement strategies.

Institutions and research teams can build trustworthiness through inclusion of diverse individuals on their research teams and the use of clinical trial navigators for both women and men. Clinical trial navigators, who often come from minoritized communities, not only provide patients with resources to address potential logistical barriers to participation but also serve as sources of hope and confidence for patients wary of research and health care.[48]

Social Determinants of Health

Although treating a disease process is at the core of providing appropriate health care, understanding the lived experience of a patient and potential barriers to care is important contributors to promoting health equity. Social determinants of care are defined in Health People 2030, a publication of the Office of Disease Prevention and Health Promotion, as *"the conditions in the environment where people are born, live, learn, work, play, worship and age that affect a wide range of health, functioning, and quality-of-life outcomes and risks."*[49] Housing, food, and financial insecurity affect a patient's experience of their treatment and the ability to follow a prescribed treatment plan. For example, if a patient has to choose between a prescription for endocrine therapy and a utility bill or a doctor's appointment and a day of work when financially unstable and supporting a family, they are placed in an impossible situation. Often times, these patients are met with questions about compliance rather than concern for how they can be supported in their care, promoting mistrust and undermining the patient–provider relationship.

Cumulative life stressors throughout daily life can lead to compromise in an individual's ability to cope and have health consequences, measured biologically as allostatic load. Measurements of allostatic load have been inconsistent in the literature but include biomarkers that measure the body's biological response to stress and downstream health outcomes.[50] In fact, an increase in allostatic load was associated with a 9% increase in cancer-specific mortality in a contemporary systematic review and meta-analysis.[51] Although this finding is compelling, it is worth noting that the heterogeneity in defining allostatic load in the literature limits this analysis.

In addition to psychosocial stressors, systemic racism, or political, legal, economic, health care, school, and criminal justice systems that lead to institutionalized race-based discrimination must be considered when contextualizing a patient's lived experience.[52]

How Can We Move the Needle?

An understanding of the complex contributing factors is critical to begin to dismantle health disparities in breast cancer care delivery. To make progress toward equitable care, concerted and intentional efforts must be made at the provider, institutional, health system, and societal levels.

Implicit bias is the result of rapid, unconscious stereotyping, and discriminatory behavior. Implicit bias can affect shared decision-making and patient–provider relationships as well perpetuate mistrust. In a study of 2535 physicians who took the Race Attitude Implicit Association Test (IAT), there was an overall preference for White Americans over Black Americans. Of note, individual self-reported bias and actual implicit bias were not concordant, with higher levels of implicit bias seen on IAT than self-report.[53] Implicit bias can also lead to microaggressions, which are subtle insults or prejudicial behavior toward a marginalized group, and in some cases to macroaggressions, which are overt prejudicial behavior. An awareness of individual bias and how it can affect patient care decisions and patient–provider interactions is critical to overcoming imbedded mistrust and promoting equitable care. A focus on contextualizing the experience of our patients and familiarizing ourselves with support services can help strengthen the patient–provider relationship. Routine screening for unmet social needs and evaluation of the patient experience during their course of treatment is gradually becoming more common via increased use of social need screens and patient-reported outcome measure tools.[54]

At the institutional and health system level, efforts to achieve a diverse workforce will help mitigate disparities in patient care. A diverse work environment leads to a better understanding of racial and culture differences that contributes to culturally competent care for all patients. Furthermore, providers who are traditionally underrepresented in medicine are more likely to provide care to minoritized and medically underserved communities.[55] Given the often complex financial, social, and medical needs of patients, especially from minoritized communities, receiving breast cancer treatment, having a robust suite of supportive services, including social work, financial counselors, and patient navigators may help overcome barriers to high-quality care delivery, including delays in care and perioperative support.

Public health interventions to address the root cause of higher rates of obesity and comorbid conditions within Black and Hispanic communities are a high-level and complex goal that is a critical piece of promoting health equity. Dismantling systemic and structural racism that are deeply embedded in the foundation of society are a crucial step in addressing inequities in care delivery for breast cancer and mitigating disparate health outcomes across all disease sites.

SUMMARY

The anatomy of health disparities is complex, and although this article addresses many of the contributing factors, it is not exhaustive. Health disparities affect the spectrum of the breast care experience, ranging from risk assessment, screening behavior, and early detection to treatment protocols and survivorship. Drivers of disparate breast cancer outcomes begin before a patient's stepping foot into the office a breast cancer specialist.[54] Attention to implicit bias, improving diversity in the work force, and providing robust supportive care services to treat patients in the context of their lived experience rather than their disease alone represent critical steps to promoting equity in breast cancer diagnosis, treatment, outcomes, and clinical trial participation.

DISCLOSURES

Dr O.M. Fayanju is supported by the National Institutes of Health, United States (NIH) under Award Numbers 7K08CA241390-03 (PI: Fayanju) and P50CA244690 (PIs: Beidas, Bekelman). The content of this manuscript is solely the responsibility of the authors and does not necessarily represent the official views of the NIH. Dr O.M. Fayanju also reports institutional grants from Gilead Sciences, United States, and Sanofi as well as support via philanthropic funds from the Haas family. Dr L.C. Elmore has nothing to disclose.

REFERENCES

1. American Cancer Society. Breast Cancer Facts & Figures 2019-2020. Accessed December 15, 2022. https://www.cancer.org/content/dam/cancer-org/research/cancer-facts-and-statistics/breast-cancer-facts-and-figures/breast-cancer-facts-and-figures-2019-2020.pdf.

2. American Cancer Society. Cancer Facts & Figure for African American/Black People 2022-2024. Accessed December 15, 2022. https://www.cancer.org/content/dam/cancer-org/research/cancer-facts-and-statistics/cancer-facts-and-figures-for-african-americans/2022-2024-cff-aa.pdf.

3. Office of Disease Prevention and Health Promotion. Health Equity in Healthy People 2030. Accessed January 21, 2023. https://health.gov/healthypeople/priority-areas/health-equity-healthy-people-2030.

4. Center for Disease Control and Prevention Office of Minority Health & Health Equity. What is Health Equity? Accessed January 21, 2023. https://www.cdc.gov/healthequity/whatis/index.html#anchor_09858.

5. Yu AYL, Thomas SM, DiLalla GD, et al. Disease characteristics and mortality among Asian women with breast cancer. Cancer 2022;128(5):1024–37.

6. Champion CD, Thomas SM, Plichta JK, et al. Disparities at the Intersection of Race and Ethnicity: Examining Trends and Outcomes in Hispanic Women With Breast Cancer. JCO Oncol Pract 2022;18(5):e827–38.

7. Swami N, Nguyen T, Dee EC, et al. Disparities in Primary Breast Cancer Stage at Presentation Among Hispanic Subgroups. Ann Surg Oncol 2022;29(13):7977–87.

8. Quinn GP, Sanchez JA, Sutton SK, et al. Cancer and lesbian, gay, bisexual, transgender/transsexual, and queer/questioning (LGBTQ) populations. CA: a cancer journal for clinicians 2015;65(5):384–400.

9. Newman LA, Kaljee LM. Health Disparities and Triple-Negative Breast Cancer in African American Women: A Review. JAMA Surg 2017;152(5):485–93.

10. Newman LA, Jenkins B, Chen Y, et al. Hereditary susceptibility for triple negative breast cancer associated with Western Sub-Saharan African Ancestry: results from an International Surgical Breast Cancer Collaborative. Annals of surgery 2019;270(3):484–92.

11. Huo D, Feng Y, Haddad S, et al. Genome-wide association studies in women of African ancestry identified 3q26.21 as a novel susceptibility locus for oestrogen receptor negative breast cancer. Hum Mol Genet 2016;25(21):4835–46.

12. Warner ET, Tamimi RM, Hughes ME, et al. Racial and Ethnic Differences in Breast Cancer Survival: Mediating Effect of Tumor Characteristics and Sociodemographic and Treatment Factors. J Clin Oncol 2015;33(20):2254–61.

13. Cho B, Han Y, Lian M, et al. Evaluation of Racial/Ethnic Differences in Treatment and Mortality Among Women With Triple-Negative Breast Cancer. JAMA Oncol 2021;7(7):1016–23.

14. Kaiser Family Foundation. Health Coverage by Race and Ethnicity, 2010-2021. Accessed December 15, 2022. https://www.kff.org/racial-equity-and-health-policy/issue-brief/health-coverage-by-race-and-ethnicity/.

15. Schueler KM, Chu PW, Smith-Bindman R. Factors associated with mammography utilization: a systematic quantitative review of the literature. J Womens Health (Larchmt) 2008;17(9):1477–98.

16. Greenup RA. Financial Toxicity and Shared Decision Making in Oncology. Surgical Oncology Clinics 2022;31(1):1–7.

17. Politi MC, Yen RW, Elwyn G, et al. Women Who Are Young, Non-White, and with Lower Socioeconomic Status Report Higher Financial Toxicity up to 1 Year After Breast Cancer Surgery: A Mixed-Effects Regression Analysis. Oncol 2020;26(1):e142–52.

18. Keating NL, Kouri EM, He Y, et al. Location Isn't Everything: Proximity, Hospital Characteristics, Choice of Hospital, and Disparities for Breast Cancer Surgery Patients. Health Serv Res 2016;51(4):1561–83.

19. Dai D. Black residential segregation, disparities in spatial access to health care facilities, and late-stage breast cancer diagnosis in metropolitan Detroit. Health Place 2010;16(5):1038–52.

20. Molina Y, Silva A, Rauscher GH. Racial/Ethnic Disparities in Time to a Breast Cancer Diagnosis: The Mediating Effects of Health Care Facility Factors. Med Care 2015;53(10):872–8.

21. Griggs JJ, Sorbero MES, Stark AT, et al. Racial Disparity in the Dose and Dose Intensity of Breast Cancer Adjuvant Chemotherapy. Breast Cancer Res Treat 2003;81(1):21–31.

22. Green AK, Aviki EM, Matsoukas K, et al. Racial disparities in chemotherapy administration for early-stage breast cancer: a systematic review and meta-analysis. Breast Cancer Res Treat 2018;172(2):247–63.

23. Chavez-MacGregor M, Clarke CA, Lichtensztajn DY, et al. Delayed Initiation of Adjuvant Chemotherapy Among Patients With Breast Cancer. JAMA Oncol 2016;2(3):322–9.

24. Fedewa SA, Ward EM, Stewart AK, et al. Delays in adjuvant chemotherapy treatment among patients with breast cancer are more likely in African American and Hispanic populations: a national cohort study 2004-2006. J Clin Oncol 2010; 28(27):4135–41.

25. Akinyemiju TF, Vin-Raviv N, Chavez-Yenter D, et al. Race/ethnicity and socioeconomic differences in breast cancer surgery outcomes. Cancer Epidemiology 2015;39(5):745–51.

26. Sarver MM, Rames JD, Ren Y, et al. Racial and Ethnic Disparities in Surgical Outcomes after Postmastectomy Breast Reconstruction. J Am Coll Surg 2022;234(5): 760–71.

27. Mets EJ, Chouairi FK, Gabrick KS, et al. Persistent disparities in breast cancer surgical outcomes among hispanic and African American patients. European Journal of Surgical Oncology 2019;45(4):584–90.

28. Dragun AE, Huang B, Tucker TC, et al. Disparities in the application of adjuvant radiotherapy after breast-conserving surgery for early stage breast cancer. Cancer 2011;117(12):2590–8.

29. Du XL, Gor BJ. Racial Disparities and Trends in Radiation Therapy After Breast-Conserving surgery for Early-stage Breast Cancer in Women, 1992 to 2002. Ethn Dis 2007;17(1):122–8.

30. Martinez SR, Beal SH, Chen SL, et al. Disparities in the Use of Radiation Therapy in Patients With Local-Regionally Advanced Breast Cancer. Int J Radiat Oncol Biol Phys 2010;78(3):787–92.

31. Smith GL, Shih YC, Xu Y, et al. Racial disparities in the use of radiotherapy after breast-conserving surgery: a national Medicare study. Cancer 2010;116(3): 734–41.

32. Keating NL, Kouri E, He Y, et al. Racial differences in definitive breast cancer therapy in older women: are they explained by the hospitals where patients undergo surgery? Med Care 2009;47(7):765–73.

33. Roberts MC, Wheeler SB, Reeder-Hayes K. Racial/Ethnic and socioeconomic disparities in endocrine therapy adherence in breast cancer: a systematic review. Am J Public Health 2015;105(Suppl 3):e4–15.

34. Advani P, Advani S, Nayak P, et al. Racial/ethnic disparities in use of surveillance mammogram among breast cancer survivors: a systematic review. J Cancer Surviv 2022;16(3):514–30.

35. Jiralerspong S, Goodwin PJ. Obesity and Breast Cancer Prognosis: Evidence, Challenges, and Opportunities. J Clin Oncol 2016;34(35):4203–16.

36. Nayak P, Paxton RJ, Holmes H, et al. Racial and Ethnic Differences in Health Behaviors Among Cancer Survivors. Am J Prev Med 2015;48(6):729–36.

37. Fayanju OM, Greenup RA, Zafar SY, et al. Modifiable Barriers and Facilitators for Breast Cancer Care: A Thematic Analysis of Patient and Provider Perspectives. J Surg Res 2023;284:269–79.
38. Taveras EM, Gillman MW, Kleinman KP, et al. Reducing racial/ethnic disparities in childhood obesity: the role of early life risk factors. JAMA Pediatr 2013;167(8):731–8.
39. Williams DR, Mohammed SA, Shields AE. Understanding and effectively addressing breast cancer in African American women: Unpacking the social context. Cancer 2016;122(14):2138–49.
40. Clarke S, Chin SN, Dodds L, et al. Racial disparities in breast cancer preclinical and clinical models. Breast Cancer Res 2022;24(1):56.
41. Stewart JH, Bertoni AG, Staten JL, et al. Participation in Surgical Oncology Clinical Trials: Gender-, Race/Ethnicity-, and Age-based Disparities. Ann Surg Oncol 2007;14(12):3328–34.
42. Fayanju OM, Ren Y, Thomas SM, et al. A Case-Control Study Examining Disparities in Clinical Trial Participation Among Breast Surgical Oncology Patients. JNCI Cancer Spectr 2020;4(2):pkz103.
43. Reverby SM. Ethical failures and history lessons: the US Public Health Service research studies in Tuskegee and Guatemala. Publ Health Rev 2012;34:1–18.
44. Rodriguez MA, García R. First, Do No Harm: The US Sexually Transmitted Disease Experiments in Guatemala. American Journal of Public Health 2013; 103(12):2122–6.
45. Clark LT, Watkins L, Piña IL, et al. Increasing Diversity in Clinical Trials: Overcoming Critical Barriers. Curr Probl Cardiol 2019;44(5):148–72.
46. Barrett NJ, Boehmer L, Schrag J, et al. An Assessment of the Feasibility and Utility of an ACCC-ASCO Implicit Bias Training Program to Enhance Racial and Ethnic Diversity in Cancer Clinical Trials. JCO Oncol Pract 2023;Op2200378. https://doi.org/10.1200/op.22.00378.
47. Duma N, Hoversten KP, Ruddy KJ. Exclusion of male patients in breast cancer clinical trials. JNCI Cancer Spectr 2018;2(2):pky018.
48. Guerra CE, Sallee V, Hwang WT, et al. Accrual of Black participants to cancer clinical trials following a five-year prospective initiative of community outreach and engagement. J Clin Oncol 2021;39(15_suppl):100.
49. Office of Disease Prevention and Health Promotion. Healthy People 2030: Social Determinants of Health. Accessed January 15, 2023. https://health.gov/healthypeople/priority-areas/social-determinants-health.
50. Obeng-Gyasi S, Tarver W, Carlos RC, et al. Allostatic load: a framework to understand breast cancer outcomes in Black women. NPJ Breast Cancer 2021;7(1):100.
51. Mathew A, Doorenbos AZ, Li H, et al. Allostatic Load in Cancer: A Systematic Review and Mini Meta-Analysis. Biol Res Nurs 2021;23(3):341–61.
52. Braveman P, Arkin E, Proctor D, et al. Systemic And Structural Racism: Definitions, Examples, Health Damages, And Approaches To Dismantling. Health Aff 2022;41(2):171–8.
53. Sabin J, Nosek BA, Greenwald A, et al. Physicians' implicit and explicit attitudes about race by MD race, ethnicity, and gender. J Health Care Poor Underserved 2009;20(3):896–913.
54. Fayanju OM, Ren Y, Stashko I, et al. Patient-reported causes of distress predict disparities in time to evaluation and time to treatment after breast cancer diagnosis. Cancer 2020. https://doi.org/10.1002/cncr.33310.
55. Walker KO, Moreno G, Grumbach K. The association among specialty, race, ethnicity, and practice location among California physicians in diverse specialties. J Natl Med Assoc 2012;104(1–2):46–52.

Lasting Impacts of the COVID-19 Pandemic on Breast Cancer Diagnosis and Treatment in the United States

Jenna L. Sturz, DO[a], Judy C. Boughey, MD[b],*

KEYWORDS

- Breast cancer • COVID-19 • Screening • Elective procedures
- Neoadjuvant endocrine therapy

KEY POINTS

- COVID-19 pandemic resulted in a decrease in the use of screening mammography in the early part of the pandemic.
- The moratorium on elective procedures early in the COVID-19 pandemic resulted in increased use of neoadjuvant endocrine therapy for hormone positive breast cancer delaying surgical resection until later in the pandemic.
- COVID-19 pandemic resulted in an increase in the utilization of telehealth and decreased enrollment in breast cancer clinical trials.
- There was an increase in same day discharge after all breast operations including mastectomy with or without reconstruction.
- Use of hypofractionated radiation regimens increased.

INTRODUCTION

Concern regarding a novel coronavirus first began in late fall of 2019 in China with the first human case of COVID-19 caused by SARS-CoV-2 reported in Wuhan City, China, in December 2019.[1] After more than 118,000 cases were reported in 114 counties and 4,291 deaths, escalation to the declaration of a worldwide pandemic by the World Health Organization (WHO)[1] occurred on March 11th, 2022.[2] Upon the declaration of a pandemic and surge of cases, countries began to close their borders to international travel and implemented stay-at-home orders. Social distancing and mask-wearing guidelines ensued in order to mitigate the spread of the novel virus.

[a] Department of Surgery, Mayo Clinic, Rochester, MN, USA; [b] Division of Breast and Melanoma Surgical Oncology, Department of Surgery, Mayo Clinic, Rochester, MN 55905, USA
* Corresponding author.
E-mail address: Boughey.judy@mayo.edu

Surg Oncol Clin N Am 32 (2023) 811–819
https://doi.org/10.1016/j.soc.2023.05.010
1055-3207/23/© 2023 Elsevier Inc. All rights reserved.
surgonc.theclinics.com

As the number of cases escalated, hospital systems became overwhelmed due to the shortage of essential medical equipment (especially PPE and ventilators), hospital beds, and health care workers. State of emergency declarations were made in order to reallocate and prioritize resources towards the COVID-19 pandemic. The reallocation of resources created unique challenges and downstream effects on many aspects of breast cancer diagnosis, treatment, and research efforts. Several medical societies collaborated in order to provide guidance on how to continue providing breast cancer care in unprecedented times. Due to the abrupt cessation of elective imaging and procedures, concern for continuing to provide appropriate screening, diagnosis, and treatment arose, especially in the oncology sector of health care. In addition, due to widespread concern about contracting the COVID-19 virus patients began to cancel or delay medical visits. In September 2020, the CDC released data in the *Morbidity and Mortality Weekly Report (MMWR)* that an estimated 41% of US adults had delayed or avoided seeking medical care due to concerns about exposure to COVID-19.[2]

IMPACT ON BREAST CANCER SCREENING

Modern modalities for breast cancer screening were developed in the late 1960s with the first official recommendations of screening mammography by the American College of Surgeons (ACS) in 1976.[3] The goal of screening is to detect and diagnose diseases at an early stage. At the time of the COVID-19 pandemic, the United States Preventive Services Task Force (USPSTF) recommended women aged 50-74 with an average risk of breast cancer have a screening mammogram every two years.[4] Since approximately 1 in 8 women will be diagnosed with breast cancer in their lifetime, early detection with screening modalities has an important impact on morbidity and mortality.[3]

At the onset of the COVID-19 pandemic in March of 2020, elective imaging and procedures, including cancer screening modalities, were put on hold in order to conserve personal protective equipment, create hospital capacity and to protect patients and medical personnel from exposure to the virus. On March 26, 2020, the American Society of Breast Surgeons (ASBrS) and the American College of Radiology (ACR) issued a joint statement recommending medical facilities to postpone all breast screening including mammography, ultrasound and MRI.[5] As a result of guidelines and patients' fear of exposure to the virus, there was a significant decrease in the number of breast cancer screening appointments during the initial months of the pandemic. In a study conducted by Grimm and colleagues[6] that utilized the National Mammography Database, screening mammograms were down 63.7% in the time period of March 1- May 31, 2020. Another study looking at the National Breast and Cervical Cancer Early Detection program, a program designed to provide treatment and screening modalities to low income or underserved populations, demonstrated a sharp decline of 87% in the number of screening mammograms in April of 2020 compared to the previous five years.[7]

Consequently, there was a decrease in the number of new breast cancers diagnosed during the moratorium of breast screening modalities.[6] Concerns arose regarding possible worsening of cancer outcomes due to delay in diagnosis. Studies conducted during the early phases of the pandemic predicted that patients would present with more advanced disease resulting in possibly worse cancer outcomes.[8] A recent study published in December 2022 evaluating the National Cancer Database reported a 12.4% deficit in the number of expected cancer diagnoses in 2020. Breast cancer was amongst the largest absolute decrease in the number of cases with approximately 34,000 fewer cases in 2020 than expected.[9]

In May 2020 the Society of Breast Imaging released guidelines on how to proceed with a safe return to imaging, followed by recommendations from the ACR in July 2020.[6] Guidelines provided strategies for health care systems and for patients to safely return to screening practices including expanding hours, spacing out appointments and sanitization strategies. Upon the cessation of elective procedure moratoriums, screening mammography rates began to rebound. According to the study by Grimm and colleagues,[6] the volume of screening mammograms, diagnostic mammograms, and breast biopsies rebounded to 85.3%, 97.8%, and 91.5%, respectively, during March-May of 2021 when compared to the pre-COVID-19 volume from March-May of 2019.

Although early studies predicted patients would present with more advanced disease, more recent retrospective studies looking at the effects of screening delays due to the COVID-19 pandemic on breast cancer stage at the time of diagnosis have shown mixed results. In a single-institution, retrospective review published in April 2021 by a university referral center in Italy, no significant difference in tumor biology was demonstrated but a significant increase in clinical stage III disease and node positive disease at diagnosis was found after a two-month interruption in breast cancer screening.[10] Another retrospective, single-site study, from the first year of the pandemic found no difference in breast cancer stage at diagnosis, method of cancer detection, or tumor biology comparing March-August 2020 (early COVID) to March-August 2019 (pre-COVID).[11] In a more recent retrospective, multi-institutional study published January 2022, there was a slight increase in presenting tumor size and positive nodal status in the newly diagnosed breast cancers during the early phase of the pandemic due to the tumors being self-detected.[12] As soon as regular screening was resumed, the significance was no longer demonstrated.[12]

The overall impact of the breast cancer screening moratorium from COVID-19 is still unknown and ongoing and given the latency in breast cancer diagnosis and mortality, it may take years to be realized.

IMPACT ON BREAST CANCER TREATMENT

In order to mitigate the viral spread and preserve medical equipment, especially PPE and ventilators, cessation of nonessential appointments and elective procedures was imposed in mid-March of 2020.[13] This resulted in the closure of many operating rooms and limitation on all procedures including operations for cancer. These unprecedented times prompted health care systems to implement creative measures and triage strategies with guidance from several medical societies in order to weigh the challenging situation of protecting patients and workers safety by decreasing exposure to the novel virus while continuing to provide medical care.

The COVID-19 Pandemic Breast Cancer Consortium, created by representatives from ACR, ACS, ASBrS, American Society for Clinical Oncology, National Comprehensive Cancer Network and the Society of Surgical Oncology, released an article in April 2020 to provide expert opinion on how to safely provide multidisciplinary breast cancer care during the COVID-19 pandemic.[14] As an effort to evaluate the impact of these expert guidelines and overall impact of the pandemic on breast cancer management in the United States, the ASBrS created a COVID-19 supplemental module to their established registry database.[15]

Conduction of outpatient visits was also changed due to the COVID-19 pandemic. Guidelines recommended implementing a triage strategy to only conduct in person visits with patients who were prioritized as high risk such as patients with a new diagnosis of breast cancer or established patients with new problems such as infections, palpable findings or suffering from severe side effects from their treatment regimens.[14]

During the early phases of the pandemic, it was widely encouraged by institutions across the United States to limit the number of treatment team members during in per-son visits along with strict visitor restrictions for in person patient encounters.[16]

IMPACT ON SURGERY

In response to the Centers for Disease Control recommending that all elective sur-geries and non-essential medical, surgical, and dental procedures be delayed during the novel COVID-19 outbreak, several medical societies published guidelines for pro-viders and health care administrators on how to categorize non-emergent surgery.[17] The COVID-19 Pandemic Breast Cancer Consortium recommendations implemented a triage strategy based on breast cancer tumor biology and disease stage. Surgical intervention was recommended in patients who were completing neoadjuvant chemo-therapy for triple-negative disease. Whereas for patients with early stage, hormone positive disease neoadjuvant endocrine therapy was recommended in order to safely delay surgery and avoid undergoing surgery during the height of the pandemic.[14,15]

Along with the implementation of prioritization strategies to determine which patients with breast cancer should undergo surgery, which surgery to offer was also influenced. To minimize the length of hospital stay and potential COVID-19 exposure along with conserving resources, outpatient, same day procedures were encouraged.[15] Patients eligible for breast conservation therapy (BCT) were discouraged from undergoing mas-tectomy to minimize operative time. In patients who were to undergo mastectomy, contralateral prophylactic mastectomy, and immediate reconstruction were discour-aged in order to reduce surgical time and risk of complications.[15,18,19] Increased health care cost due to multiple surgical interventions along with long-term patient psycholog-ical effects were acknowledged as possible consequences.[15] All prophylactic surgery as well as breast surgery for benign or high-risk lesions, such as fibroadenoma or atypia were also postponed.

Given the focus on minimizing exposure of patients and health care workers to the virus and shortage of PPE many centers shifted from routine 23-hour observation or admission of patients after mastectomy to same day discharge.[20] This was not only for patients undergoing total mastectomy but also those that underwent mastectomy with immediate reconstruction. Although the COVID-19 pandemic placed unprece-dented emphasis on outpatient breast cancer surgery, the initial shift to home recov-ery after mastectomy began in the early 2000s with literature supporting that home recovery is a safe option for appropriately selected patients without increased risk of complications.[21] A recent study published in January 2023 looked at outcomes of same-day discharge mastectomy pre- and post-COVID19 pandemic and showed no difference in complication rates including hematomas, readmissions or surgical site infections.[20] These studies support the continued effort of enhanced recovery af-ter surgery practices which will likely continue to grow in both the number and types of procedures that will be performed as an outpatient.

IMPACT ON CHEMOTHERAPY

Treatment of breast cancer requires a multidisciplinary approach with medical oncol-ogists providing expertise in hormonal, chemotherapy, and/or targeted therapy regi-mens. In response to the delays or cancellations of non-emergency surgery in March 2020, the medical management of breast cancer changed, especially the utili-zation of neoadjuvant endocrine therapy.

The standard of care for early stage, estrogen positive (ER+) breast cancer was generally upfront surgery with partial or total mastectomy with or without axillary staging, followed by adjuvant endocrine therapy with or without adjuvant radiation or chemotherapy. Prior to the COVID-19 pandemic, the use of neoadjuvant endocrine therapy in ER + breast cancer was recommended to downstage disease in patients with large or locally advanced tumors in order to potentially allow patients to become breast conservation surgery candidates and was used for elderly patients or patients with significant comorbidities contraindicating operative intervention.[22] In response to mandated surgical delays during the early phase of the COVID-19 pandemic, guidelines recommended that patients with ER+/HER2-disease can safely defer surgery and receive neoadjuvant endocrine therapy for 6-12 months without any clinical compromise.[14]

Although the widespread use of neoadjuvant endocrine therapy in early-stage ER + breast cancers has only been widely adopted in the US due to the unprecedented nature of the COVID-19 pandemic and implemented guidelines, this strategy has been used commonly in the UK even prior to the pandemic. Pre-pandemic neoadjuvant endocrine treatment in ER+/HER2-breast cancer use in the US was increasing in patients where the clinical team wanted to decrease tumor size and enable breast-conserving surgery. The pandemic resulted in a significant boost in the use of neoadjuvant endocrine therapy as a bridge until surgery could be safely performed.[15] As we move forward it can also be used post-pandemic when treatment teams anticipate delays in surgery for patients (such as those with comorbidities, or those needing to stop smoking prior to mastectomy with reconstruction) and to assess responsiveness to endocrine therapy.

Medical oncologists were also faced with considering alternative treatment schedules and regimens to minimize the risk of virus exposure in their immunocompromised patient population. Chemotherapy schedules were encouraged to be modified in order to reduce clinic visits by changing dosing intervals.[14] In addition, an increased use of genomic testing on core needle biopsies at diagnosis occurred to aid in medical decision making regarding neoadjuvant chemotherapy versus neoadjuvant endocrine therapy or upfront surgery.[15] While the data on genomic assays were developed using surgical specimens from upfront surgery, genomic assays are now frequently performed on percutaneous core needle biopsy.

IMPACT ON RADIATION THERAPY

As with the medical and surgical treatment of breast cancer, a triaged and personalized approach was recommended for the utilization of radiotherapy in patients with breast cancer. Patients with symptomatic disease who would benefit from palliative regimens and patients progressing on neoadjuvant therapy were considered high priority.[14] Current literature supports that adjuvant radiotherapy initiation can be delayed safely up to 3-6 months in select patients,[18] so the priority of radiotherapy was for high-risk patients, palliative treatment or patients already initiated on a treatment regimen.

In a similar manner to systemic treatment, changes to radiotherapy schedules in order to minimize exposure to the virus were also recommended. Guidelines recommended the use of moderate hypofractionation and ultra-hypofractionation for appropriate patients. In patients with breast cancer without positive regional lymph node disease, moderate hypofractionation was already widely used but the pandemic accelerated the use of ultra-hypofractionation in patients with early-stage breast cancer.[23] As a result of the COVID-19 pandemic, utilization of telemedicine and hypofractionation modalities are likely to remain part of the radiotherapy treatment of breast cancer.

IMPACT ON CLINICAL TRIALS

The COVID-19 pandemic had a significant impact on the recruitment and conduct of clinical trials due to multiple factors. A survey conducted at the beginning of the pandemic suggested that at least 60% of investigators halted or delayed enrollment of patients into clinical trials with 50% reporting prioritizing enrollment to higher priority trials.[24] At the beginning of the pandemic, health care systems were overwhelmed which required the reprioritization of health care resources across the nation. Research efforts including institutional review boards prioritized efforts in the investigation and creation of therapies and vaccinations against the novel virus. The US Food and Drug Administration also issued specific guidelines in order to address situations in which to consider withdrawal of participation in trials in regard to their safety as the pandemic evolved.[25] Although appropriate, this led to a significant backlog in study startups and delay in the opening of new cancer-related clinical trials. Funding for cancer research, including grant funds from large organizations such as the American Cancer Society, were also considerably decreased due to the economic unrest from the pandemic.[3]

In addition to the reallocation of research resources, transmission mitigation strategies including stay at home mandates and transition to working in a remote setting had significant impacts on the conduction of clinical trials. In order to protect health care workers from unnecessary COVID-19 exposure, many "non-essential" personnel were transitioned to working remotely which created challenges in the conduction of trial operations. Even during the initial pandemic recovery phase, on-site research staff continued to be limited causing a decrease in clinical trial enrollment and slowing trial conduction.[26] The cessation of elective procedures also interrupted many aspects of clinical trials such as screening, diagnostic imaging, and research biopsies as these were placed on hold.

Patients enrolled in clinical trials also faced challenges both with the worry of exposure risk, especially amongst immunocompromised patients with cancer, and also with long distance travel to tertiary centers during times of mandated quarantine. Due to this, many patients opted for treatment options that required fewer visits to medical centers which prevented the consideration of some clinical trials.[26] The National Cancer Institute provided interim guidance for enrolled patients which included allowing patients to transfer care to local health care providers and use of local laboratories for blood tests etc. when they could not travel to the enrolling study site.[27]

Despite the initial shutdown and challenges of conducting clinical trials, restarting resumed in a stepwise approach beginning with patients in phase 1 trials, moving on to other treatment trials and observation cohort studies, tissue collection studies, and quality of life studies as the last to resume.[26] The COVID-19 pandemic was an incredibly challenging time for the recruitment and conduction of cancer clinical trials that required the adaptation of a hybrid system of virtual and in person visits. As an unintended consequence, the pandemic may have provided meaningful improvement in the utilization of telehealth and virtual communication platforms in many aspects of the trial process including informed consent.

IMPACT ON MENTAL HEALTH

The COVID-19 pandemic resulted in a significant impact on both breast cancer patient and health care provider mental health. In addition to stay-at home mandates creating social isolation, strict hospital visitor restrictions for hospital stays and appointments incurred additional anxiety for patients during the pandemic. According to the COVID-19 Mental Disorder Collaborator, there was a 27.6% increase in the cases of major depressive disorder and 25.6% increase in the cases of anxiety disorders globally throughout 2020.[28]

Impacts of the pandemic on physician well-being were studied via the CROWN study which surveyed over 800 breast specialists in the United States. The study aimed to evaluate the effect of delayed patients' treatment on physician emotional wellness. Nearly 80% of breast physicians reported some sort of delay in either screening, surgical interventions, or systemic treatment for their patients. The survey also found that mean anxiety and COVID-19 burnout scores were higher in physicians whose patients experienced delays in their cancer treatments.[29]

DISCUSSION

The COVID-19 pandemic was an unprecedented time with lasting impacts on the diagnosis, treatment, and research of breast cancer in the United States. As a result of the pandemic there have been advancements in the utilization of telehealth methods in patient care and clinical trials, increase in the use of genomic testing on core needle biopsy to guide upfront surgery versus neoadjuvant therapy, increase in the use of neoadjuvant endocrine therapy in patients with early-stage ER + and increase in outpatient surgery for breast disease. Further research is ongoing and necessary to determine the long-term outcomes and psychological impact of the COVID-19 pandemic on patients with breast cancer.

CLINICS CARE POINTS

- Outpatient surgery for patients undergoing mastectomy without and with reconstruction will continue to grow as evidence supports home recovery after mastectomy has no difference in adverse outcomes
- Increased use of neoadjuvant endocrine therapy treatment in ER+/HER2-breast cancer during the pandemic as a bridge to surgery may also be more commonly used post-pandemic to assess responsiveness to endocrine therapy and as a bridge to surgery while awaiting genetic testing or smoking cessation
- The pandemic resulted in an improvement in the infrastructure and increase in the utilization of telehealth and virtual communication with patients.
- The pandemic resulted in the acceptance of telehealth for informed consent and accepting more laboratory testing to be performed locally which will improve access for patients to clinical trials
- Hypofractionation modalities are likely to remain part of the radiotherapy treatment of appropriately selected patients with breast cancer post-pandemic

DISCLOSURES

Dr J.C. Boughey receives research funding from Eli Lilly & Co, United States and SymBioSis paid to her institution and is on DSMB for CairnsSurgical. She has spoken for EndoMag, PER, PeerView and receives royalties from UpTo Date.

REFERENCES

1. World Health Organization. Origin of SARS-COV-2. World Health Organization. Available at: https://www.who.int/publications/i/item/origin-of-sars-cov-2. Access January 21, 2023.

2. Centers for Disease Control and Prevention. CDC Museum Covid-19 Timeline. Centers for Disease Control and Prevention. Available at: https://www.cdc.gov/museum/timeline/covid19.html. Accessed January 21, 2023.

3. American Cancer Society. COVID-19 and 2020 ACS Grants. Available at: https://www.cancer.org/research/we-fund-cancer-research/apply-research-grant/grant-types/covid-19-and-2020-acs-grants.html. Accessed January 12, 2022.

4. US Preventive Services Taskforce. Breast Cancer: Screening. Recommendation: Breast Cancer: Screening | United States Preventive Services Taskforce. Available at: https://www.uspreventiveservicestaskforce.org/uspstf/recommendation/breast-cancer-screening. Accessed: January 11, 2016.

5. The American Society of Breast Surgeons and The American College of Radiology. Joint Statement on Breast Screening Exams During the Covid-19 Pandemic. Available at: https://www.breastsurgeons.org/news/?id=45. Accessed September 24, 2021.

6. Grimm LJ, Lee C, Rosenberg RD, et al. Impact of the COVID-19 pandemic on breast imaging: an analysis of the national mammography database. J Am Coll Radiol 2022;19(8):919–34.

7. DeGroff A, Miller J, Sharma K, et al. COVID-19 Impact on screening test volume through the national breast and cervical cancer early detection program, January-June 2020, in the United States. Prev Med 2021;151:106559.

8. Maringe C, Spicer J, Morris M, et al. The impact of the COVID-19 pandemic on cancer deaths due to delays in diagnosis in England, UK: a National, Population-based, Modelling Study. Lancet Oncol 2020;21(8):1023–34.

9. Nogueira LM, Palis B, Boffa D, et al. Evaluation of the Impact of the COVID-19 Pandemic on Reliability of Cancer Surveillance Data in the National Cancer Database. Ann Surg Oncol 2023;30(4):2087–93.

10. Toss A, Isca C, Venturelli M, et al. Two-month stop in mammographic screening significantly impacts on breast cancer stage at diagnosis and upfront treatment in the COVID era. ESMO Open 2021;6(2):100055.

11. Tonneson JE, Hoskin TL, Day CN, et al. Impact of the COVID-19 pandemic on breast cancer stage at diagnosis, presentation, and patient management. Ann Surg Oncol 2022;29(4):2231–9.

12. Mason H, Friedrich AK, Niakan S, et al. The influence of screening mammography cessation and resumption on breast cancer presentation and treatment: a multi-hospital health system experience during the early COVID-19 pandemic. Eur J Breast Health 2022;18(4):306–14.

13. Meredith JW, High KP, Freischlag JA. Preserving Elective Surgeries in the COVID-19 Pandemic and the Future. JAMA 2020;324(17):1725–6.

14. Dietz JR, Moran MS, Isakoff SJ, et al. Recommendations for prioritization, treatment, and triage of breast cancer patients during the COVID-19 pandemic. the COVID-19 pandemic breast cancer consortium. Breast Cancer Res Treat 2020;181(3):487–97.

15. Wilke LG, Nguyen TT, Yang Q, et al. Analysis of the impact of the COVID-19 pandemic on the multidisciplinary management of breast cancer: review from the american society of breast surgeons COVID-19 and mastery registries. Ann Surg Oncol 2021;28(10):5535–43.

16. Centers for Medcare & Medicaid Services. Hospital Visitation – Phase II Visitation for Patients Who are Covid-19 Negative. Available at: https://www.cms.gov/files/document/covid-hospital-visitation-phase-ii-visitation-covid-negative-patients.pdf. Access January 21, 2023.

17. American College of Surgeons. Covid-19: Elective case Triage Guidelines for Surgical Care. Available at: https://www.facs.org/for-medical-professionals/covid-19/clinical-guidance/elective-case/. Accessed January 21, 2023.
18. Petropoulou Z, Arkadopoulos N, Michalopoulos NV. Breast cancer and COVID-19: challenges in surgical management. Cancers 2022;14(21):5360.
19. Rocco N, Montagna G, Di Micco R, et al. The impact of the COVID-19 pandemic on surgical management of breast cancer: global trends and future perspectives. Oncol 2021;26(1):e66–77.
20. Olimpiadi Y, Goldenberg AR, Postlewait L, et al. Outcomes of the same-day discharge following mastectomy before, during and after COVID-19 pandemic. J Surg Oncol 2023;127(5):761–7.
21. Ludwig KK, Rao R. ASO author reflections: homing in on safety-home recovery after mastectomy. Ann Surg Oncol 2022;29(9):5809–10.
22. Weiss A, King TA, Mittendorf EA. The landmark series: neoadjuvant endocrine therapy for breast cancer. Ann Surg Oncol 2020;27(9):3393–401.
23. Knowlton CA. Breast cancer management during the COVID-19 pandemic: the radiation oncology perspective. Curr Breast Cancer Rep 2022;14(1):8–16.
24. Waterhouse DM, Harvey RD, Hurley P, et al. Early impact of COVID-19 on the conduct of oncology clinical trials and long-term opportunities for transformation: findings from an american society of clinical oncology survey. JCO Oncol Pract 2020;16(7):417–21.
25. US Food and Drug Administration. FDA Guidance on Conduct of Clinical Trials of Medical Products during COVID-19 Public Health Emergency: Guidance for Industry, Investigators, and Institutional Review Boards. Available at: https://www.fda.gov/regulatory-information/search-fda-guidance-documents/fda-guidance-conduct-clinical-trials-medical-products-during-covid-19-public-health-emergency. Accessed September 13, 2020.
26. Boughey JC, Snyder RA, Kantor O, et al. Impact of the COVID-19 pandemic on cancer clinical trials. Ann Surg Oncol 2021;28(12):7311–6.
27. National Cancer Institute. Additional Guidance Regarding Alternative Procedures for Clinical Trials Supported by the NCI Cancer Therapy Evaluation Program (CTEP) and NCI Community Oncology Research Program (NCORP) Affected by the Spread of the Novel Coronavirus. Available at: https://ctep.cancer.gov/investigatorResources/docs/Memorandum_on_Additional_Guidance_for_Clinical_Trial_Activities_Affected_by_the_Novel_Coronavirus_3-23-2020.pdf. Accessed January 4, 2023.
28. Daly M, Robinson E. Depression and anxiety during COVID-19. Lancet 2022; 399(10324):518.
29. Yao KA, Attai D, Bleicher R, et al. Covid-19 Related Oncologist's Concerns about Breast Cancer Treatment Delays and Physician Well-being (The CROWN Study). Breast Cancer Res Treat 2021;186(3):625–35.

UNITED STATES POSTAL SERVICE ® Statement of Ownership, Management, and Circulation (All Periodicals Publications Except Requester Publications)

1. Publication Title	2. Publication Number	3. Filing Date
SURGICAL ONCOLOGY CLINICS OF NORTH AMERICA	012 – 565	9/18/2023

4. Issue Frequency	5. Number of Issues Published Annually	6. Annual Subscription Price
JAN, APR, JUL, OCT	4	$335.00

7. Complete Mailing Address of Known Office of Publication (Not printer) (Street, city, county, state, and ZIP+4®)

ELSEVIER INC.
230 Park Avenue, Suite 800
New York, NY 10169

Contact Person
Malathi Samayan

Telephone (Include area code)
91-44-4299-4507

8. Complete Mailing Address of Headquarters or General Business Office of Publisher (Not printer)

ELSEVIER INC.
230 Park Avenue, Suite 800
New York, NY 10169

9. Full Names and Complete Mailing Addresses of Publisher, Editor, and Managing Editor (Do not leave blank)

Publisher (Name and complete mailing address)

Dolores Meloni, ELSEVIER INC.
1600 JOHN F KENNEDY BLVD. SUITE 1600
PHILADELPHIA, PA 19103-2899

Editor (Name and complete mailing address)

JOHN VASSALLO, ELSEVIER INC.
1600 JOHN F KENNEDY BLVD. SUITE 1600
PHILADELPHIA, PA 19103-2899

Managing Editor (Name and complete mailing address)

PATRICK MANLEY, ELSEVIER INC.
1600 JOHN F KENNEDY BLVD. SUITE 1600
PHILADELPHIA, PA 19103-2899

10. Owner (Do not leave blank. If the publication is owned by a corporation, give the name and address of the corporation immediately followed by the names and addresses of all stockholders owning or holding 1 percent or more of the total amount of stock. If not owned by a corporation, give the names and addresses of the individual owners. If owned by a partnership or other unincorporated firm, give its name and address as well as those of each individual owner. If the publication is published by a nonprofit organization, give its name and address.)

Full Name	Complete Mailing Address
WHOLLY OWNED SUBSIDIARY OF REED/ELSEVIER, US HOLDINGS	1600 JOHN F KENNEDY BLVD. SUITE 1600 PHILADELPHIA, PA 19103-2899

11. Known Bondholders, Mortgagees, and Other Security Holders Owning or Holding 1 Percent or More of Total Amount of Bonds, Mortgages, or Other Securities. If none, check box ▶ ☐ None

Full Name	Complete Mailing Address
N/A	

12. Tax Status (For completion by nonprofit organizations authorized to mail at nonprofit rates) (Check one)
The purpose, function, and nonprofit status of this organization and the exempt status for federal income tax purposes:
☒ Has Not Changed During Preceding 12 Months
☐ Has Changed During Preceding 12 Months (Publisher must submit explanation of change with this statement)

PS Form **3526**, July 2014 (Page 1 of 4 (see instructions page 4)) PSN: 7530-01-000-9931   PRIVACY NOTICE: See our privacy policy on www.usps.com

---

13. Publication Title	14. Issue Date for Circulation Data Below
SURGICAL ONCOLOGY CLINICS OF NORTH AMERICA	JULY 2023

15. Extent and Nature of Circulation		Average No. Copies Each Issue During Preceding 12 Months	No. Copies of Single Issue Published Nearest to Filing Date
a. Total Number of Copies (Net press run)		97	99
b. Paid Circulation (By Mail and Outside the Mail)	(1) Mailed Outside-County Paid Subscriptions Stated on PS Form 3541 (Include paid distribution above nominal rate, advertiser's proof copies, and exchange copies)	63	71
	(2) Mailed In-County Paid Subscriptions Stated on PS Form 3541 (Include paid distribution above nominal rate, advertiser's proof copies, and exchange copies)	0	0
	(3) Paid Distribution Outside the Mails Including Sales Through Dealers and Carriers, Street Vendors, Counter Sales, and Other Paid Distribution Outside USPS®	22	17
	(4) Paid Distribution by Other Classes of Mail Through the USPS (e.g. First-Class Mail®)	6	11
c. Total Paid Distribution (Sum of 15b (1), (2), (3), and (4))	▶	91	99
d. Free or Nominal Rate Distribution (By Mail and Outside the Mail)	(1) Free or Nominal Rate Outside-County Copies included on PS Form 3541	6	0
	(2) Free or Nominal Rate In-County Copies included on PS Form 3541	0	0
	(3) Free or Nominal Rate Copies Mailed at Other Classes Through the USPS (e.g. First-Class Mail)	0	0
	(4) Free or Nominal Rate Distribution Outside the Mail (Carriers or other means)	0	0
e. Total Free or Nominal Rate Distribution (Sum of 15d (1), (2), (3) and (4))	▶	6	0
f. Total Distribution (Sum of 15c and 15e)	▶	97	99
g. Copies not Distributed (See Instructions to Publishers #4 (page #3))	▶	0	0
h. Total (Sum of 15f and g)	▶	97	99
i. Percent Paid (15c divided by 15f times 100)		93.32%	100%

* If you are claiming electronic copies, go to line 16 on page 3. If you are not claiming electronic copies, skip to line 17 on page 3.

16. Electronic Copy Circulation		Average No. Copies Each Issue During Preceding 12 Months	No. Copies of Single Issue Published Nearest to Filing Date
a. Paid Electronic Copies	▶		
b. Total Paid Print Copies (Line 15c) + Paid Electronic Copies (Line 16a)	▶		
c. Total Print Distribution (Line 15f) + Paid Electronic Copies (Line 16a)	▶		
d. Percent Paid (Both Print & Electronic Copies) (16b divided by 16c × 100)	▶		

☒ I certify that 50% of all my distributed copies (electronic and print) are paid above a nominal price.

17. Publication of Statement of Ownership

☒ If the publication is a general publication, publication of this statement is required. Will be printed
in the ____ OCTOBER 2023 ____ issue of this publication.   ☐ Publication not required.

18. Signature and Title of Editor, Publisher, Business Manager, or Owner

Malathi Samayan

Malathi Samayan - Distribution Controller

Date 9/18/2023

I certify that all information furnished on this form is true and complete. I understand that anyone who furnishes false or misleading information on this form or who omits material or information requested on the form may be subject to criminal sanctions (including fines and imprisonment) and/or civil sanctions (including civil penalties).

PS Form **3526**, July 2014 (Page 3 of 4)   PRIVACY NOTICE: See our privacy policy on www.usps.com

Printed and bound by CPI Group (UK) Ltd, Croydon, CR0 4YY

03/10/2024

01040470-0020